# Speech Science Primer

## Physiology, Acoustics, and Perception of Speech

### SIXTH EDITION

**Lawrence J. Raphael, Ph.D.**
*Department of Communication Sciences and Disorders*
*Adelphi University*
*Emeritus, Department of Speech and Theatre*
*Lehman College, City University of New York*
*Bronx, New York*
*Emeritus, The Graduate School, City University of New York*
*New York, New York*

**Gloria J. Borden, Ph.D.**
*Emerita, Department of Speech*
*Temple University*
*Philadelphia, Pennsylvania*

**Katherine S. Harris, Ph.D.**
*Emerita, Ph.D. Program in Speech-Language-Hearing Sciences*
*The Graduate Center, City University of New York*
*New York, New York*
*Haskins Laboratories*
*New Haven, Connecticut*

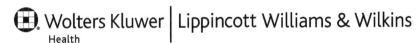
Wolters Kluwer | Lippincott Williams & Wilkins
Health
Philadelphia • Baltimore • New York • London
Buenos Aires • Hong Kong • Sydney • Tokyo

*Acquisitions Editor:* Peter Sabatini
*Managing Editors:* Tiffany Piper, Kristin Royer
*Marketing Manager:* Allison M. Noplock
*Designer:* Terry Mallon
*Compositor:* Aptara, Inc.
*Printer:* Strategic Content Imaging

351 West Camden Street
Baltimore, MD 21201

Two Commerce Square
2001 Market Street
Philadelphia, PA 19103

Printed in the United States of America

First Edition, 1980
Second Edition, 1984
Third Edition, 1994
Fourth Edition, 2003
Fifth Edition, 2007

**Library of Congress Cataloging-in-Publication Data**

Raphael, Lawrence J.
   Speech science primer : physiology, acoustics, and perception of
speech / Lawrence J. Raphael, Gloria J. Borden, Katherine S. Harris. – 6th ed.
      p. ; cm.
   Includes bibliographical references and index.
   ISBN 978-1-60831-357-0
   1. Speech.   I. Borden, Gloria J.   II. Harris, Katherine S.   III. Title.
   [DNLM:   1. Speech–physiology.   2. Speech Acoustics.   3. Speech
Perception. WV 501]
   P95.B65 2011
   612.7'8–dc22                                              2010041933

To purchase additional copies of this book, call our customer service department at (800) 638-3030 or fax orders to (301) 223-2320. International customers should call (301) 223-2300.

**Visit Lippincott Williams & Wilkins on the Internet: http://www.LWW.com. Lippincott Williams & Wilkins customer service representatives are available from 8:30 am to 6:00 pm, EST.**

11   12   13   14

*To our students, past, present, and future.*

# Preface

The purpose of this primer has remained constant through six editions: to satisfy the need for a comprehensive but elementary book on speech science that is easy to understand and that integrates material on the production, acoustics, and perception of speech. We hope that the popularity of the first five editions and the demand for a sixth is an indication that we have been successful in meeting that need.

A primer in any discipline is, by nature, resistant to certain types of change. Because it is intended to explicate fundamental concepts, it will not be likely to discuss either information that is too advanced for the beginning student or untested hypotheses, no matter how interesting or potentially influential such information or theories may be. Moreover, the resistance to change is dictated by the stability of the fundamental concepts and data that the primer contains. Basic information concerning acoustics, the acoustic analysis of speech, speech anatomy and physiology, and speech perception, although not immutable, changes very slowly over time.

## NEW TO THIS EDITION

Although primers may be resistant to changes in basic information, by their nature they must be extremely receptive to changes that make the text more interesting and easier to read for beginning students. Thus, the reader will find that many sections of the text have been rewritten for clarity. The reader who is familiar with the earlier editions of the book will undoubtedly notice that the current edition contains a new, separate chapter on the prosody, a topic which has been, perhaps, too long underemphasized in this and other basic books dealing with speech science.

As in the design of the previous edition, we have continued to present subject matter in shorter segments to allow readers to identify coherent units of information that were not as evident when they were included in longer chapters.

Students will find information about normal communication processes that will serve as a basis for comparison with the disorders that they will soon be treating in the clinic. Each chapter of the present edition includes a section on some potential clinical applications of the material presented. These "Clinical Notes" are not intended to be exhaustive. Rather, we hope that they may stimulate readers to think about other ways that the information in any chapter might be put to work in a clinical setting. The need for such information and the role of speech science in providing it will be made amply clear throughout the text.

## ORGANIZATION

Throughout the text we have tried to retain the style of those sections that faculty and students have found to be clear and easy to read, and we have tried to improve the style of sections that some students and instructors have found to be less clear. We continue to preserve many of the classic illustrations from the research literature in their original form because we think their presence increases the value of the book.

With one exception, the organization of the book remains as it was in previous editions. Section I now contains only one chapter, intended to set speech in the larger framework of language and thought. The chapter on the Pioneers in Speech Science, formerly in Section I, has been relocated. It is now the first chapter of Section V, the section that treats instrumentation. Because many of the accomplishments of the pioneers described in the chapter centered on the development and innovative use of instruments for the study of speech, we feel that it provides a useful introduction to the description and use of modern instrumentation in the final two chapters of the book. .

Section II (Chapter 2) contains a discussion of basic acoustics, the foundation on which the structure of speech science is built. Section III (Chapters 3 through 8) deals with speech acoustics and speech production. The new chapter on prosody is in this section. We have attempted to integrate physiology and acoustics, as we have found that the physiology of speech production is better understood and remembered when the sound-producing mechanisms and processes are closely associated with the acoustic output. Section IV (Chapters 9 to 11) treats speech perception, including material on hearing, acoustic cues, and models of speech perception. Section V, as noted above, contains our

discussion of instrumentation. Although we have placed most of the emphasis on the instruments and techniques that may be generally available to students in most college and university laboratories, we also describe the instruments and techniques that are found in larger speech science laboratories as well, so that students will be familiar with them when they study the research literature.

As we have suggested above, because this book is a primer and serves as an introduction to a large body of information, we do not presume to have covered every topic of importance or to have dealt with the topics included in depth. An updated selected bibliography concludes each chapter, however, to encourage the student to pursue each subject further and to fill in the necessary gaps. In an undergraduate course, the text may be used as presented; in a graduate course, many of the references might be added as required readings.

## ANCILLARIES

We have revised and expanded the selection of audio illustrations that can be accessed through the World Wide Web. These audio illustrations are referenced in the text: wherever the reader sees the marker in the margin, he or she will be able to hear the sounds being described by going online to the book's Web site. We trust that the updated version of the audio illustrations will make the book substantially more useful and informative. Words about sounds are severely limited in how much they can convey. Technology has allowed us to move beyond printed words so that the *Speech Science Primer* is no longer analogous to a book about art history that contains no illustrations of the art being discussed.

Instructors can also access PowerPoint slides and chapter outlines as aids to the planning and presentation of the material included in the book.

The primary audience to whom this text is addressed consists of students of speech and language pathology and audiology. The book will also be of interest to students of medicine, psychology, education, and linguistics, as each of these disciplines includes some aspects of the material that we have presented. Moreover, the text provides an opportunity for students in other disciplines to obtain a comprehensive view of speech science. Although this book is clearly introductory, it can also serve as a graduate text for students who never had a survey course in speech science as undergraduates.

It is only relatively recently that speech science has emerged as a unified discipline, although many of its components have been studied for centuries. Acoustics has long been an aspect of physics and engineering, speech physiology a part of biology, speech perception an outgrowth of both biology and sensory psychology, and speech in its relation to language in general has long been included in the study of phonetics and linguistics. This book embraces each of these components and attempts to integrate them into a unified treatment.

**Lawrence J. Raphael**
**Gloria J. Borden**
**Katherine S. Harris**

# Acknowledgments

The comments and suggestions made by many colleagues and students (too numerous to mention here) who have used this book in class have been most helpful in its revision. There is no greater corrective to the mistaken idea that one has written a sentence or a paragraph as clearly as possible than the puzzled question of a student who asks what that sentence or paragraph might mean.

The glossary remains largely the work of Jolie Bookspan, whose efforts in compiling it continue to enrich the text for future students. Throughout the process of revising the text for the fifth and sixth editions, the first author received support from Adelphi University in the form of the access to laboratory and computing facilities and from the encouragement and interest of the faculty of the Department of Communication Sciences and Disorders of the School of Education. We also thank the Ph.D. Program in Speech-Language-Hearing Science of the City University of New York for the use of its facilities. We probably would not have written the text in its present form had we not had the common experience of working at Haskins Laboratories in New Haven, where researches in speech production and

speech perception are viewed as natural complements of one another.

Several people have been of great assistance in locating and supplying sound recordings for use on the Web site that accompanies this book. We thank Fredericka Bell-Berti of St. Johns University, New York; Winifred Strange and James Jenkins, formerly of the Graduate Center of the City University of New York; Valeriy Shafiro of Rush University Medical Center, Chicago; and Alice Faber of Haskins Laboratories, New Haven. Without their help, our inventory of audio samples would be far less extensive.

Thank you also to those who helped us create the PowerPoint slides: Laura L. Koenig, Ph.D., Long Island University and Senior Scientist at Haskins Laboratories, and Nassima Abdelli-Beruh, Ph.D., C. W. Post Campus of Long Island University.

We are grateful to our spouses, children, and grandchildren for cheering us on: to John, Becky, Julie, Tom, and Sam Borden; to George, Maud (White), and Louise Harris; and to Carolyn Raphael, Melissa, Frank, Andrew, and Gabriel Zinzi, David, Nina, and Nathan Raphael. Finally, our many questions have been answered with patience by the editor for the first edition, Ruby Richardson, the editor for the second edition, William R. Hensyl, the editor for the third edition, John P. Butler, the editors for the fourth edition, John Butler and Tim Julet, the editors for the fifth edition, Pamela Lappies and Peter Sabatini, and, finally, the editor for this edition, Peter Sabatini. The guidance, advice, and encouragement sup-

plied for the third, fourth, fifth, and sixth editions by our managing editors, Linda Napora and Andrea Klingler, Tiffany Piper, and Kristin Royer were of value beyond measure. We thank them all.

**Lawrence J. Raphael**
**Gloria J. Borden**
**Katherine S. Harris**

# Contents

# SECTION I   Introduction

# Speech, Language, and Thought

# 1

*O chestnut tree, great rooted blossomer,*
*Are you the leaf, the blossom or the bole?*
*O body swayed to music, O brightening glance,*
*How can we know the dancer from the dance?*

                                                  —W. B. Yeats, "Among School Children," 1928

This book is about speech. It is about spoken English in particular. It is not about language or thought. But before we isolate speech and consider it separately from thought and language, we need to recognize that speech is the most common way in which we express our thoughts and that when we do so, we organize our speech by using the rules of language. If we were to study wine grapes without mentioning vineyards, it would be a little like the study of speech with no recognition of its origins in thought and language. We also need to recognize that speech is only one of the ways in which humans communicate with each other. It is unique to humans.

The animal kingdom offer many examples of nonlinguistic signs that communicate various conditions within and across species. For instance, a dog will growl and bare its teeth to keep an intruder from entering its territory. Or a female ape will assume a sexually submissive and presumably inviting posture to indicate that she is willing to mate with a male ape. Presumably, communications of this sort reflect thought, but the thoughts are not expressed in speech and the forms of the messages are not determined by the rules of language.

Humans also use many other methods of communication that are not classified as speech. We signal to others by waving flags, by sending messages in Morse Code, by raising an eyebrow, by sending e-mail and text messages, by writing blogs, by playing musical instruments, by putting our hands on our hips, by painting pictures, by sticking out our tongues, by kissing, by blushing, and by dancing. But mostly, we speak.

There are many reasons humans use speech as their primary mode of communication. Most of those reasons relate to the fact that speech was selectively advantageous in the evolution of our species. First, the vocal–auditory channel of speech permitted communication under conditions in which a different channel, such as the gestural–visual, would fail. Using speech, messages could be sent in the dark, around corners, or when visibility was limited for other reasons. Second, using speech allowed communication to occur at the same time that manual tasks, such as tool making or food gathering, were being performed. Third, as we shall see, because of the way speech is produced by the human vocal tract, it is both efficient and redundant. The efficiency of speech allows conveyance of information more quickly than with other channels of communication; the redundancy of the speech signal allows listeners to understand messages even when they are not completely heard, because of either external interference or momentary lapses of attention. Fourth, there is evidence that human beings are genetically equipped to respond to the speech signal.

The use of speech as a means of conveying thought and language is thus not accidental or arbitrary, and it is not surprising that we use speech naturally and with great frequency. We speak in our homes, at work, at school, and at play. We speak to our babies, to our pets, and to ourselves. But what is speech and how does it relate to language and to thought? If you have ever known an adult with brain damage sufficient to impair speech, you have probably observed that the speech impairment is accompanied by some effects on language and on some aspects of thought. Speech, language, and thought are closely related, but we can consider them separately because they are qualitatively different.

## SPEECH

If you have ever been to a foreign country and heard everyone around you speaking a language that you do not understand, especially a language unrelated to your own, you are likely to have had three impressions. The first is that the spoken language seems like a long stream of complex and constantly changing sounds without separations. You have no way of knowing when one word ends and the next begins. The second impression is that this strange language sounds extremely complex. The third impression is that the speakers, even the young children, seem to talk much faster than speakers of your language.

These impressions of a foreign language are more accurate as a description of speech in general than they are as a description of our own speech. We take our own speech for granted. It seems simple to us, but the sounds change just as quickly as those spoken in a foreign language and require complex articulatory gymnastics on the part of the speaker. Despite this complexity, children are quite good at learning to speak, and by 3 or 4 years of age, they have mastered most of the difficulties of producing speech in their native language. Although some children eventually encounter problems learning to read or write, all normal children learn to speak and to understand speech. They do this with virtually no formal instruction, acquiring speech simply by hearing those around them speak. And of course, at the same time, they acquire language.

## LANGUAGE

The reason we fail to understand the strange speech of an unknown language is that we do not know the words, the sounds, or the rules of that language. Any *language* is a rule-governed communication system composed of meaningful elements that can be combined in many ways to produce sentences, many of which have never been uttered by a speaker or heard by a listener. Our knowledge of English permits us to say and understand something as prosaic as, "I have a headache." This sentence has undoubtedly been said many times, but our language also permits us to say and understand something completely new, something we have never heard said before, such as the following passage.

Speech–language pathologists and audiologists are trained to provide therapy for people who have communication disorders. Sometimes these disorders prevent people from producing speech normally; sometimes the problems prevent listeners from understanding hearing a spoken message. Providing therapy for either type of disorder requires professional training in more than one specialty and, on occasion, may demand the services of more than one type of therapist.

Whether we hear these sentences read aloud or read them from the printed page, we can understand them, even though have never heard them before, because we share with the author the knowledge of the rules of English. The rules of *semantics* enable us to associate words or phrases with meanings. We and the author have a common understanding of words such as "therapy" and "disorder." The rules of *syntax* enable us to have common expectations of word order. When we read "Speech language pathologists and audiologists," we realize recognize the phrase as the potential subject of the first sentence and so expect a verb to follow. When the verb "are" appeared after the end of the phrase, we also expected that "train," the verb immediately after "are" would have an "-ed" ending to mark it as a past participle. The author and readers know the same rules; they share a language, as we have seen, they can create and understand sentences never read or heard before.

Speech, as you probably realize, is a physical event. As you will discover in following chapters, we can analyze speech as an acoustic signal and specify its components in terms of frequencies, amplitudes, and durations. Language, unlike speech, is intangible.

It is our knowledge of a creative communication system, and that knowledge is in our minds. How is language related to speech? Noam Chomsky has called this knowledge of language *linguistic competence* to distinguish it from the use of language, *linguistic performance.* Speech, then, is one of the ways in which we use language; it is the conversion of language to sound. There are, however, other modes of communication into which we can convert language. American Sign Language (Ameslan or ASL), used by the deaf, is an example of gestural language.

The syntactic rules of ASL differ from those of English. Word order is often determined by the chronology of events or by emphasized words. For example, in ASL one would sign "Sun this morning. I saw. Beautiful." rather than "It was a beautiful sun I saw this morning." If the word "movies" should have the greatest emphasis in "I like the movies," an Ameslan user indicates that by signing "Movies I like," with the most stressed word appearing at the end of the sentence.

The semantic rules are also different from those of English because the ASL user associates meanings with signs made by the hands, face, and arms. The shape of hands making the sign, their movements or how the movements change, and their position relative to the rest of the body are all meaningful. Again, in the case of ASL, one's competence (knowledge of the system) can be called *language*, in contrast to the use of it–the physical production of gestures or signs–which is called *performance.*

As with speech, performance usually falls short of the user's competence. Signs are sometimes indicated quickly and incompletely. Mistakes are made, but the user's competence remains. When we speak, we often use fragments of sentences rather than complete ones. We think of something else in midsentence and start a new sentence before we have completed the first. Yet when a teacher says, "Put your answer in a complete sentence," the student knows how to do it. He or she knows the language, even though that knowledge may be inconsistently reflected in speech. How does this linguistic knowledge relate to thought?

## THOUGHT

*Thought* may be defined as an internal or mental representation of experience. Jerome Bruner has suggested that the representation can be in the form of images, action, or language. We presumably use all available representations of our experiences, but some people report the use of some forms more than others. We may think via internal images, vaguely visual, when we are solving a problem such as how many suitcases we think we can fit into the trunk of a car. Architects and artists often think in visual images. Thought can also be represented by internal action or muscle imagery. In solving the problem of the direction and force needed to place a tennis shot out of reach of an opponent, we think in terms of action. Choreographers, athletes, and some physicists think this way. Albert Einstein, describing his understanding of how he thought, wrote:

*The words of the language, as they are written or spoken, do not seem to play any role in my mechanism of thought. The psychical entities which seem to serve as elements in thought are certain signs and more or less clear images which can be "voluntarily" reproduced and combined . . . . But taken from a psychological viewpoint, this combinatory play seems to be the essential feature in productive thought—before there is any connection with logical construction in words or other kinds of signs which can be communicated to others. The above mentioned elements are, in my case, of visual and some of muscular type.*

–Quoted in Ghiselin, B., *The Creative Process.* New York: Mentor Books, 1955, p. 43.

Representation of thought in language seems to be important in the mental activities of language users. Although it is apparent that we can think without any formal language, it is equally apparent that those who do know a language use it to aid their thinking. But what if a thinking individual does not have access to a language? Let us consider the ramifications of thought without language before going on to discuss the more usual situation, thought with language.

### Thought Without Language

We have all had an idea that was difficult to put into words. Indeed, words often seem inadequate. Our ideas, as we express them, sometimes seem to be only a rough sketch of our thoughts. People with aphasia (language impairment caused by brain damage) demonstrate that thought is independent of language. Often an aphasic person seems to have an idea to express but lacks the linguistic ability to express the thought.

Some deaf children who have not been exposed to sign language are quite delayed in learning the language of their community because of the difficulties they encounter in learning oral speech. Hans Furth has shown, however, that the cognitive abilities of these children develop almost normally. Helen Keller, who was blind and deaf from the age of 18 months, wrote that she did not understand the first important concept of language learning, that symbols stand for elements of our experience, until she was 9 years old. As her teacher, Annie Sullivan, was communicating the word "water" by having the child feel her lips and face with one hand as she spoke the word and having her feel the water with the other hand, the child suddenly made the association. Keller soon learned the names of everything in her environment. Language learning had begun, yet Keller surely was not an unthinking child before that experience. Her thoughts must have been represented by images.

The Swiss psychologist Jean Piaget concluded from his observations of normal children that cognition develops on its own. Language interacts with it and certainly reflects the child's thinking, but language does not determine the thinking. According to his view, it does no good to train a child in language to develop cognition. Rather, he held, stages of cognitive development are reflected in the child's use of language.

Lev Vygotsky, a Russian psychologist, also observed evidence of nonverbal thought in children. Infants demonstrate their understanding of relationships and their problem-solving abilities independently of their use of language, even while they make speech-like babbling sounds that seem to lack intellectual content. Later in the child's development, speech and thought unite.

## Thought and Language

Vygotsky's great contribution was his idea of "inner speech." Although he viewed early language as being essentially externally communicative, he maintained that some early language use was egocentric. That is, children talk to themselves. From approximately 3 to 7 years of age, the vocal egocentric speech gradually becomes subvocal inner speech, a way of talking to oneself. Such a process, which obviously involves language, lies somewhere between thought and speech but is not quite either. When we think by using language, we think in linguistic fragments, in abbreviated phrases, the words fading quickly or only partly formed.

Piaget agreed with Vygotsky's description of inner speech, having observed its beginnings in the egocentric speech of the children in his studies. Preschool children echo words and phrases they hear around them (*echolalia*) and incorporate them into their own *monologues*. They talk about what they are doing, the toys they are playing with, the pictures they are painting. A roomful of kindergarten children can be talking, sometimes taking turns as in conversation, but each one is talking about his or her own experiences in a *collective monologue*. Piaget's point was that this use of language reflected a stage of thinking in which children seldom include the point of view of others. They see things primarily from their own viewpoint, hence the *egocentric speech*. The frequency of the egocentric speech gradually decreases as the frequency of socialized speech increases. If in some sense we "speak" to ourselves as well to others, does this inner speech aid in thinking?

## Language and Speech as Carriers for Thought

Thoughts are not always formed in orderly sequences. Sometimes a thought is formed as a set of associations internally "seen" as a whole. We necessarily distort it when we string it out on the timeline of language and speech. Despite this distortion, there are many advantages in using language to represent thought. For one thing, language helps make an idea or an experience available. Expressing a thought verbally allows it to be recorded in various forms for analysis. Then, too, language also aids thinking by providing a frame to hold information in memory. It enables us to communicate ideas about people, places, activities, qualities, or things when they are not present.

Throughout this discussion, we have viewed language as a means of expressing thought and as a reflection of thought but not as something that determines thought. The linguists Edward Sapir and his student Benjamin Whorf proposed the theory of linguistic determinism (also called the *Sapir–Whorf hypothesis*), which proposes that the way human beings think about their world is determined, in part, by the particular language that they speak. In its strongest version the hypothesis maintains that language determines thinking. It was based on the notion that when languages differ in the number of terms available for categories such as "color" and "snow," the speakers of languages with more words available to describe such categories will think differently about colors or types of snow than people speaking a language with fewer words for snow and color. The reasoning was that people who know many words for "snow" actually perceive distinctions that people with fewer words fail to perceive. Analogously, people who speak a language with no color term for "gray" or "blue" will not be able to perceive those colors. This strong version of the hypothesis is not generally accepted today. Steven Pinker maintains that "...there is no scientific evidence that languages dramatically shape their speakers' ways of thinking." A weaker, less controversial version of linguistic determinism holds that it may be easier for an Eskimo to talk about snow than it is for a Guatemalan but that there is no significant difference between their abilities to perceive or think about snow. The interests and needs of one language group may simply differ from those of another—which explains the differences in vocabulary.

Instead of comparing languages, one can look at a particular language and observe differences based on social group membership. Basil Bernstein, a sociolinguist, used cultural differences as an explanation of linguistic differences he observed between middle-class and working-class children in Great Britain. When children were asked to describe a picture, for example, the typical middle-class child would be fairly explicit, using many nouns. One would not need to see the picture to imagine it. The typical working-class child, in describing the same picture, would use far fewer nouns, substituting such words as "he," "it," or "they," so that it would be difficult to imagine the picture from the description alone. Bernstein attributed this difference to cultural differences: the hierarchy of relationships in a working-class family in England has an authoritarian structure, so that children are expected not to express themselves creatively but to listen to the head of the family, whereas the middle-class family is less authoritarian and each member has a say. In addition, the working-class family member usually talks about shared experiences, so the context is understood, whereas the middle-class family member is more apt to talk about experiences of his or her own and not to assume so much knowledge on the part of the listener. Bernstein's choice of terms, *restricted code* (in the working-class case) and *elaborated code* (in the middle-class case) is unfortunate, as it has been used to support the notion that members of the working class suffer from cognitive deficits, an idea that has been generally discredited by more recent research and that Bernstein himself eventually rejected. His studies, do, however, point out the influence of cultural habits, if not differences in thinking, on language.

Despite small differences in the use of language by different people who share a language and despite the larger differences among languages in their structure and vocabularies, there may be some universal features of human languages. To the extent that this is true, one ought to be able to learn something about the human mind, as Chomsky suggests, by studying the rules of human language.

> *There are any number of questions that might lead one to undertake a study of language. Personally, I am primarily intrigued by the possibility of learning something, from the study of language, that will bring to light inherent properties of the human mind.*
> —Chomsky, N., *Language and Mind* (enlarged edition). New York: Harcourt Brace Jovanovich, 1972, p. 103.

If we define language as a set of rules that speakers apply to generate an infinite number of sentences, using a set of words that constantly expands to cover all the concepts they may choose to express, then humans are the only creatures known to have a command of language. In addition, the ability to talk about language also seems to be unique to humans. Humans may well be the only creatures on Earth who use their brains in an attempt to understand brains and use language in an attempt to understand languages. The interaction of thinking, language, and speech may seem clearer if we look further at language development in normal children.

## DEVELOPMENT OF LANGUAGE AND SPEECH

At birth, normal children have the potential to walk and talk, although as babies, they can do neither. They are genetically endowed with the appropriate neurophysical systems, but time is needed for these systems to develop and mature. Their brains are approximately 40% of the size they will be when they are fully grown; peripheral areas such as the vocal tract and the legs must still undergo anatomic change and the development of motor–sensory associations appropriate to talking and walking. At 6 months, children sit up and *babble* in meaningless vocal play. By the first birthday, they may have started to walk and name things. By the

second birthday, they may be putting two words together for rudimentary telegraphic sentences, and by the fourth, they have mastered the basic rules of the language of their elders.

The rapidity and apparent ease with which children learn language is a phenomenon of childhood that cannot be repeated with such ease by adults. Adults, especially those who already know several languages, can learn new ones, but the age of puberty seems to be the dividing line between the ability to acquire a new language with relative ease and learning a new language with more difficulty. In fact, some researchers reserve the term "language acquisition" to refer to the critical time period during which language is learned easily and without formal instruction; they use the term "language learning" refer to the methods and techniques, including formal instruction, that speakers must employ if they want to add a second language to their repertoire. There is, however, considerable controversy about the seriousness of the limitations imposed on the language learner who is beyond the so-called critical period. Lenneberg and others who base their arguments on neurobiologic data suggest that natural language acquisition abilities cease to exist after the "critical period." Others, including those who observed Genie, a child who did not begin to acquire language until after puberty, argue that the native ability to learn language is never completely extinguished.

What children universally accomplish with spontaneity and speed, speech scientists, linguists, and psychologists have laboriously analyzed with only partial success. The question they ask is, how do children acquire language? Theorists on this subject can be generally divided into two groups. One group of theorists analyzes language development in terms of learning principles. The other group analyzes language development in terms of an innate ability to acquire language. Perhaps the most popular view is that the details or individual items of a particular language are learned, whereas the rule-building abilities that underlie the structure and meaning of language, and thus the ability to create novel utterances, are innate.

## Learning Theory and Language

Learning in the classic sense is the formulation of a new bond or association between a stimulus and a response. The classic experiment performed by Pavlov in Russia in the 1920s resulted in an association or bond between the sound of a bell and a dog's salivation. This bond was new and therefore considered to be learned, because before the experiment, the dog did not salivate at the sound of a bell. The learned behavior, or conditioned response, was produced by pairing an unconditioned stimulus, in this case, meat powder, with the conditioned stimulus, the bell. Since meat powder reflexively causes increased salivation (an automatic physiological response to food), the presentation of meat powder together with the sound of the bell produced a neural bond between the two, so that finally the bell alone would produce salivation.

In classic conditioning of this type, the unconditioned response (e.g., changes in perspiration, heart rate, or salivation) is involuntary and its cause is known (e.g., fear or food). In another model of learning, the unconditioned response is under voluntary control (the subject pushes a lever or makes a sound) and the cause is not evident. In this case, the learning is caused not by the pairing of stimuli but by reinforcement or reward, a method called *operant conditioning*. If the operant response is rewarded with food, praise, or some other positive experience, the behavior is strengthened, but if it is punished with electric shock, criticism, or some negative experience, the behavior is weakened. B. F. Skinner, who presented his theory of language learning in the book *Verbal Behavior*, developed the operant conditioning model. Skinner proposed that language is learned by selective reinforcement provided to the child as he or she uses language to operate on the environment.

Another learning theorist, O. H. Mowrer, has suggested that the reinforcement or reward may not always produce an observable response but that responses may occur within the child. In the observable instance, the association of the utterance "mama" with the rewarding presence of the mother with food and comfort establishes "mama" as a learned response. In the case of an internal response, the child finds that just the word "mama" produces positive feelings or rewards even if the word is not said aloud. In what Mowrer has termed his *autistic theory*, words that children have heard but never uttered are rehearsed subvocally. This rehearsal evokes internal rewards that are sufficient for the words to become learned or conditioned behavior. Mowrer's theory thus accounts for the sudden production of new words that children have not previously spoken.

Learning theories are consistent with facts about much of children's semantic acquisition, especially the learning of word meanings. They may even explain the initial stages of adopting the syntax or word order of a particular language. The shaping of the correct sounds of speech may also be dependent on the reward of being understood and perhaps obeyed. If a child who has said /tuti/ ("tootie") without getting the desired response but then finds that "cookie" produces the food that was wanted, he or she is amply rewarded and will say /kuki/ in the future.

## Innateness Theory

There is much about language development that learning theories cannot explain. Human language users are creative in their use of the system. Children, after they have heard sufficient utterances in their language, construct rules governing the generation of sentences. Those rules allow them to both understand and produce sentences that they have never heard before and therefore cannot have learned. They may first learn an irregular past tense verb form such as "ran" by conventional learning methods. However, once they have figured out the regular past tense rule of adding /d/ to a present tense form as in "turned," "hugged," or "closed," they are apt to cease using "ran" and to say "runned" instead because their rule-building ability leads them to regularize language forms and ignore the models that they have heard and initially learned. Many psycholinguists think that this ability to abstract the rules of the language is innate; some think that certain aspects of linguistic structure are innate.

## Linguistic Competence

Noam Chomsky has written most persuasively on this subject. As we have seen, he is careful to distinguish between one's competence in a language—the set of rules a person knows and used to produce and understand language—and performance, which is the speech, however fragmented, that a person utters. One has only to contrast a skilled speaker with an inarticulate one to realize the differences that can occur in performance. Nonetheless, all normal individuals possess basic linguistic competence. It is this fundamental knowledge that many linguists believe humans have an inborn ability to acquire.

Eric Lenneberg, Phillip Lieberman, and others have presented evidence that certain features of human anatomy and physiology evolved in such a way that they are now specialized for the production of speech and language. If this is so, then the potential to acquire language is not only innate but also species specific, as *Homo sapiens* alone displays such specialized anatomic and physiological adaptations.

Thinking provides a foundation for language; children can talk only about what they know, but they may know more than they can express with their incompletely developed language. Psycholinguists find that children are pattern seekers. On the basis of the language they hear around them, they seem to form hypotheses about linguistic rules and apply them in their own way. The language of children is not a poor imitation of adult language but rather a different language system with its own rules. The syntac-

tic rule system, vocabulary, and phonology (sound system) of child language are each comparatively undifferentiated. Young children's syntactic rules for the negative may include the use of "no" with an affirmative sentence, as in "No go home," despite the fact that they have never heard adults produce a negative sentence in such form. In the vocabulary of children, "doggie" may at first refer to any four-legged animal; only later will they narrow the meaning of the term. Children's phonological systems may specify the use of stop consonants wherever stops, fricatives, or consonant clusters appear in adult speech. For example, they might pronounce the words "two," "Sue," and "stew" as /tu/ ("two").

As they develop their language systems, they are enlarging their knowledge of *semantics*, the meanings associated with words and phrases. At the same time, they are discovering the rules by which their particular language is governed. The rules are of three sorts: *syntactic* rules, which account for the structure of sentences, including the relationships among simple declarative sentences and questions; *morphological* rules, which account for contrasts in meaning caused by differences between meaningful sequences of sounds ("cut" vs. "cat" vs. "cats") or by intonation ("Yes!" vs. "Yes?"); and *phonological* rules, which account for the occurrence of particular sounds in the stream of speech.

We can illustrate these various rules by inspecting a simple declarative sentence such as "The eggs are in the basket." Children, well before they reach adolescence, come to understand that there is a relationship between the syntax of this sentence and that of "Are the eggs in the basket?" They are evidently able to construct a rule that enables them to create questions by exchanging the positions of the noun phrase ("the eggs") and the verb (are) to create a question. They also learn that the prepositional phrase, "in the basket," must stay in its original position so that the anomalous sentence "*Are in the basket the eggs?" is not produced. (The asterisk, *, is used by linguists to denote anomalous or unattested utterances.) And, finally, they become aware that the rule cannot be applied to establish the relationship between just any declarative sentence and its associated question: The interrogative form of "The eggs simmered in the pan," is not "*Simmered the eggs in the pan?" In other words, children must be able to formulate a variety of rules associating questions with statements, rules that are based on the syntactic structure and the lexical content of the declarative form of the sentence.

Children must also construct rules that enable them to manipulate the morphemes contained in sentences. A *morpheme* is the smallest linguistic segment that means something. The word "cats" comprises two morphemes, "cat," the singular form of the noun, and "-s," (articulated as /s/), which means "more than one." There are two morphemes in "eggs" for the same reason. When morphemes are combined, as in "cats" or "eggs," the nature of the combination sometimes depends on the sound that occurs at the end of the singular. Notice that the form of the morpheme meaning "more than one" in cats is /s/, whereas in "eggs" it is /z/. If children wish to make a word such as "wish" plural, they must precede the /z/ by a very weakly stressed vowel. Formal rules can be stated for many such combinations of morphemes, but not for all of them. The structures of some combinations are determined on a word-by-word basis, and, in such cases, rules will not apply generally. For example, a child who has learned to make plurals only by using the rules exemplified above for "cats, eggs," and "wishes," will not produce the expected plural of the word "child," and might say "*Two childs were playing in the room." And, indeed, children often do produce such regularized plurals until they learn the exceptions to the general rules for combining morphemes.

Finally, children who are acquiring language must construct rules for dealing with the *phonemes* of their native language. A *phoneme* is a family of sounds that functions in a language to signal a difference in mean-

ing. The fact that "pat" and "bat" differ in meaning demonstrates that /p/ and /b/ are different phonemes in English. A phoneme by itself is meaningless. It cannot be described as a sound, either, for a phoneme can be produced only as one of several sounds. Thus, the sounds of /p/ in "*p*ie," "s*p*oon," and "to*p*" differ from one another: the first is produced with a vigorous burst of air as the lips are parted, the second with a minimal burst of air, and the third often with no burst of air at all if the lips remain in contact as when the word occurs at the end of an utterance. These sounds, when they are being discussed as variants of the phoneme, are called *allophones*. The production of specific allophones in specific contexts is often, but not always, rule-governed. Any actual sound discussed without relation to its phonemic affiliation is a *phone*.

The term "phoneme" is used when one wishes to refer to the function of a sound family in the language to signal differences in meaning, whereas the term "allophone" or "phone" is used when one wishes to refer to a particular sound that is articulated or heard. Slashes are used to enclose symbols intended to represent phonemes: /p/. Brackets are used to enclose symbols intended to represent allophones or phones: [p]. Ordinary alphabetic characters can be used to symbolize some sounds unambiguously, but there are many sounds for which this is not possible. In our sample sentence "The eggs are in the basket," the last sound, /z/ in the word "eggs," is represented by the spelling "s," which is ambiguous because the same letter is used to represent the final /s/ in the words "cats," the medial /ʒ/ in the word "leisure," and the initial consonant, /ʃ/ in the word "sure." Thus, the same alphabetic symbol is being used to represent four different phonemes. To make the transcription of sounds unambiguous, phoneticians and linguists have devised the International Phonetic Alphabet, which appears in Appendix A.

Spoken language is the end product of a process that connects knowledge of meanings (semantics) with formal structures (syntactic units, morphemes, phonemes) and that encodes the structures into the sounds of speech. We conclude this chapter with a model of this process, as we view it, that links thought to speech.

## FROM THOUGHT TO SPEECH

Two young women in the Philadelphia Museum of Art pause before a painting by Henri Matisse, entitled *Odalisque Jaune* (Fig. 1.1). One woman says to the second, "Look at this picture. There's something about the face and the patterns that reminds me of some Japanese prints I saw in a museum in New York." We cannot presume to know how this utterance was derived from the young woman's linguistic knowledge and originally from her thought processes, but we must assume that some reference was made to her stored visual experiences of Japanese prints and that associations were made between the highly patterned areas of the Japanese woodcuts (Fig. 1.2) and the arrangement of patterns in the Matisse painting. A sense of plea-

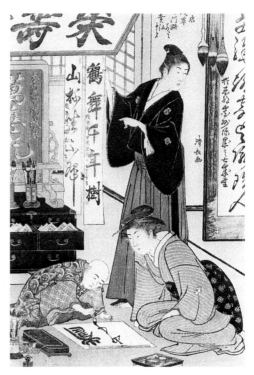

**FIGURE 1.2** Japanese woodcut. Kiyonaga: *Shigeyuki Executing Calligraphy,* 1783. Philadelphia Museum of Art: Given by Mrs. John D. Rockefeller.

sure and a positive attitude toward the effects produced must have also been a part of the process.

A model of thought, language, and speech conversions is presented in Figure 1.3. The circles overlap to suggest both the interrelationships involved and their simultaneity. The young woman's visual and aesthetic experiences, both in the present and the past, relate to ideas she has about their similarities and to her feelings about the pictures. The woman chose to represent her thought in language to communicate her response to the pictures to her companion.

There are a number of ways the woman could have framed her ideas and feelings, but on the basis of certain semantic, syntactic, morphological, and phonological decisions, she expressed her thought in words that were recorded earlier. She was constrained by the rules of her language and by the rules of

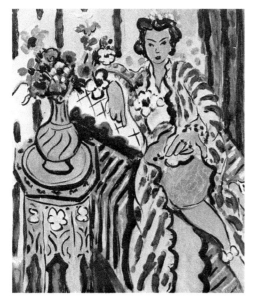

**FIGURE 1.1** Matisse painting, *Odalisque Jaune.* Philadelphia Museum of Art: Samuel S. White, III, and Vera White Collection.

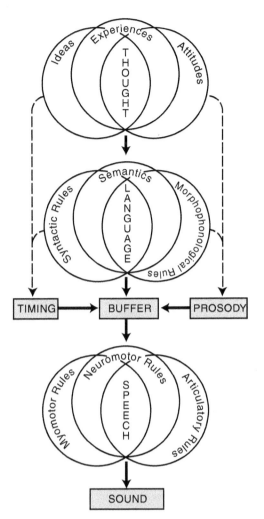

**FIGURE 1.3** Model showing contributions of various factors to output at the thought, language, and speech stages. It is conceived that thought can be embodied in language and expressed aloud by transforming dynamic representations of chunks of speech from a buffer into audible pressure waves via a stream of coordinated movements.

her speech-producing mechanism. We shall make no attempt to suggest how the intended meaning was converted into a form ready for speaking. We recognize, too, that the delivery of the message could have been in writing or in some gestural language and in speech. Choosing speech, however, the young woman somehow readied the message for delivery to her friend.

It seems probable that chunks of the message were briefly stored in a buffer (temporary storage) ready for output. The chunks were perhaps of sentence length or phrase length. Sentences and phrases can be relatively lengthy, at least compared with individual words, and we might ask whether there is any evidence for the storage of such substantial stretches of planned utterances. Such evidence exists in the form of studies of slips of the tongue. Consider Victoria Fromkin's example in which the planned utterance "He cut the salami with the knife," is actually produced as "He cut the knife with the salami." The timing and other *prosodic* aspects (e.g., intonation and stress patterns) of the utterance are viewed in our model (Fig. 1.3) as superimposed on the message as it is converted into speech. For example, the prosody remains constant despite slips of the tongue. The heaviest stress in the sentence is placed on the last word, whether the speaker says "He cut the salami with the KNIFE" or "He cut the knife with the SALAMI." This suggests that prosodic features of the entire sentence or phrase are stored in advance of its production and that the instructions for intended word order are generated independently of the prosodic instructions. Consider, also, that the utterance can be said at a variety of rates, from fast to slow, which suggests independent generation of timing commands. The timing of articulatory movements within and across phonetic segments that differentiates phonemes (e.g., the timing of laryngeal vibrations and lip movements that distinguish /p/ from /b/) is thought to be intrinsic to specifications stored in the buffer.

At the level of production, there may be a transformation from a relatively abstract representation of speech sounds to the actual neuromotor activity that controls the muscle activity, cavity changes, and air pressure modifications heard as speech. The language conversions are mediated by linguistic rules; in the speech conversions (Fig. 1.4), neuromotor, myomotor, and articulatory rules are used. The abstract representations of the intended phonemes that make up the input

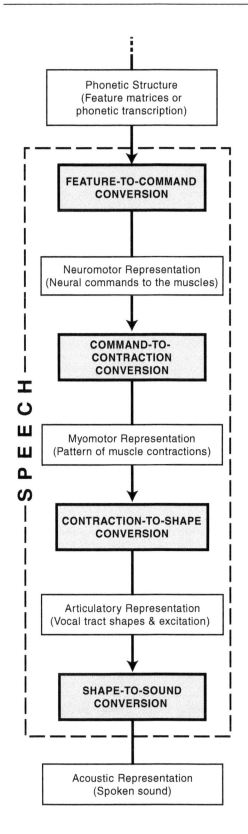

to this model are stored in the buffer, perhaps in the form of distinctive (phonological) features of speech production, such as manner and place of articulation and whether or not each sound is intended to be voiced or voiceless. Four conversions are shown in Figure 1.4: (1) from the internal abstract representation to nerve impulses, (2) from nerve impulses to muscle contractions, (3) from muscle contractions to vocal tract shape and air pressure changes, and (4) from these changes to an acoustic signal. These conversions result in an acoustic signal in which the phonetic realizations of phonological features overlap and in which the abstract phonemes no longer exist as separate entities.

The same speech rules are used in our model (Fig. 1.3), although here they are simultaneously interrelated and simultaneously applied to the input of the buffer. In the buffer, the utterance exists as an abstract internal representation of the speaker's acoustic and physiological goals. These internal representations include specifications of both the three-dimensional space in which the articulators must move and the relative timing of movements of the individual articulators. The speaker knows the intended sounds and the rules that must be applied to produce them. She unconsciously knows what cavity shapes and air pressure changes are required for the transition from the end of the word "Japanese" to the beginning of the word "prints" and from the /n/ to the /i/

**FIGURE 1.4**  Model of speech production. It is assumed that each speech sound can be represented as a complex of abstract phonetic features. The features are actualized as neural commands to the articulatory muscles, which shape the vocal tract. The shape of the vocal tract determines the output sound. (Reprinted with permission from Cooper, F. S., How Is Language Conveyed by Speech? In *Language by Ear and by Eye.* J. F. Kavanagh and I. G. Mattingly (Eds.). Cambridge, MA: MIT Press, 1972, p. 34.)

in /ʤæpəniz/ "Japanese." By applying these rules, she produces a stream of sound.

We are far from understanding the details of how this process works. Neither do we fully understand how a listener processes speech to arrive at the intent of the speaker. Speech science is the study of these issues: the production of speech, the acoustics of the signal, and the perception of speech by a listener. If the buffer is considered to hold the intended message, speech scientists concern themselves with everything downstream of that stage. The transformations from an intended phrase to its acoustic realization by a speaker and the transformations from acoustics of speech to the decoding of the intended phrase by a listener are what the speech scientist studies.

## REFERENCES AND SUGGESTED READING

Bernstein, B., A Socio-Linguistic Approach to Socialization: With Some Reference to Educability. In *Directions in Sociolinguistics*. J. J. Gumperz and D. Hymes (Eds.). New York: Holt, Rinehart & Winston, 1972, pp. 465–497.

Bickerton, D., *Language and Human Behavior*. Seattle: University of Washington Press, 1995.

Bruner, J. S., *Studies in Cognitive Growth*. New York: Wiley & Sons, 1966.

Chomsky, N., *Language and Mind* (enlarged edition). New York: Harcourt Brace Jovanovich, Inc., 1972.

Cooper, F. S., How Is Language Conveyed by Speech? In *Language by Ear and by Eye*. J. F. Kavanagh and I. G. Mattingly (Eds.). Cambridge, MA: MIT Press, 1972, pp. 25–45.

Crain, S., and Lillo-Martin, D., *An Introduction to Linguistic Theory and Language Acquisition*. Oxford: Blackwell Publishers, 1999.

Fromkin, V., and Rodman, R., *An Introduction to Language*, 7th ed. Boston: Heinle, 2003.

Furth, H., *Thinking Without Language: Psychological Implications of Deafness*. New York: Free Press, 1966.

Jusczyk, P. W., *The Discovery of Spoken Language*. Cambridge, MA: MIT Press, 1997.

Knowles, G., *A Cultural History of the English Language*. London: Arnold, 1997.

Krashen, S., The Critical Period for Language Acquisition and Its Possible Bases. *Ann. N.Y. Acad. Sci. 263*, 1975, 211–224.

Lenneberg, E. H., *Biological Foundations of Language*. New York: Wiley, 1967.

Levelt, W. J. M. *Speaking: From Intention to Articulation*. Cambridge, MA: MIT Press, 1989.

Liberman, A. M., The Grammars of Speech and Language. *Cognit. Psychol. 1*, 1970, 301–323.

Lieberman, P., Crelin, E., and Klatt, D., Phonetic Ability and Related Anatomy of the Newborn and Adult Human, Neanderthal Man and the Chimpanzee. *Am. Anthropol. 74*, 1972, 287–307.

Macaulay, R., *The Social Art: Language and Its Uses*. New York: Oxford University Press, 1994.

Mowrer, O. H., *Learning Theory and Personality Dynamics*. New York: Ronald Press, 1950.

Piaget, J., *The Language and Thought of the Child*. Atlantic Highlands, NJ: Humanities, 1959. (Translation of *Le Langage et la Pensée chez L'Enfant*. Neuchâtel and Paris: Delachaux et Niestlé, 1923).

Pinker, S., *The Language Instinct*. New York: William Morrow and Company, 1994.

Pinker, S. *Words and Rules*. New York: Basic Books, 1999.

Skinner, B. F., *Verbal Behavior*. New York: Appleton-Century-Crofts, 1957.

Vygotsky, L. S., *Thought and Language*. Cambridge, MA: MIT Press, 1962.

Whorf, B. L., *Language, Thought, and Reality*. Cambridge, MA: MIT Press, 1956.

# SECTION II    Acoustics

# Acoustics

2

*Holla your name to the reverberate hills,*
*And make the babbling gossip of the air cry out.*

—William Shakespeare, Twelfth Night

The study of sound is called acoustics. Because speech is a continuously changing stream of sound, it is necessary to have a clear understanding of the nature of sound in general to understand the production and perception of speech.

Sound has no physical substance. It has no mass or weight but is, rather, an audible disturbance in a medium caused by a vibrating source such as a tuning fork or the vocal folds. Such disturbances are characterized as waves. A sound wave can exist in a gas, such as air; in a liquid, such as water; or in a solid, such as a water pipe or a railroad track. The medium in which speech is most usually transmitted is air; therefore, sound waves traveling in air are the major focus of this chapter.

One of the problems students encounter in their first attempt to understand sound is the fact of its invisibility. Because molecules of air are not visible to the human eye, the waves of disturbance moving through air cannot be seen. Another obstacle is the fact that most sound waves consist of complex patterns of air molecule disturbance. To overcome these barriers to understanding, we must make the invisible visible and begin our discussion with the simplest of all sounds, the *pure tone*.

## PURE TONE: AN EXAMPLE OF SIMPLE HARMONIC MOTION

One seldom hears a pure tone. Most of the sounds we hear—street noises, speech, and music—are complex. That is, they consist of two or more tones or frequencies heard simultaneously. A pure tone, in contrast, consists of only one frequency. It is the result of a vibration that repeats itself in exactly the

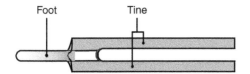

**FIGURE 2.1**   A typical tuning fork. When struck, it produces a pure tone.

same way at an unchanging rate. Each individual vibration is called a cycle and the number of cycles completed in one second is the *frequency of vibration*. A tuning fork, for example, creates a sound wave that consists of a single frequency. That is, the tuning fork vibrates only at one specified frequency, and the result of the vibration is a pure tone, the simplest of all sound waves and therefore the easiest to describe.

When it is struck, the tines or prongs of the tuning fork vibrate in *simple harmonic motion* (SHM; Fig. 2.1). That is, they move back and forth a fixed number of times per second, no

matter how hard the tuning fork is struck. The initial impact forces both tines of the fork to move away from their rest positions (Fig. 2.2). Because of the elasticity of the fork, however, the tines stop moving at a point of maximum displacement and then turn back toward their original rest positions. Elasticity is the restoring force that causes an elastic medium to bounce back when stretched or displaced. Push your finger into the fatty part of your arm or leg and you will find that the tissue restores itself quickly because of its elasticity. In SHM, however, the movement does not stop with the elastic recoil of the tines. That is, the tines of the tuning fork continue to move through their rest positions because of *inertia*, the tendency for motion or lack of motion to continue. In the case of the tuning fork tines, which are in motion at their rest positions, it takes less energy for them to continue moving than to stop. Thus, the tines of the tuning fork pass through their original

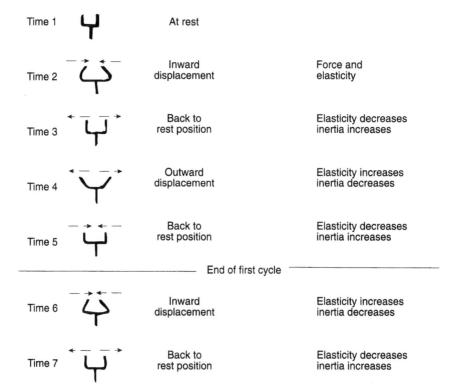

**FIGURE 2.2**   Tuning fork displacements in 1.5 cycles of vibration.

rest positions. When they do so, the elastic force begins to increase, slowing the motion of the tines until they stop at their point of maximum displacement on the other side of their rest positions. The elastic force then returns the tines once more to and through their rest positions. At the moment when the tines reach their rest positions, they have completed one cycle of vibration and begin another as they pass through.

The forces of elasticity and inertia are almost always simultaneously at work, although at any moment one of them may be dominant. Elasticity causes a decrease in the velocity of movement of the tines as they approach their points of maximum displacement. The more the tines move away from their rest positions in either direction, the greater the elastic force becomes until it overcomes the force of inertia and the tines come to their momentary rest at their points of maximum displacement. Then, the elastic force begins to move the tines back toward their rest positions. This movement imparts an inertial force to the tines that increases as they approach their rest positions and causes them to overshoot them. The overshoot reintroduces the elastic force (neutralized at the rest positions) so that it continues to increase again as the tines continue to move away from their rest positions. The repeated cycles of movement are thus generated by a simultaneous interplay of the two forces, not by their alternation.

We have described one cycle of vibration in SHM, but it should be illustrated further for clarity. Figure 2.2 illustrates the motion and positions of the tines of a tuning fork during its first one and one-half cycles of vibration.

## The Swing Analogy: Velocity Gradation in Simple Harmonic Motion

Consider the SHM of a swing hanging from the branch of a tree. When you displace the swing from its resting position by pulling it back and then releasing it, it not only returns to its original position but also goes past it. This back and forth movement, although different in some respects, is analogous to the movement of the tuning fork tines and to the movement of air particles that are set into vibration during the transmission of a sound. The swing illustrates an important property of SHM, which is the continuous manner in which the displaced object changes velocity. Velocity is the speed of an object, in this case the seat of the swing. In Figure 2.3, the spot on the ground over which the swing seat hangs when at rest is point 2. Assume a given force will displace

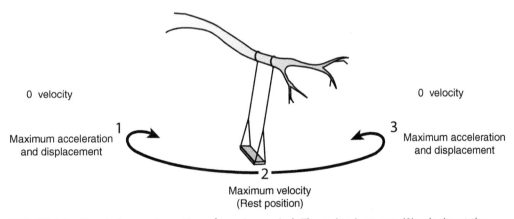

0 velocity

0 velocity

1

Maximum acceleration and displacement

3

Maximum acceleration and displacement

2

Maximum velocity
(Rest position)

**FIGURE 2.3** Simple harmonic motion of a swing period. The swing is at zero (0) velocity at the extremes of its excursion (points 1 and 3) as it changes direction and at maximum velocity at point 2, in the middle of its excursion.

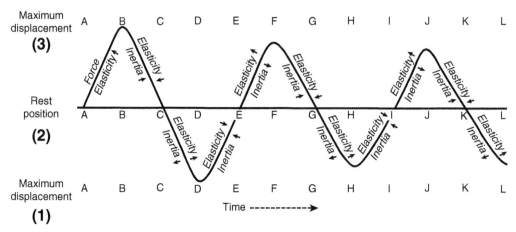

**FIGURE 2.4** Waveform produced by graphing the simple harmonic motion of a swing.

the swing to point 3; then it will swing back and forth between points 1 and 3 until its motion dies down. While swinging, the velocity changes, gradually diminishing as it approaches 1 and 3, where it drops for an instant to zero before the swing changes direction. Maximum velocity is reached each time the swing seat passes over its original resting position. Because the swing comes to a momentary standstill at each end of the excursion, the maximum acceleration, the rate of change in velocity, is at these extreme points where the swing changes direction.

If the movement of the swing were graphed as it changes position in time, it would look like Figure 2.4. The velocity is graded, with zero velocity and maximum acceleration at *B*, *D*, *F*, *H*, *J*, and *L* and maximum velocity at the zero crossings *C*, *E*, *G*, *I*, and *K*. The extent of the motion, called the *amplitude*, is also decreasing gradually because of the loss of energy from friction. That is, on each successive cycle, the points of maximum displacement are closer together—less distant from the rest position. This decrease in the amplitude of displacement over time is called *damping*. Although the distance between the rest position of the swing and its points of maximum displacement is decreasing, the frequency of the swing's motion does not change. Frequency is the number of completed cycles per second, expressed as *Hertz*

(Hz). As Figure 2.4 shows, the time it takes for the swing to complete its first cycle (*A* to *E*) is equal to the time it takes to complete the second cycle (*E* to *I*). The time taken for each cycle is called the *period of vibration*. If the frequency of a vibrating body were 20 Hz, the period would be 1/20 second, or 50 milliseconds (ms). The movement of a body vibrating in SHM can be graphically represented as a *sine wave*. The pattern of movement is simple because there is only one frequency of vibration and, because it repeats itself, is periodic.

## Particle Movement in Sound

Individual air molecules move in SHM in response to the SHM movement of a pure tone vibrator. They do not, however, move along an arc as the seat of a swing or a pendulum does. Rather, they move, alternately, in the same or opposite direction that the sound wave moves as it is propagated from the source of vibration. We will discuss this motion in some detail later in this chapter.

You can illustrate SHM for yourself by placing your pencil or finger on the middle dot marked *B* in Figure 2.5a. Move it to *C*, then *A*, then *C*, and continue at a fixed, relatively slow frequency without stopping. Try moving your finger at the same frequency

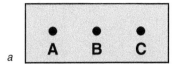  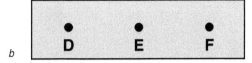

**FIGURE 2.5**  Simulate simple harmonic motion by moving finger rhythmically from *B* to *C* to *A* to *C*, oscillating with gradually and continuously changing velocity. Repeat with *EFDF* at same frequency.

but with a larger excursion from the resting place, using Figure 2.5b to set the range. The movements you make with your pencil or finger could be displayed as an amplitude-by-time graph called a *waveform* (Fig. 2.6).

Return to Figure 2.5 and practice SHM at a constant frequency for both *a* and *b*, but this time make the movements at a relatively high frequency (an increased number of cycles per second). The waveforms look more like those in Figure 2.7.

These movements back and forth over the resting place are magnified versions of the movement of a single air molecule when a pure tone is sounded. When a tuning fork specified to vibrate at 440 Hz (A above middle C on the piano) is sounded in the middle of a room, every molecule of air in the room soon moves in place. Each particle initially moves away from the tuning fork because of the force exerted against it by a neighboring particle, then back to the resting place because of elasticity, then closer to the fork because of inertia, then back to the resting place because of elasticity, and so on as long as the vibration lasts. Each particle completes 440 of these cycles per second.

## Pressure Wave Movement in Sound

We have been analyzing the movement of individual molecules during the generation of a pure tone. If each molecule is moving back and forth over its rest position, how does the disturbance move from one location to another? Molecules nearest the source of vibration start moving before molecules that are farther away. The molecules of air oscillating in SHM disturb adjacent molecules, and thus the disturbance is transmitted away from the source. This disturbance takes the form of a pressure wave radiating outward, much like the ripples emanating from a point in still water after a pebble has been tossed in. Because the pure tone is periodic, the pressure wave is repeated and is followed by evenly spaced pressure waves. Figure 2.8 shows 10 individual air molecules. At time 1, before the pure tone vibrator is set into motion, the molecules are shown at rest, equidistant from one another. At time 2, the outward movement of one of the tines of the tuning fork has forced molecule A to move away from the fork, approaching molecule B. At time 3, molecule A has bounced back to its resting place because of elasticity, but molecule B

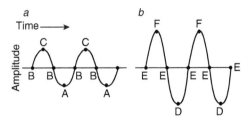

**FIGURE 2.6**  Waveform of simple harmonic motion traced in Figure 2.5; *a* and *b* differ in amplitude but are equal in frequency.

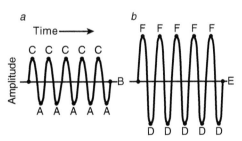

**FIGURE 2.7**  Waveforms *a* and *b* differ in amplitude but are equal in frequency.

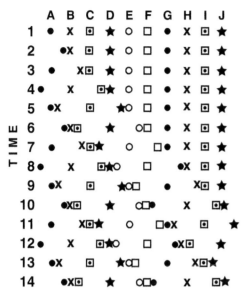

**FIGURE 2.8** Schematic drawing of 10 air particles in simple harmonic motion at 14 moments. The sound source is conceived to be to the left. Pressure waves move to the right. Time runs from top to bottom. Although the pressure wave, indicated by a clustering of three adjacent particles, moves from left to right, each individual particle moves relatively little around a rest position.

has been displaced by the influence (during time 2) of the impinging molecule A. Notice that as time proceeds, areas of compression, in which molecules are closer together and the air pressure is higher, alternate with areas of rarefaction, in which molecules are farther apart and the air pressure is lower. For example, in time 7, a high-pressure area formed by the juxtaposition of molecules B, C, and D is surrounded by relatively low-pressure areas. By time 10, the first area of high pressure has moved farther from the sound source and now consists of particles E, F, and G. At the same time, an area of high pressure, consisting of molecules A, B, and C is emanating from the vibrator.

It is helpful to visualize compression waves moving through a medium by a simple demonstration using a coiled wire. A toy called a Slinky serves well. Spreading the coil along a tabletop between your hands, hold one hand steady and move the other back and forth in SHM until waves can be seen to flow through the coil. Observe that the waves move in the same direction as your hand when it moves toward your stationary hand. This type of wave, in which particle movement is in the same direction as wave movement, is called a *longitudinal wave*. Sound waves are longitudinal whether in air or in liquid. Waves seen radiating from tossing a stone or dipping a finger into water are called *transverse waves* because although the waves move out from the source of disturbance, the water molecules move at right angles to the wave: up and down, as any cork-watching fisherman will attest.

If all the air molecules in a room were colored gray, a tuning fork vibrating in the center of the room would be surrounded by a sphere of relatively dark gray (an area of compression of air particles) that would move away from the vibrator. Although each molecule moves back and forth in place, the disturbance moves throughout the room. Each compression area is followed by a pale gray area (rarefaction area), then another compression area (Fig. 2.9). The alternating

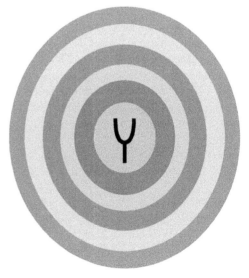

**FIGURE 2.9** Pressure wave emanating from a sound source. The areas of compression encircle the vibrator as a globe, not indicated in this two-dimensional figure.

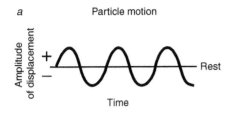

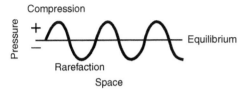

**FIGURE 2.10** Waveform of a pure tone (*a*) and a graph of pressure variations as a function of distance from the source (*b*). The waveforms look alike, although they have different coordinates.

areas of compression and rarefaction constitute a pressure wave that moves away from the tuning fork in all directions and that can be represented as a sine wave in the same way as the motion of individual molecules (Fig. 2.10).

Waveforms are common representations of sound signals. A waveform is a display of how amplitude varies with time and therefore can represent molecular motion, as in Figure 2.10a, but it can also represent the pressure variation in the medium as a whole, as in Figure 2.10b. Several acoustic analysis programs can be used to display waveforms on computer monitors (see Chapter 13, Figure 13.3). Remember that the movement of any particular molecule, were it visible, would not look like that waveform. Rather, the waveform is an abstract representation of the molecule's displacement from rest during a certain time or of the variations in air pressure generated by the vibrating source and the air molecules. The *amplitude* of displacement indicates the intensity or power of the sound, and so the *ordinate* (*y*, or vertical axis) of a waveform is often scaled in units of in-

tensity. Time is represented along the *abscissa* (*x*, or horizontal axis).

## Essential Constituents of Sound

The discussion so far allows us to identify three prerequisites for the production of sound. They are (1) *a source of energy* that is applied to, (2) *a vibrating source*, such as a tuning fork, that will generate an audible pressure wave in, and (3) *a medium of transmission*, such as air. But do the transmitted pressure waves constitute sound, or must we add a fourth prerequisite: a receiver—someone to hear the sound? This raises an old question: If a tree falls in the forest and there is no one to hear it, does it make a sound? Notice that this is more of a philosophical or metaphysical question than a question about physics. Also notice that we have been describing sound in purely physical terms. Therefore, unless someone can supply a reason why the laws of physics in the forest have been suspended, we can assert that the tree does, indeed, make a noise when it falls, and we can limit the number of prerequisites for sound production to the three we have named.

Let us arbitrarily define *sound*, then, as a potentially audible disturbance of a medium produced by a vibrating source. The source may be a guitar string energized by the pluck of a finger or human vocal folds energized by air from the lungs. The medium may be gas, liquid, or solid; any elastic medium can carry an acoustic signal. The disturbance must be such that it will be capable of causing corresponding vibrations in a receiver, if one is present. The optional receiver can be the auditory system of any creature to whom the signal is audible.

## Interference Patterns

It is remarkable that the air can be filled with many sounds, all transmitted simultaneously. Because air molecules vibrate in place, they can be responsive to many signals at once. Signals of the same frequency, however, can interfere with one another. This occurs when the frequency is generated from two sources or, more often, when the signal is reflected from a barrier such as a wall to compete, in a sense, with itself.

The waveforms of two signals having a common frequency sum in a straightforward way. The resulting summed waveform depends on the *phase* relationship between the signals. To understand phase relationships, it helps to conceive of a cycle of vibration as a circle. Every circle has a total of 360°, so that half of a cycle would be 180°, one fourth of a cycle would be 90°, and three fourths, 270°. Although sine waves are not actually made up of semicircles, we have depicted them as circles twisted open in the middle at the top of Figure 2.11 to illustrate the concept of phase.

If two signals of the same frequency are *in phase*, their pressure waves crest and trough

at the same time, and if their amplitudes are identical, the sum of the signals has twice the amplitude of each component signal. Figure 2.11 illustrates pure tone signals that are in phase (a), 90° out of phase (b), and 180° out of phase (c). When signals are 90° out of phase, one signal is one fourth of a cycle ahead of the other. At each instant, the amplitudes of the two waveforms are simply added. When two acoustic signals having the same frequency and amplitude of vibration are 180° out of phase, the result is silence, for each molecule is subjected to equal forces that act in opposite directions. Each molecule then remains at rest.

The problem of interference patterns is especially important in concert halls, which must be designed by experts trained in architectural acoustics. If halls are poorly

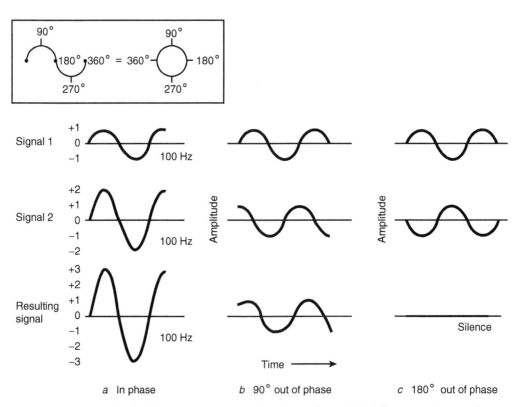

**FIGURE 2.11** Results of adding two pure tones (*signal 1* and *signal 2*), differing in phase and amplitude but of the same frequency. In all cases, the *resulting signal* is a pure tone of the same frequency, but phase and amplitude vary. The addition of two pure tones of the same frequency and amplitude but 180° out of phase produces silence, as shown in c.

designed acoustically, any sound produced in them may be repeatedly reflected by the hard walls in such a way that it *reverberates* excessively. This means that the sound will persist for too long a period of time as it bounces back and forth and interferes with listeners' perception of the following sound. Also, because of the interference patterns, a sound may be louder in some places and softer in others. The presence of a large audience dressed in sound-absorbing clothing will reduce reverberation, as will absorbent materials used in wall, ceiling, and floor coverings and in chair upholstery. On the other hand, too much absorption dulls the power of the sounds by causing insufficient reverberation. The right balance is difficult to achieve, yet none of us wants to have the misfortune of sitting in an acoustically dead spot in an auditorium where interference patterns caused by reflected sound and sound absorption create partial sound cancellation.

## COMPLEX TONES

Most sound sources, unlike the tuning fork, produce complex vibrations. Rather than vibrating in SHM, they move in a complex manner that generates more than one frequency. When these movements are graphed, a more complex waveform replaces the sine wave of the pure tone. To understand the derivation of a *complex tone*, simply add two sine waves of different frequencies. If many waves of the same frequency and phase relationship are added to each other (Fig. 2.11), the result is always a sine wave: a representation of a pure tone. If two or more pure tones of different frequencies are added, however, the result is a complex tone.

Figure 2.12 shows an instance of the addition of two pure tones (waves X and Y) to form a complex tone (wave XY). The frequency of wave Y is twice that of wave X. That is, wave Y completes two full cycles in the time that wave X completes one. The values of the amplitudes of waves X and Y have been measured at nine points in time

(A through I) and have been entered into the table in the figure. The amplitude values at each time have been added to each other and entered into the right-hand column in the table. The summed values have then been plotted in the bottom graph of the figure (labeled wave XY). Note that the waveform representing the combined pure tones is not a simple sine wave. It is more complex. Also note that if we were to extend wave X to two cycles and wave Y to four cycles, sum their amplitude values and plot them, then wave XY would display two identical cycles. That is, wave XY in Figure 2.12 would repeat itself exactly over time. It would be an example of a complex *periodic* sound wave: Periodic sound waves are those in which the pattern of vibration, however complex, repeats itself exactly over time. A second type of complex wave is termed *aperiodic*: An *aperiodic* sound wave is one in which the vibration is random and displays no repeatable pattern.

Play a note on the piano or sing "ah" and the resulting sounds will be complex but periodic in their waveforms. Drop a book on the floor or hiss through your teeth and the resulting sounds will be complex (having more than one frequency) but aperiodic (having no repeatable pattern) in their waveforms.

Table 2.1 displays the possible combinations and characteristics of wave types: simple versus complex and periodic versus aperiodic. Note that all aperiodic waves are complex. That is, they comprise more than one component frequency. We distinguish periodic from aperiodic complex waves on the basis of the mathematical relations among the frequencies of their components. To understand this distinction, we will first need to consider the nature of the harmonic structure of complex periodic sounds.

### Harmonics: Characteristics of Periodic Complex Tones

Periodic complex vibrations produce signals in which the component frequencies are integral (whole-number) multiples of the lowest frequency of pattern repetition, or the

**TABLE 2.1**   Possible Wave Types and Their Characteristics

| | Periodic | Aperiodic |
|---|---|---|
| Simple | One component frequency<br>A pure tone | –<br>– |
| Complex | Two or more component frequencies that are harmonically related: a fundamental frequency plus harmonics<br>A complex tone | Two or more component frequencies not harmonically related: no fundamental frequency, no harmonics<br>Noise |

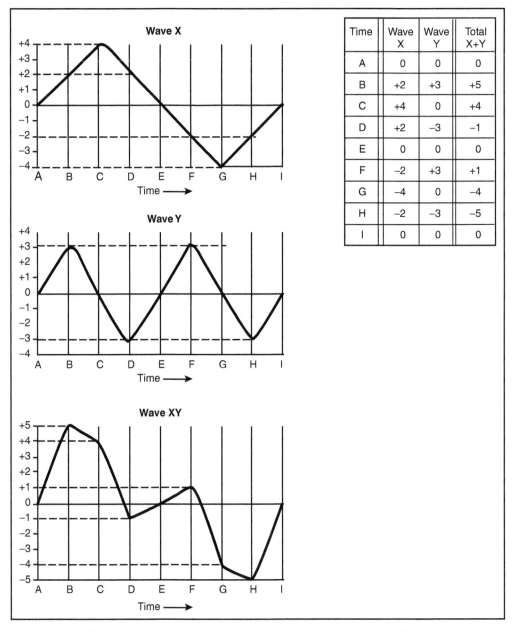

| Time | Wave X | Wave Y | Total X+Y |
|---|---|---|---|
| A | 0 | 0 | 0 |
| B | +2 | +3 | +5 |
| C | +4 | 0 | +4 |
| D | +2 | −3 | −1 |
| E | 0 | 0 | 0 |
| F | −2 | +3 | +1 |
| G | −4 | 0 | −4 |
| H | −2 | −3 | −5 |
| I | 0 | 0 | 0 |

**FIGURE 2.12**   Waveform of a complex tone derived from two pure tones of differing frequency.

fundamental frequency. This fundamental frequency derives from the rate at which the sound source produces its vibratory cycle. As an example, consider a vibrating source, such as a string on a guitar or a violin. When the string is plucked or bowed, it vibrates along its entire length at a given rate, say 100 Hz. This is the fundamental frequency of vibration of the string. If the string were vibrating in SHM, 100 Hz would be the only frequency generated, and the resulting sound would be a pure tone. But strings, reeds, vocal folds, and most other sound sources do not vibrate in SHM. At the same time that the whole string is vibrating at 100 Hz, both halves of the string are vibrating at 200 Hz–twice the string's fundamental frequency. The string therefore simultaneously generates frequencies of 100 and 200 Hz. But the complexity of the string's vibration goes well beyond that, for just as the entire string and each of its halves are vibrating at 100 and 200 Hz, each third of the string is vibrating at 300 Hz, each quarter at 400 Hz, each fifth at 500 Hz, and so on in ever-decreasing fractions of the string's length and ever-increasing frequencies of vibration. Each of the tones generated by this  complex vibration is called a *harmonic*, and the full set of harmonics is called a *harmonic series*.

As you have probably noticed, the frequency of each harmonic is a whole-number multiple of the fundamental frequency, which is also called the first harmonic. In the example above, the harmonic series comprises the following frequency components:

| Harmonic | Frequency |
| --- | --- |
| First | 100 Hz (100 × 1) |
| Second | 200 Hz (100 × 2) |
| Third | 300 Hz (100 × 3) |
| Fourth | 400 Hz (100 × 4) |
| Fifth | 500 Hz (100 × 5) |

There is a tendency for the harmonics in a series to decrease in amplitude as their

frequency increases. Therefore, although there is no theoretical limit to the number of harmonics a vibrating source can produce, the effect of very high-frequency harmonics on the overall quality of a sound is considered to be negligible for most common sources of sound, including the human voice.

This whole-number multiple relationship between the frequency of the fundamental and frequencies of the higher harmonics holds for all complex periodic waves. So if the fundamental frequency of a complex periodic wave were 200 Hz, the second, third, fourth, and fifth harmonics would have frequencies of 400, 600, 800, and 1,000 Hz, respectively. The bottom of Figure 2.13 shows the waveform of just such a wave. It is actually the waveform generated by a female speaker saying the vowel [ɑ]. If we compare this waveform with the 200-Hz pure tone at the top of the figure, we can see that both patterns repeat themselves at the same frequency.

A complex periodic wave does not have to consist of a complete harmonic series. The only requirement for periodicity is that every component present in the wave has a frequency that is a whole-number multiple of the fundamental frequency of the wave. That is, it must be part of a harmonic series. So, for example, combining components whose frequencies are 100 Hz, 300 Hz, 500 Hz, . . . will produce a wave that is complex and periodic,

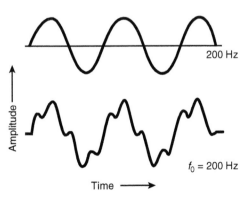

**FIGURE 2.13** Waveforms of a pure tone and a complex tone, each with a frequency of 200 Hz.

even though the even-numbered harmonics (200 Hz, 400 Hz, . . .) are missing.

Waveforms supply a fair amount of information about the sound signal: We can determine the fundamental frequency of the sound the waveform presents by counting the number of times its pattern is repeated each second; once we have determined the fundamental frequency, we can calculate the period of vibration and the frequencies of the individual harmonics. We cannot, however, directly discover the amplitudes of the *individual* harmonics (although variations in the *overall* amplitude of the signal over time are apparent in the waveform).

To depict harmonic amplitude we must turn to a different sort of display, the line (or amplitude) *spectrum* (plural, *spectra*). In a line spectrum, the ordinate (the vertical axis) represents amplitude, as in a waveform, but the abscissa (the horizontal axis) represents frequency. It is thus possible, using a spectral display, to indicate the frequency and amplitude of each harmonic in a complex periodic wave. Figure 2.14 pairs several of the wave-

forms previously presented with their corresponding spectra. Notice that a line spectrum does not depict the dimension of time. The information it presents is thus valid only for a particular instant in time. If we want to see how harmonic amplitude varies over time, we must make a sequential series of line spectra or resort to alternative types of displays, some of which are described in later chapters.

The sort of analytic process that produces a line spectrum reverses the synthetic process of adding sine waves to each other (Fig. 2.12). In the synthetic process of addition, as long as the simple waves being added are harmonically related, the summed wave will be periodic (and, of course, complex). Applying the analytic process to a periodic wave allows us to discover the frequencies and amplitudes of the simple waves—the harmonic components—of which it is composed. This process, called Fourier analysis, was first devised by J. B. Fourier, a French mathematician, during the first quarter of the 19th century. Originally a long and complex

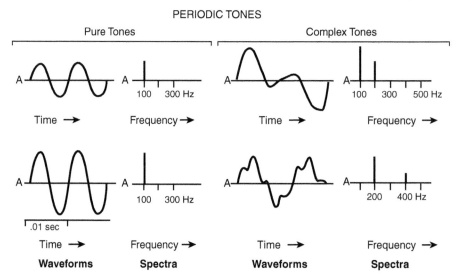

**FIGURE 2.14** Waveforms shown as a function of amplitude and time and corresponding spectra shown as a function of amplitude and frequency. The two signals on the *left* are vibrations at a single frequency (pure tones); the two signals on the *right* represent different complex vibrations, analyzed as a fundamental frequency and higher harmonics.

mathematical procedure, Fourier analysis is today performed directly and rapidly by a number of commercially available electronic analytic devices.

## Aperiodic Complex Signals

The sound of a book dropped on a table or of a hiss made between the teeth is complex, consisting of more than one frequency, but the frequencies are not harmonically related, as they are for periodic sounds. In both cases, the air molecules are set into random vibration within a broad range of frequencies. The waveforms of such vibrations are aperiodic, because there is no regular repetition in the molecular displacement patterns. The sound of the book hitting the tabletop is, however, transient, producing a burst of noise of short duration, whereas the hiss is continuous for as long as the airstream is made turbulent as it passes through a narrow constriction. Amplitude spectra can be made for aperiodic as well as periodic signals. Figure 2.15 shows the waveforms and spectra of typical aperiodic sound signals.

## FREQUENCY AND PITCH

We have stated that frequency is the number of vibratory cycles per second. The notations 100 Hz, 100 cps, and 100~, all mean the same thing: 100 cycles per second. The abbreviation Hz is preferred in the speech and hearing literature, and prevails in virtually all recently published material. The other two notations (cps and ~) are found only in writing that dates back 35 years or more.

## The Relationship Among Frequency, Hearing Acuity, and Vocal Production

People differ in the frequency range to which their hearing mechanism will respond, but in general, young, healthy human listeners can detect vibrations as low as 20 Hz and as high as 20,000 Hz. Vibrations too low in frequency to be audible are called subsonic, and those too high, ultrasonic. We may not hear extremely low frequencies as sound, but we can often feel them. The frequencies most important for the comprehension of the speech signal are within the 100- to 5,000-Hz range. Contrasting this frequency range with that used by bats, which emit sound between 20,000 and 100,000 Hz, one sees that sound can be used for different purposes. Human beings use sound to communicate thoughts and feelings, whereas bats use it to locate insects for food. Whether sound emission is used for localization or for communication,

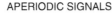

APERIODIC SIGNALS

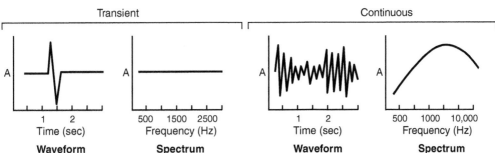

**FIGURE 2.15**  Noise signals. The graphs to the *left* are the waveform and spectrum of a sound similar to a book hitting a tabletop. The graphs to the *right* are the waveform and spectrum of a hissing noise. The envelope of the amplitude as a function of frequency is indicated. Because many frequency components are not harmonically related, continuous lines indicate the amplitudes.

however, it is important that the frequency response of the auditory system be matched to the frequency characteristics of the sound-producing mechanism. Human vocal folds normally vibrate between about 80 and 500 Hz during speech, but some of the speech noises made in the mouth contain frequencies that extend to several thousand cycles per second. The human auditory system, then, is responsive to the appropriate range of frequencies.

## The Distinction Between Frequency and Pitch

Frequency relates directly to *pitch*. Pitch is a sensation. In general, when the frequency of vibration is increased, we hear a rise in pitch, and when the frequency is decreased, we hear a lowering of pitch. The relationship is not linear, however. A constant interval of frequency increase does not result in a constant change in pitch. Frequency is a fact of physics, an event that can be measured by instruments: the number of cycles in a specified time. Pitch, in contrast, is a psychological phenomenon. It is the listener's perception of frequency changes and differences. It can be measured only by asking listeners to make judgments.

The human auditory system is more responsive to some frequency changes than to others. In the frequencies less than 1,000 Hz, perceived pitch is fairly linear in relation to frequency, but as the frequencies get higher, it takes a larger change in frequency to cause a change in the sensation of pitch. The relation between the physical property of frequency and the psychological sensation of pitch is illustrated in Figure 2.16. The units of frequency are cycles per second; the units of pitch are *mels*. Testing listeners at various frequencies, the pitch of a 1,000-Hz tone is used as a reference and is arbitrarily called 1,000 mels. Whatever frequency is judged to be half that pitch is 500 mels; twice that pitch is 2,000 mels. The mel curve shown by

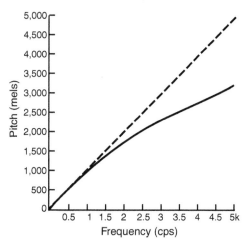

**FIGURE 2.16**   Replotting of the Stevens and Volkmann mel scale. The *solid line* indicates the way pitch (measured in mels) increases with frequency in cycles per second (Hz). The *broken line* shows the relationship if correlation were perfect. (Adapted from Stevens, S. S., Volkmann, J., and Newman, E. B., et al., A Scale for the Measurement of the Psychological Magnitude Pitch. *J. Acoust. Soc. Am. 8*, 1937, 185–190.)

the *solid line* in Figure 2.16 is the result of this scaling procedure.

Another way of looking at the effect of frequency changes on pitch is to consider the Just Noticeable Difference (*JND*) for frequency. This is often given nominally as 3 Hz, although as you can see in Figure 2.17, the JND can be considerably larger at higher frequencies. Nonetheless, the existence of a JND, no matter what its size, means that (1) there are some changes in frequency, those smaller than the JND, that will not affect pitch perception and (2) the terms frequency and pitch are not synonyms.

## The Pitch of Complex Tones

We have seen that frequency refers to the physical measure of cycles per second and that pitch is reserved for the perception of frequency. The mel scale was plotted by having listeners judge the pitch of pure tones.

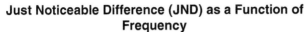

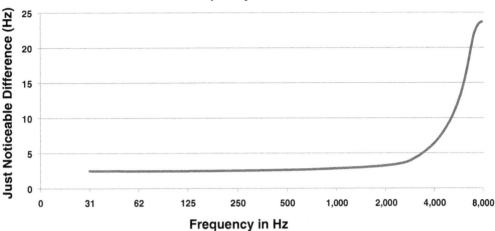

**FIGURE 2.17**   Values of the Just Noticeable Difference for frequencies between 31 and 16,000 Hz.

But how do listeners judge the pitch of complex tones, sounds containing more than one frequency? Listeners judge the pitch of a complex periodic tone to correspond to the fundamental frequency of the harmonic series. Surprisingly, even if the fundamental frequency of a harmonic series is not present, the auditory system compensates for the loss of the lower harmonics and "hears" the fundamental frequency ($f_0$). For example, a complex tone composed of 600, 900, and 1,200 Hz is judged to have the pitch of a 300-Hz tone, because 300 Hz, the largest divisor, is the rate at which the basic pattern of the complex wave repeats itself. Judgments of pitch for aperiodic sounds are more generally influenced by the center of the frequency band or the frequency at which the amplitude is highest.

## THE DECIBEL: A MEASURE OF RELATIVE INTENSITY

The amplitude of vibration (the extent of particle displacement) is an indication of the intensity or power of the sound. To describe the relative intensity of two sounds,

we use a unit of measurement called a *decibel* (dB), literally one tenth of a bel, a unit named in honor of Alexander Graham Bell (1847–1922), the American inventor of the telephone and educator of the deaf (see Chapter 12). The decibel scale of intensity is an example of a logarithmic scale. In a *linear scale*, such as a measuring stick, there is a zero, and each increment is equal to the next, so you can sum units by addition. A *logarithmic scale*, as you can see on the chart below, is based on "exponents" of a given number called the base. For decibels the base is 10, and the scale is constructed with increments that are not equal but represent increasingly larger numerical differences.

---

**Linear Scale**

---

1,000
  >diff. = 1,000
2,000
  >diff. = 1,000
3,000
  >diff. = 1,000
4,000

---

## Logarithmic Scale

$10^2 = 100$
 >diff. = 900
$10^3 = 1,000$
 >diff. = 9,000
$10^4 = 10,000$
 >diff. = 90,000
$10^5 = 100,000$

10 = base; 2, 3, 4, and 5 are logarithms.

Why use a logarithmic scale for sound intensity? There are two reasons: First, the human ear is sensitive to a large intensity range, as many as $10^{13}$ (10 followed by 12 zeros, or 10 trillion) units of intensity in a linear scale. That number is unmanageably large, but on a condensed logarithmic scale, the number is reduced to 130 dB.

The second reason is that the logarithmic scale more nearly approximates the way human ears judge loudness. It has been known since the 19th-century writings of German scientists Ernst Weber (1834) and Gustav Lechner (1860) that equal increases in sensation (in this case loudness) are obtained by multiplying the stimulus by a constant factor. This principle does not work for every intensity of sound to which the ear is sensitive, but it is accurate enough to be practical. Each step in the decibel scale, then, corresponds roughly to an equal growth in loudness, although the sound power differences are large.

The power of a sound is proportional to the square of the pressure, or to put it in reverse, the pressure is the square root of the power. Just as an inch or a centimeter is a unit of measurement used for length, the units of measurement used in acoustics are *watts* (for power) and *dynes* (for pressure). In physics, *intensity level* (IL) refers to the power of the signal as measured in watts per square centimeter. In the acoustics of speech and hearing, *sound pressure level* (SPL) has customarily been used as the measure, and the pressure unit is dynes per square centimeter. Either power or pressure units can be converted to decibels.

You may have heard that a certain airplane takes off with a sound level of 100 dB *SPL* or that the average intensity of conversational speech is about 60 dB *IL*. The first measure uses pressure as the reference; the sound pressure of the airplane noise is $10^5$ more than a barely audible sound (100,000:1 ratio). Were it to be measured by using a power reference, it would still be 100 dB, but the intensity ratio would be $10^{10}$ to 1 (10 billion to 1), because the power increments are the square of the pressure increments. The second measure, the speech intensity, uses a power reference. This relationship between power and pressure makes it necessary to use separate formulas to compute the decibel, one when using a power reference (watts) and the other for use with a pressure reference (dynes).

The important thing about measuring the intensity of a sound is that there is always a standard. The decibel is a unit of intensity that is really a ratio, a comparison of the sound in question with a reference sound. The power reference is $10^{-16}$ watts/cm$^2$, and the pressure reference is 0.0002 dyne/cm$^2$, both signals at the threshold of human audibility. The formula for decibels using an intensity (power) reference is:

$$\text{dB IL} = 10(\log_{10} W_o / W_r) \qquad (2.1)$$

where IL is the intensity level (reference is $10^{-16}$ watts/cm$^2$), $W_o$ is the output power in watts (power of signal to be measured), $W_r$ is the reference power in watts (power of the reference signal $10^{-16}$ watts/cm$^2$), and $\log_{10}$ is the logarithm of the ratio $W_o$ to $W_r$. The base is 10. The log is the exponent. For example, if the ratio is 100:1, the log is 2, because $10^2 = 100$, and the exponent is 2.

The formula used to compute decibels using an SPL reference for comparison is:

$$\text{dB SPL} = 20(\log_{10} P_o / P_r) \qquad (2.2)$$

In this formula, $P_o$ is the output pressure you wish to measure and $P_r$ is the reference pressure you use for comparison. For example, if the sound measured has a pressure level of 20 dyne/cm$^2$, that sound is 100,000 times the reference pressure

$$\frac{20 \text{ dynes/cm}^2}{0.0002 \text{ dynes/cm}^2} = \frac{100,000}{1} \quad (2.3)$$

Because the ratio is 100,000:1, the logarithm to the base 10 of the ratio is 5 (count the zeros). The formula instructs us to multiply the log of the ratio by 20. Because 20 × 5 = 100, the answer is 100 dB SPL. The expression:

$$\log_{10} P_o / P_r \quad (2.4)$$

is one small number, the exponent; in this case, 5.

To take another example, if a sound with 10 times as much pressure as a barely audible sound is measured, how many decibels SPL would it be? The log of 10 is 1 (only one zero) and 20 × 1 = 20; therefore, it is 20 dB SPL.

You should also be able to compute the ratio or the pressure in dynes when given the decibels. A 60-dB SPL conversation, as an instance, is how much more sound pressure than what is barely audible?

$$\begin{aligned} 60 \text{ dB SPL} &= 20x \\ (x &= \log_{10} P_o / P_r) \quad (2.5) \\ x &= 3 \end{aligned}$$

Because the log is 3, the ratio must be 1,000:1 (3 zeros).

So the sound pressure of an average conversation is 1,000 times greater than the SPL of a barely audible sound, or, to be exact, 0.2 dyne/cm$^2$.

$$\frac{0.0002 \text{ dynes/cm}^2 \times 1000}{0.2000 \text{ dynes/cm}^2} \quad (2.6)$$

What does 0 dB mean? If a sound is measured to have an intensity of 0 dB, does it

mean that there is no sound? Not at all.

$$\frac{\text{dB} = 20 \text{ (log of the ratio)}}{0 \text{ dB} = 20 \times 0} \quad (2.7)$$

The log is zero. Because there are no zeros in the ratio, the ratio is equal to 1, which means that the output is equal to the reference pressure.

| Ratio | Log | dB (20 × Log of Ratio) |
|---|---|---|
| 1,000:1 | 3 | 60 dB SPL |
| 100:1 | 2 | 40 dB SPL |
| 10:1 | 1 | 20 dB SPL |
| 1:1 | 0 | 0 dB SPL |

Thus, 0 dB means the sound in question is equal to the reference sound rather than to silence.

The SPLs of certain familiar sounds are approximated here:

| 0 dB | Threshold of Hearing |
|---|---|
| 20 dB | Rustling of leaves |
| 30 dB | Whisper (3 feet) |
| 35 dB | Residential area at night |
| 45 dB | Typewriter |
| 60 dB | Conversation |
| 75 dB | Shouting, singing (3 feet) |
| 100 dB | Approaching subway train, for people on a waiting platform |
| 120 dB | Jet airplane, for a person on the runway; amplified rock music (6 feet) |
| 130 dB | Painfully loud sound |

All sound within a few feet of the listener.

## INTENSITY AND LOUDNESS

*Intensity*, or sound pressure, like frequency, is a physical property of the acoustic signal that can be measured by a sound level meter. The loudness of a signal is directly related to

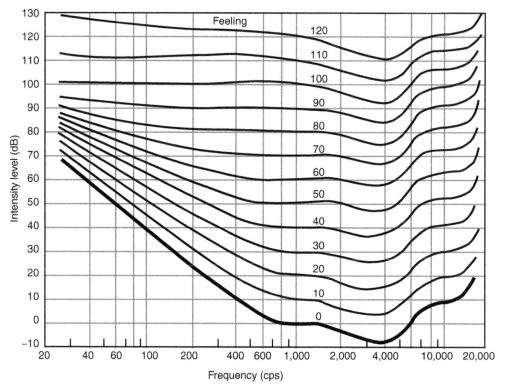

**Frequency (cps)**

**FIGURE 2.18** Loudness level contours derived by Fletcher and Munson. Each curve sounds equally loud at all frequencies. The loudness in phons is indicated on each curve. (Adapted from Fletcher, H. and Munson, W. A., Loudness: Its Definition, Measurement, and Calculation. *J. Acoust. Soc. Am. 5,* 1933, 82–108.)

its intensity. As the intensity increases, the sound is judged by listeners to be louder. *Loudness* is the subjective psychological sensation of judged intensity. Like frequency and pitch, intensity and loudness are not linearly related. Again, the human auditory system acts on the signal, so that sensations of equal loudness for different frequencies require very different intensities.

A *phon* is a unit of equal loudness. Figure 2.18 is a plot of equal loudness levels at different frequencies. The *heavy line* at the bottom of the figure is the *absolute threshold of audibility*, the intensities at each frequency that are just audible by young, healthy listeners. It is clear that the human auditory system is designed to receive the middle frequencies (1,000–6,000 Hz) with much less intensity than is needed for the extremely low and high frequencies. This information is used

in the specifications for manufacturing audiometers (instruments used to test hearing) to compare any person's threshold hearing with that of a young healthy person. The zero setting on an audiometer is simply the *heavy line* in Figure 2.18, straightened out on the graph paper that is used to chart the results of the test, the audiogram.

The *lighter lines* are the phon curves of equal loudness, referenced to tones of 1,000 Hz. Thus, the 20-phon line is as loud at all frequencies as a 1,000-Hz tone is at 20 dB, whereas a 70-phon line is as loud at all frequencies as a 1,000-Hz tone at 70 dB. Tracing the 20-phon line to the left reveals that a 200-Hz tone at 40 dB will be perceived to be as loud as the 1,000-Hz tone at 20 dB; similarly, we can see that a 70-Hz tone at 80 dB will be perceived to be as loud as a 1,000-Hz tone at 70 dB.

**TABLE 2.2** The Relationship Between the Physical and Psychological Properties of Frequency and Pitch

| Physical Properties Name and Units | | Psychological Properties Name and Units | |
|---|---|---|---|
| Frequency | Hz | Pitch | Mel (scaling) |
| Intensity | dB | Loudness | Phon (equal) |
| | | | Sone (scaling) |

For quiet sounds, there is a large difference between the middle and extreme frequencies in the amount of intensity needed to cause equal loudness judgments, but at higher loudness levels, the large intensity differences disappear.

When listeners are asked to judge relative loudness (half as loud, twice as loud) in a scaling procedure similar to that used to obtain the mel scale for pitch, the unit of loudness is called a *sone*, with 1 sone equal in loudness to a 1,000-Hz tone at 40 dB. This method demonstrates that the sensation of loudness increases more slowly than the actual increase in intensity.

Table 2.2 summarizes the relationship between the physical and psychological properties of frequency and pitch.

## VELOCITY OF SOUND THROUGH SPACE

Velocity is simply speed in a certain direction. Light travels faster than sound, or has greater velocity, as we know from our experience with thunderstorms: We see a flash of lightning some time before we hear the crash of thunder it caused. At normal atmospheric conditions, sound travels through air at about:

344 meters per second
or
1,130 feet per second
or
758 miles per hour

It travels much faster through liquids and fastest along solids, because the greater elasticity and density of these media increase the velocity of conduction. Velocity is independent of pressure as long as the temperature remains the same. A faint sound travels just as fast as a loud one, but it does not travel as far because of the *inverse square law* (intensity varies inversely as the square of the distance from the source). Temperature does make a difference, however, and sounds travel faster on a hot summer day than on a cold winter day.

The velocity of sound wave propagation must not be confused with velocity of molecular movement. Particles vibrating in SHM constantly change velocity, moving with maximum velocity over their resting places (Fig. 2.8). The velocity of the sound wave moving through space, that is, the speed with which the disturbance moves from one place to another, is, by contrast, a constant.

## WAVELENGTH

The length of a sound wave is the distance in space that one cycle occupies. For periodic waves, the *wavelength* is the distance from any point in one cycle to the corresponding point in a neighboring cycle. The symbol used to denote wavelength is the Greek letter lambda ($\lambda$). Figure 2.19 illustrates the wavelengths of complex and pure tone signals.

Wavelength depends on two factors, the frequency of the vibration and the velocity of sound wave propagation in the medium.

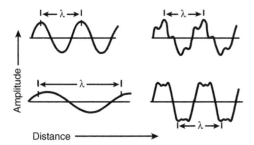

**FIGURE 2.19** Wavelength (λ) is the distance occupied by one complete cycle of vibration.

Observe wavelength changes by taking a small pan of water and dipping your finger into the water repeatedly, first at a slow frequency and then at a higher frequency. At the low frequency, the crests of the ripples are farther apart than at the high frequency. High-frequency sounds occupy less space per cycle–have a shorter wavelength–than do low-frequency sounds.

We can further illustrate the factor of frequency-conditioned wavelength using a speech sound. Imagine a man and a woman each saying the vowel [ɑ]. The woman is likely to produce the sound with a fundamental frequency of around 200 Hz, and the man with a fundamental frequency of about 100 Hz. Wavelength (λ) equals the velocity of sound (c) divided by the frequency (f):

$$\lambda = c/f \tag{2.8}$$

Placing the fundamental frequency of 200 Hz into the formula and solving the equation for λ reveals that the wavelength of the woman's voice is almost 2 meters; placing the fundamental frequency of 100 Hz into the formula reveals that the man's voice has the wavelength of more than 3 meters (a meter is 39.37 inches, or 1.1 yards):

$$\lambda = c/f$$
$$\lambda = 344 \text{ meters per second}/200 \text{ Hz}$$
$$= \text{about } 1.75 \text{ meters or } 67 \text{ inches} \tag{2.9}$$
$$(5'7'')$$
$$\lambda = 344 \text{ meters per second}/100 \text{ Hz}$$
$$= 3.4 \text{ meters or } 11'3''$$

The second factor, the medium through which the sound travels, is also important. Sound waves are conducted through solids faster than through liquids and through liquids faster than through gases. Given the formula for the wavelength:

$$\lambda = c/f \tag{2.10}$$

a sound of a certain frequency would have a longer wavelength in water, for example, than in air, because the higher velocity increases the numerator of the fraction, c.

When a speaker articulates an aperiodic sound, such as [ʃ] ("sh"), to quiet someone, the high-energy frequencies are closer to 2,500 Hz, which makes the wavelength of such a sound as short as 14 cm (5.5 inches).

$$\lambda = 34{,}400 \text{ cm per sec}/2{,}500 \text{ Hz}$$
$$= \sim 14 \text{ cm} \tag{2.11}$$

Sounds of high frequency and short wavelengths are more directional than low-frequency sounds. Long wavelengths radiate more and go around corners more easily than short ones. This is why the high-frequency (ultrasonic) sounds emitted by bats are useful in helping them to locate the small flying insects on which they prey. The sound from the bat reflects from any object in its path with more intensity than from neighboring objects, thereby localizing the prey for the kill. Only a signal with a short wavelength and little radiation could localize such a small target. Bats, even if blind, can analyze the reflected sound for information on size and distance of either obstacles or food.

Variation in wavelength also explains why we often hear voices in an adjoining room quite clearly but fail to understand what they are saying. Speech contains both high- and low-frequency components. The low-frequency sounds with longer wavelengths diffract around the wall and enter through the door. The high-frequency components of speech, having shorter, more

## CLINICAL NOTE

Although the discussion of basic acoustics may seem to be somewhat abstract, we want to make it clear that the concepts and principles presented here have very real and specific clinical applications. For instance, the distinction between periodicity and aperiodicity can be used in cases of voice disorders as a diagnostic tool and as a method of tracking progress in treatment. The same is true of the harmonic series, which will present irregularities in cases of disorders of phonation. The properties of simple waves (pure tones) are of great interest to audiologists who frequently use them to test hearing acuity. In the following section on *Resonance*, we find another aspect of acoustics that has relevance in the clinic. Studying the resonances of the vocal tract (see Chapters 5 and 6) allows clinicians to infer a great deal about the movement and placement of the articulators during the production of both normal and disordered speech. Inspecting the acoustic record of resonance may provide information that cannot be obtained simply by listening. Many features of articulation and phonation are highly complex and occur too rapidly for aural identification. The acoustic analysis of recorded speech signals allows speech scientists and clinicians to inspect those features at length, at any time after the speech has been produced and recorded.

directional wavelengths, radiate less widely and are largely unheard. Receiving only part of the signal, we often cannot understand what is being said.

## RESONANCE

If you have ever pushed a child in a swing, you know that you must time each push to coincide with the harmonic motion of the swing. If you run forward and push the swing while it is still moving toward you, you will simply shorten its arc. You may also be knocked to the ground if you attempt to push the swing as it passes at maximum velocity through its rest position. The frequency with which the swing completes a cycle during 1 second is the *natural resonant frequency* of the swing. This frequency is independent of amplitude. If you push a child with less force, then with more force, the arcs will vary in amplitude, but the frequency will remain the same. But what if the swing breaks and a piece of rope is removed from each side, making the swing shorter? Will the natural resonance frequency of the shorter-roped swing be the same as the swing with

longer ropes? We know by experience that this new swing would have a higher natural frequency (complete more cycles per second) than when the ropes of the swing were longer. In general, smaller things vibrate at higher frequencies than larger versions of the same thing. Shortening the vibrating portion of a guitar string by pressing down will, for example, cause it to vibrate at a higher frequency when it is plucked than when the string is free to vibrate along its entire length.

Everything that vibrates has a natural, or *resonant*, frequency, or as in the case of the guitar or violin string discussed above, produces many frequencies when it is plucked or bowed and left to vibrate freely (set into *free vibration*). These frequencies are those of a harmonic series. A machine could be attached to a string, forcing it to vibrate at any frequency (*forced vibration*), but under the condition of forced vibration, the string would vibrate at maximum amplitude only if forced to vibrate at its own natural resonant frequency. The resonant frequency of a vibrating source depends on its physical characteristics, as we know from the design of tuning forks.

Everything can vibrate and therefore can resonate, whether at audible frequencies or not. A *resonator* is something that is set into forced vibration by another vibration. That is, resonators do not initiate sound energy. Rather, resonators vibrate in sympathy to sounds created externally to them. If a such an externally generated sound is at or near the resonator's natural frequency (or the frequency one of its harmonic components), it will be set into vibration. Further, the resonator will generate all the frequencies that it would if it had been set into free vibration.

Take the damper off a piano string by pressing the key gently down so that there is no sound, then loudly sing the note that corresponds with the depressed key, and you will demonstrate sympathetic resonance for yourself as the string vibrates in response to your singing. The piano string, the swing, and the tuning fork are examples of mechanical resonators. An *acoustic resonator* is something that contains air. A body of air will resonate in response to sound containing frequencies that match the natural resonant frequencies of the volume of air. We can understand this principle by thinking about the construction of musical instruments. It is not enough to have strings of various lengths and thickness mounted on a board to achieve the various qualities of sound associated with a violin, cello, or guitar. Although the energy for the sound is provided by a bow or a pluck, and the source of the sound is in the vibration of the strings, it is the air-filled boxes behind the strings that serve to resonate certain frequencies that make the instruments distinctive. The small volume of air in the box of a violin will naturally vibrate at higher frequencies than the large volume of air in the box of a cello.

Listen to the pitch of the sound that is produced as you blow across the neck of an empty soft drink bottle and compare it with the pitch of the sound that is produced when the bottle is half full. You will notice that the pitch is higher when the bottle is half full because the size of the airspace above the level of the liquid is smaller than the size of the airspace in the empty bottle. The pitch that you perceive when the bottle is half full will be the same whether you hold the bottle vertically or tilt it, thus changing the shape of the airspace above the liquid. This is because the shape of the air cavity is not as important as the volume in determining the frequencies to which it will resonate.

The acoustic resonators that are of the greatest interest to us are, of course, the vocal tract and the ear canal. Both are air-filled tubes, and their resonance characteristics can be modeled on the basis of their similarity to any uniformly shaped tube that is open at one end and closed at the other. (The vocal folds are considered to form the closed end of the vocal tract, and the eardrum closes off the ear canal.) The air within such a tube vibrates at frequencies that depend on the length of the tube. The wavelength of the lowest resonant frequency in the tube is four times the length of the tube. To put it another way, only a quarter of the wave can fit into the tube at any one pass. Figure 2.20 contrasts the resonator length with the waveform of the resonant frequencies. Quarter-wave resonators vibrate only at odd multiples of the lowest resonant frequency because of the

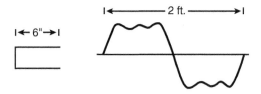

Given tube 6" long, open at one end:

$$f = \frac{c \text{ (constant velocity)}}{4 \times L \text{ (length of tube)}}$$

$$f = \frac{1130 \text{ ft}}{4 \times 1/2 \text{ ft}} = \frac{1130}{2} = 565 \text{ Hz}$$

$$3f = 1,695 \text{ Hz}$$

$$5f = 2,825 \text{ Hz}$$

**FIGURE 2.20**  A tube open at one end and closed at the other resonates at odd multiples of its lowest resonant frequency. The lowest frequency has a wavelength that is 4 times the length of the tube.

**TABLE 2.3** Types of Resonators and Their Characteristics

|  | Narrowly Tuned Resonators | Broadly Tuned Resonators |
|---|---|---|
| Natural tendency to vibrate | Very great | Very little |
| Number of resonant frequencies | One | Many |
| Rise and fall time | Relatively slow | Relatively fast |
| Damping | Lightly damped | Highly damped |

closure at one end. These resonators are discussed more fully in later chapters.

Resonators vary with respect to the range of frequencies to which they respond. We can divide them roughly into two types. Sharply (or narrowly) tuned resonators respond to a very limited number of frequencies, and broadly tuned resonators respond to a relatively large number of frequencies. Another difference correlates with sharp tuning versus broad tuning: Sharply tuned resonators are slow to reach maximum amplitude and, analogously, slow to cease vibrating once they are no longer being driven by a sound source; broadly tuned resonators, in contrast, reach maximum amplitude quickly and stop vibrating very quickly after the sound to which they are responding has ceased. These characteristics of resonator types are summarized in Table 2.3.

A tuning fork is a good example of a sharply tuned resonator: Ideally, it vibrates only in response to one particular frequency; it responds very slowly when resonating (as opposed to when it is set into free vibration by being struck); it takes a long time for its vibrations to die out. A telephone earpiece provides a good example of a broadly tuned resonator: it responds to much of the broad range of frequencies found in the human voice; it responds almost immediately to the electrical current that drives it; and it ceases vibrating almost immediately once that electrical current ceases. Because the electrical current is ultimately controlled by a human voice, we can hear a person speak from the very beginning of his or her utterance and are not troubled by the persistence of vibra-

tions after the person has stopped talking. Of course, the air molecules in a room and the mechanical components of the hearing mechanism also constitute broadly tuned resonating systems.

## ACOUSTICS AND SPEECH

This chapter will serve as a foundation for much of the rest of the book. The marvel of speech is the way in which the distinctive sounds that can be produced by the human vocal folds and vocal tract are varied and combined with one another to serve as a code for communication. In the following chapters, the general way in which humans make and perceive these significant sounds will be explored.

## REFERENCES AND SUGGESTED READING

### Textbook Treatments of Acoustics

Benade, A. H., *Horns, Strings, and Harmony*. Garden City, NY: Doubleday Anchor Books, 1960.

Denes, P., and Pinson, E., *The Speech Chain*, 2nd ed. New York: W. H. Freeman and Company, 1993.

Fry, D. B., *The Physics of Speech*. Cambridge, UK: Cambridge University Press, 1979.

Kent, R. D., and Read, C., *The Acoustic Analysis of Speech*. San Diego: Singular Publishing Group, 1992.

Ladefoged, P., *Elements of Acoustic Phonetics*, 2nd ed. Chicago: University of Chicago Press, 1996.

Pierce, J. R., and David, E. E., Jr., *Man's World of Sound*. Garden City, NY: Doubleday, 1958.

Speaks, C. E., *Introduction to Sound*. San Diego: Singular Publishing Group, 1992.

Stephens, R. W. B., and Bate, A. E., *Acoustics and Vibrational Physics*. New York: St. Martin's Press, 1966.

Van Bergeijk, W. A., Pierce, J. R., and David, E. E., Jr., *Waves and the Ear*. Garden City, NY: Doubleday Anchor Books, 1960.

Wood, A., *Acoustics*. New York: Dover Publications, 1966.

## Classic References

Fletcher, H., and Munson, W. A., Loudness, Its Definition, Measurement, and Calculation. *J. Acoust. Soc. Am. 5,* 1933, 82–108.

Fourier, J. B. J., *Théorie Analytique de la Chaleur*. Paris, France: F. Didot, 1822.

Rayleigh, J. W. S., *Theory of Sound*. New York: Dover Publications, 1960. First published by Macmillan in London, 1878.

Stevens, S. S., Volkmann, J., and Newman, E. B., A Scale for the Measurement of the Psychological Magnitude Pitch. *J. Acoust. Soc. Am. 8,* 1937, 185–190.

# SECTION III — Speech Production

# The Raw Materials—Neurology and Respiration

3

*Breath's a ware that will not keep.*

—A. E. Housman, "A Shropshire Lad"

Under ordinary circumstances, a speaker is conscious of the meaning of his or her message, of the search for appropriate words to express that meaning, and, perhaps, of feelings about the topic or listener. Only under circumstances of change or novelty, such as using unfamiliar words or speaking with a new dental appliance, does the speaker become conscious of the processes involved in sound production. Beginning students of phonetics are surprised at their inability to describe what they are doing when they produce certain speech sounds. The fact that skilled speakers can effortlessly produce such a complex and rapidly changing articulatory–acoustic stream misleads some students into the assumption that the study of phonetics must be equally effortless. They think that if speech is so easy, then the study of speech should be equally easy.

We do, in fact, know a substantial amount about the sounds that emerge from the mouth of a speaker as a result of physiological, articulatory, and acoustic analyses. We know something about the movements of the speaker's articulators and the muscle activity that underlies some of these movements. From information about muscle activity we can infer something about the nerve impulses that fire the muscles. We need to know more, however, about the organization and coordination of these impulses in the brain and about how these impulse patterns are derived from stored linguistic knowledge and ultimately from thought.

We will not attempt here to explore the poorly understood processes of conceptualization or memory as they relate to the formulation of messages. Neither will we speculate on how a speaker makes necessary decisions with regard to phonology, syntax, or semantics as he or she prepares to say something. Nevertheless, although we consider the act of speech as a more or less

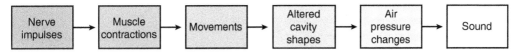

**FIGURE 3.1**  Chain of events leading to speech sound production.

isolated phenomenon, we have a wealth of topics to address: the neurophysiology of speech production, the physiology and physics of respiration for speech, the dynamics of phonation, the articulation of speech sounds, the resonances of the vocal tract, the feedback mechanisms used to monitor speech, and some of the theories of how the speech production mechanisms work. In this chapter, the emphasis is on the neurophysiology and the dynamics of respiration. Our discussion of anatomy is minimal; only the most important nerves, muscles, cartilages, and bones are mentioned.

Any speaker's goal is to produce meaningful sound combinations. Ultimately, it is an acoustic goal. To achieve that goal, the speaker uses exhaled air to make a number of sounds that are adapted to the contexts in which they occur with one another. The sounds are produced by regulating the airstream, as it passes from the lungs to the atmosphere, by moving the jaw, lips, tongue, soft palate, walls of the pharynx, and vocal folds to alter the shape of the vocal tract. The movements are mainly the result of muscle contractions, which are caused by nerve impulses, and, of course, the entire process is controlled by the nervous system. Figure 3.1 shows the sequence of neurologic, muscular, articulatory, and acoustic events underlying the production of speech.

## NEUROPHYSIOLOGY OF SPEECH

The brain and the nerve fibers that extend from the brain are constantly active. As long as there is life, nerve impulses are fired throughout the nervous system. When a signal, such as a sound, is received by the brain, the activity in certain areas sharply increases. Activity also increases as a person prepares to engage in any motor activity, including

speech. The nervous system is a network of specialized cells called *neurons*. The neurons are supported by other protective and nourishing cells and receive oxygen from a generous blood supply.

The nervous system can be divided into the central nervous system (*CNS*) and the peripheral nervous system (*PNS*). The CNS consists of the brain and the spinal cord. The PNS consists of the nerves that emerge from the base of the brain (*cranial nerves*) to serve the head region and from the spinal cord (*spinal nerves*) to serve the rest of the body (Fig. 3.2). Some neurons are *motor* or *efferent* neurons, which means that they carry impulses only from the CNS to the periphery. Other neurons are *sensory* or *afferent*, which means they carry information only from the peripheral sense organs to the CNS. For example, when a person decides to close the lips, efferent neurons (motor nerve fibers) carry the impulses from the brain to the lip muscles, which contract. When the lips touch each other, they stimulate receptors near the surface of the skin. The receptors are connected to afferent neurons which carry sensory information to the brain indicating that lips have made contact. Although neurons within the body and the spinal cord can generally be uniquely classified as afferent or efferent, the nerve fibers that make up the higher centers of the brain itself are interconnected in a compact, three-dimensional mesh. Thus, they are not easily classified as afferent or efferent. We will discuss the respective roles of the CNS and the PNS in the control of speech production after a brief review of the brain and the activity of the neurons that make up both systems.

### The Brain

The brain (Fig. 3.3) comprises a central brainstem, on top of the spinal cord, the

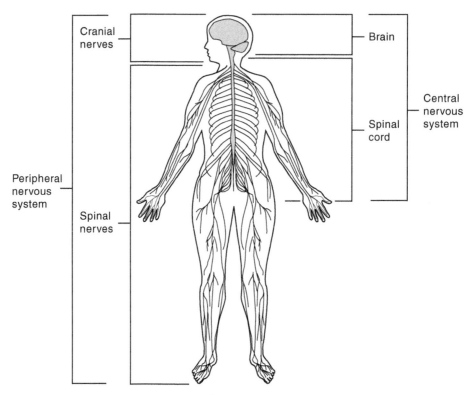

**FIGURE 3.2**   Divisions of the nervous system, anterior view.

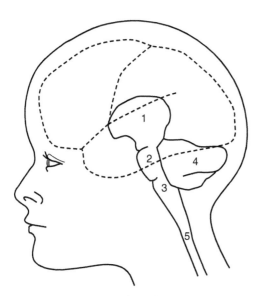

**FIGURE 3.3**   Brain in lateral view. Two cerebral hemispheres are shown as *dotted structures* lying over the higher brainstem (*1*), pons (*2*), medulla (*3*), and cerebellum (*4*). The medulla narrows into the spinal cord (*5*).

cerebellum, which is behind the brainstem, and two cerebral hemispheres, which partly obscure the brainstem, at the top. The higher brainstem includes the thalamus and basal ganglia. The lower brainstem includes the pons and medulla oblongata. The medulla narrows into the spinal cord. Figure 3.3 is a lateral view of one hemisphere showing the position of the brainstem under the cover of the cerebrum. The human brain weighs approximately 1.5 kg, or about 3 lb. The surface of the cerebrum, the cortex, is made up of billions of individual nerve cells. It is the general function of these nerve cells, or neurons, to which we now turn our attention.

## The Neuron

Neurons assume many shapes and lengths, but they always have a cell body and extensions that receive and transmit impulses. Each neuron leads an independent biologic life and on adequate stimulation, generates

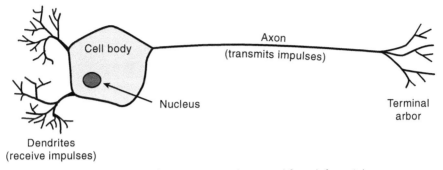

**FIGURE 3.4**  Single neuron. Impulses travel from left to right.

its own electrical activity. A type of neuron is illustrated in Figure 3.4. Neural activity approaches the cell body of the neuron via dendrites. The impulse leaves the cell body by way of the axon. The neurons of the nervous system work on an all-or-none principle of firing. For an impulse to be conducted along an axon, the first part of the axon beyond the cell body must be stimulated to its threshold. If the stimulation falls below the particular threshold for that neuron, the axon does not fire. If it reaches its threshold, however, the axon fires at full capacity no matter how high the stimulation (Fig. 3.5). A strong group of impulses arriving at the cell body can increase the frequency of impulses but not the amplitude of each impulse. Within the nervous system, then, intensity is coded in terms of frequency: The greater the stimulation, the more frequently a neuron will fire.

What happens when a neuron fires? The excitation is conducted along the axon leading away from the cell body. The critical change that takes place at the point of excitation is an increase in the permeability of the membrane that encases the axon or nerve fiber. At the point of stimulation, a momentary increase in permeability of the membrane allows an exchange of ions that depolarizes the nerve fiber for an instant.

Imagine a cross section of an axon (Fig. 3.6). The interior of the nerve fiber is filled with a jellylike substance rich in potassium ions ($K^+$). Outside the membrane that sheaths the axon is a seawater-like fluid rich in sodium ions ($Na^+$). Before a neuron fires, most of the sodium ions are excluded from the axon by the nature of the membrane itself and by complex metabolic interactions. Potassium ions, however, are free to cross the membrane.

When a neuron is at rest, the electrical charge in the interior of the nerve fiber is negative by some 50 to 80 millivolts (mV; thousandths of a volt) relative to the electrical charge outside the neuron. If the stimulus reaching the neuron is at or above threshold, the membrane surrounding the axon becomes more permeable, allowing the $Na^+$ to

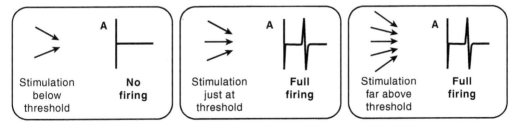

**FIGURE 3.5**  All-or-none principle. Left to right, stimulation of a nerve below threshold, at threshold, and above threshold. If the neuron fires, it fires with a fixed amplitude (A).

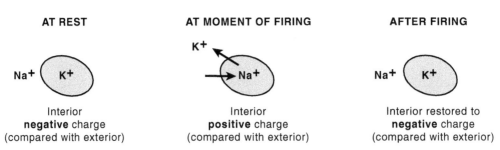

**FIGURE 3.6** Electrochemical events at the cell membrane before, during, and after a nerve cell fires.

enter. $K^+$ then starts to leave the neuron, and for the brief moment (0.5 ms) when the neuron fires, the interior of the axon is more positively charged than the exterior by about 30 to 50 mV. Immediately after the moment of firing, the chemistry of the neuron is restored to that of the resting state until another nerve impulse comes along. As each point along the axon is depolarized, it stimulates the next point, which, in turn, passes the stimulation further along. Thus, once it begins to fire, the neuron is self-stimulating. Although the nervous impulse travels along the nerve fiber longitudinally, the actual movement of particles is across the membrane and therefore is perpendicular to the nerve fiber (Fig. 3.7).

The velocity with which each impulse travels along a nerve fiber depends on the diameter of the nerve fiber and on its myelinization. Conduction velocity in mammals is proportional to about six times the diameter of the neuron. For example, a small neuron of 10 μm (micrometers) diameter conducts an impulse at a velocity of approximately 60 meters per second (m/s), whereas a 20-μm neuron, the largest in the human body, conducts an impulse at a velocity of about 120 m/s. The rate of nerve impulse conduction also depends on the presence or absence of *myelin*, which encases most human nerve fibers. Myelin's fatty, whitish appearance accounts for the term *white matter* used to describe some parts of the nervous system. The myelin coats each axon, with periodic discontinuities along the neuron that expose the axon. The nervous impulse skips along from one exposed area to the next at high velocities. The cell bodies, by contrast, are not coated with a white myelin sheath and are therefore called *gray matter*.

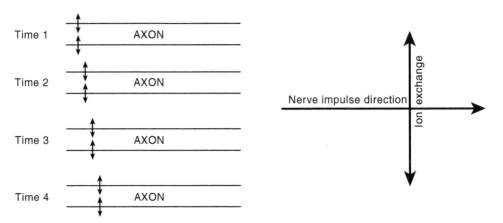

**FIGURE 3.7** Transmission of an impulse along an axon. *Left,* the position of ion exchange at successive moments. *Right,* the nerve impulse travels perpendicular to the direction of the ion exchange.

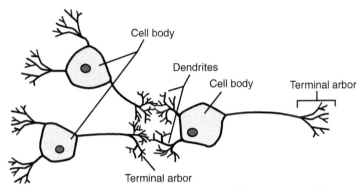

**FIGURE 3.8**   Three neurons. The two at the left synapse with the one at the right. Impulses travel from left to right.

Conduction from one neuron to another involves the release of chemicals at the *synapse*, the juncture of the neurons (Fig. 3.8). The chemicals act to bridge the small space between the fibers of the terminal arbor of the transmitting neuron and the dendrites of the receiving neuron. There are approximately 1 trillion such synapses in the human brain.

Some chemicals facilitate the firing of the next cell, whereas other chemicals inhibit firing. Many neurons can converge to fire on a single neuron, and conversely, a single neuron can stimulate many other neurons simultaneously. This arrangement of convergences and divergences of neurons combines with the chemical variations that can inhibit or facilitate synaptic transmission. Together, they account for the enormous flexibility of the nervous system. A myriad of three-dimensional patterns of nerve fiber networks can be established in both the CNS and the PNS.

A bundle of neuron fibers is called a *nerve*. Each neuron fires independently, but a nerve often serves a particular area of the body. The auditory nerve, for instance, is a bundle of some 30,000 fibers, most of them sensory, carrying information from the inner ear to the brain.

Frequency of neuronal firing is limited by the fact that an axon must restore itself after each firing to its state of rest before it can fire again. Some neurons can fire about 200 times a second. Others, in some highly specialized nerve cells, can fire more than 1,000 times a second.

With this basic review of nerve fiber function as a background, let us consider what is known about how the CNS controls spoken language.

## Control of Speaking in the CNS

Although we are far from understanding the nerve networks that may govern speech, we have obtained information about certain general areas of the brain that are related to the production of speech. It has long been known that when a gunshot wound or other trauma is inflicted on the brain, or when a person suffers a stroke—damage to the cells of the brain caused by a ruptured blood vessel or a blood clot (cerebral vascular accident, or CVA)—language disturbances often result. The language impairment, called aphasia, can take many forms: disabilities in forming utterances, in comprehension, in articulation, in writing, in reading, or in naming things. There may, of course, be multiple combinations of these disabilities in varying degrees of severity.

Long known, too, is the fact that the left cerebral hemisphere of the brain controls movement and sensation on the right side of the body, whereas the right cerebral hemisphere controls movement and sensation on the left side of the body. Thus, a victim of

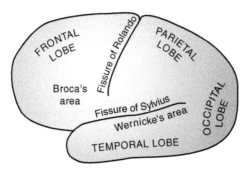

**FIGURE 3.9** Lateral view of the cerebral cortex with the major divisions marked. Lateral surface of the cortex is divided into four lobes: frontal, parietal, temporal, and occipital. The fissure of Rolando divides the frontal lobe from the parietal, and the fissure of Sylvius separates the temporal lobe from the parietal and frontal lobes. Areas believed by Broca and Wernicke to be implicated in speech production and speech understanding are indicated.

a CVA in the right hemisphere may be partially or completely paralyzed on the left side, depending on the location and extent of the brain damage.

In 1861 the Parisian neurosurgeon and anthropologist Paul Broca discovered by autopsy of a formerly aphasic patient that speech production was controlled in the third convolution of the *frontal lobe* of the left cerebral hemisphere (Fig. 3.9). Not long after, in 1874, Carl Wernicke localized the understanding of speech in the first convolution of the left *temporal lobe*. Such strict localization of function has given way in recent times to a view of the brain as more flexible in its assignment of function. Neurologists agree, however, that the left hemisphere is dominant for the control of speech in almost all right-handed people and most left-handed people. They also agree that the area around the temporal–parietal juncture is critical for language in general and that although the exact site known as Broca's area can sometimes be removed without affecting speech, the production of the motor impulses for speech muscles involves some portion of the posteroinferior area of the left frontal lobe.

Broca and Wernicke performed autopsies on a few patients to develop and substantiate their theories, which have been confirmed in part. The important areas of the cerebral cortex for speech have been further delineated by Wilder Penfield, a neurosurgeon who used an entirely different approach. While treating epilepsy by surgical methods, Penfield and his colleague Lamar Roberts (1959) electrically stimulated the exposed areas of the brains of more than 70 patients to map the cortex before surgery. The simulations were used to locate areas contributing to the epileptic seizures, but as a byproduct, the surgeons learned a great deal about brain function.

Because the brain contains no pain receptors, electrical stimulation can be conducted without general anesthesia, permitting patients to be fully conscious and to speak during the procedure. A small electrical current was applied to various locations on the surface of the exposed cortical cells via a fine wire. Stimulation at one location might cause a patient to respond with a muscle contraction, whereas at other locations the response to the stimulus might be the report of a tingling sensation, vocalization, the reexperiencing of past auditory and visual experiences, or a sudden inability to speak. Locations for each type of response were numbered using tiny pieces of paper that were placed on the sites. The cortex was then photographed. Figure 3.10*a* shows a photograph of such a mapped cortex with the locations of the positive responses to each stimulation numbered. Figure 3.10*b* indicates the area in relation to the entire side of the cerebrum.

A glance at Figure 3.9 or 3.10*b* shows the *fissure of Rolando* creating a vertical division between the *frontal lobe* and the *parietal lobe*. Stimulations applied to the posterior portion of the frontal lobe usually resulted in motor responses: muscle contractions and resulting movements of body parts. This area is called the motor strip, although a few of the responses were sensory. Behind the Rolandic fissure, in the parietal lobe, almost all of the

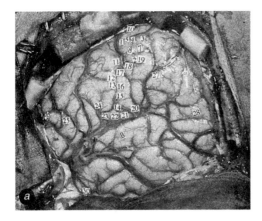

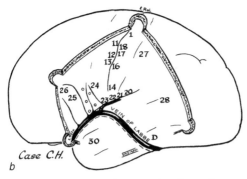

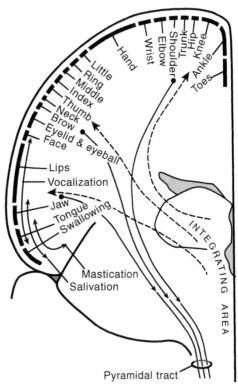

**FIGURE 3.10**  (a) Left cortical surface of case CH after speech mapping. *Numbers* indicate points stimulated. (*b*) Penfield's drawing of case CH on a standard chart. Aphasia (aphasic arrest) was produced by the stimulating electrode placed at *points 26, 27,* and *28.* Anarthria (motor speech arrest) was produced at *points 23* and *24.* (Reprinted with permission from Penfield, W., and Roberts, L., *Speech and Brain-Mechanisms.* Princeton, NJ: Princeton University Press, 1959.)

**FIGURE 3.11**  Frontal cross section through the motor strip of the right hemisphere showing the location of response to electrical stimulation. (Modified with permission from Penfield, W., and Roberts, L., *Speech and Brain-Mechanisms.* Princeton, NJ: Princeton University Press, 1959.)

responses to stimulation were sensory. In both motor and sensory strips of the cortex, the body is represented upside down, as illustrated in a cross section of the motor strip in the right hemisphere (Fig. 3.11). The motor responses of the toes and lower limbs are represented at the top of the cortex, whereas the motor responses of the head are represented on the inferior surface of the frontal lobe. Notice the relatively large area of cortical representation assigned to the lips, tongue, jaw, and laryngeal mechanism in both the motor and sensory areas of the cerebrum. Along

with the hand, the body parts implicated in speech have the highest representation of associated gray matter along the motor and sensory strips of both cerebral hemispheres. It is as if most of the rest of the body were meant to nourish and transport the head and hands, which act on and receive information from the environment.

Although some of the strictly motor and sensory aspects of the speech production mechanism seem to be controlled from both hemispheres, the overall control of organized spoken language resides in one hemisphere, usually the left. When Penfield stimulated certain regions of the cortex, patients were unable to name pictures or answer questions. At other sites they spoke but with slurred articulation. It was possible, on a single stimulation in the temporal–parietal region, to elicit a sequential auditory and visual experience. One patient reported that she was in her kitchen and could hear the sounds of the neighborhood outside. It was more than a memory of an event. The subject relived and reheard the event while simultaneously being conscious of being in Montreal with Dr. Penfield. These experiences could, on occasion, be elicited several times by consecutive stimulation. Another stimulation in the temporal–parietal region interrupted the naming of pictures. When a picture of a butterfly was shown to the subject, he could not elicit its name. After the stimulation stopped, the patient reported that he had also tried unsuccessfully to recall the word "moth." Figure 3.12 summarizes the areas found by

Penfield and Roberts to be important for speech, on the basis of stimulation evidence. The anterior area in the lower frontal lobe coincides with Broca's area, and stimulation here most often resulted in slurred speech or temporary *dysarthria*. The large posterior area includes part of the temporal lobe, an extension of Wernicke's area, and part of the parietal lobe. Penfield considered this region to be most critical for language and speech. Stimulations in this region not only produced sequential experiences of past events but also interfered with the ability to use language. The patient sometimes could not say what he wanted to say or failed to understand what was said to him, thus simulating aphasia. The superior speech cortex was considered to be least important but supplemental to the motor area.

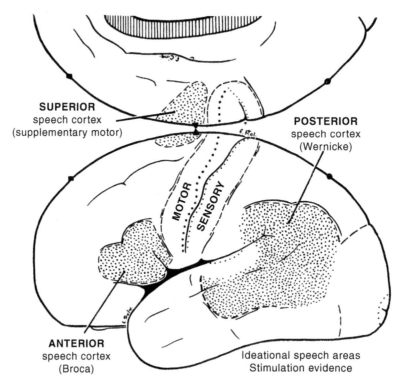

**FIGURE 3.12** Summary map of the areas of the surface of the left cerebral hemisphere found by Penfield to be important for speech. The lower drawing shows the lateral surface; the upper drawing shows continuation of the areas on the medial cortical surface. (Modified with permission from Penfield, W., and Roberts, L., *Speech and Brain-Mechanisms*. Princeton, NJ: Princeton University Press, 1959.)

Twenty years later, Lassen and his Scandinavian colleagues (1978) suggested, on the basis of blood flow studies, that the supplementary motor area is involved in the planning of sequential motor tasks. It seems that the planning and execution of speech may be physiologically as well as behaviorally separate. Behavioral evidence for the separation of planning from execution lies in the symptoms of certain forms of brain damage. Speech motor planning problems (apraxia) and speech motor execution problems (dysarthria) have long been differentiated by speech and language pathologists working on the communication difficulties associated with aphasia. The work of Lassen and others on the role of the supplementary motor cortex has revived interest in this area of the brain, largely neglected by speech scientists since the work of Penfield. Although three general areas of the cortex were cited by Penfield and Roberts as important to speech, the functions of the areas were not found to be as discrete as they had expected. They attribute the overlaps to subcortical connections among the areas. They were careful to point out that an electrical stimulus would disrupt whole systems and networks, implicating nerve cells far from the site of the stimulating electrode.

The Penfield and Roberts evidence is rich in implications about CNS control of speech, language, sequential memory, and even thought. It is worth our attention that the simple responses of vocalization and the contraction of speech muscles were bilaterally induced in their studies, whereas the more complex responses of recounting experiences or aphasic interruptions of speech were limited to one side of the brain. No stimulation resulted in a spoken word. For example, at no point did a stimulation result in the patient involuntarily saying something like "chair." Speech involves simultaneous activity in many parts of the brain and is apparently too complex to be elicited by a single stimulus, although its production can be interrupted by stimulation.

Clearly, it is important to know which cerebral hemisphere is dominant for speech and language, particularly if surgery becomes imperative for a patient. Physicians are reluctant to operate on the brain unless they know which areas control language. Medical decisions about the extent of an operation depend on assessing the potential degree of disruption to the patient's ability to communicate. A physician can remove more tissue on the side of the cerebrum that is not dominant for speech. To determine which hemisphere is dominant for speech and language, Penfield's group developed the *Wada test*. To administer this test, the investigator injects sodium amobarbital into the *carotid artery* on one side of the neck. The carotid artery conducts the blood supply to the brain, and sodium amobarbital produces a temporary effect on the side in which it is injected. Normal function returns quickly, so there is little time for elaborate testing. The patient often lies on a table with arms extended toward the ceiling and knees flexed. The effect of the injection is immediate and dramatic. The leg and the arm on the side opposite the affected cerebral hemisphere collapse. The patient is asked to count, to name pictures, and to answer questions. The patient is then injected on the other side of the neck and the procedure is repeated.

Usually, the sodium amobarbital injection has a much more disruptive effect on speech and language for one side of the brain than for the other. Brenda Milner of McGill University in Montreal found that in 140 right-handed and 122 left-handed people, 96% of the right-handers and 70% of the left-handers had speech represented on the left side of the brain. When speech was represented bilaterally, as it was in a few subjects, naming was stronger on one side and the ability to order words was stronger on the other. All of the evidence for lateralization of speech production, whether from the autopsies performed by Broca or Wernicke, from the electrical stimulation work by Penfield and Roberts, or from the sodium amobarbital test as described by Wada and Rasmussen

(1960), is derived from studies of the cerebral hemispheres. Although many neurophysiologists view the cerebrum as the source of voluntary motor activity, Penfield believes that the origin of voluntary motor impulses is in the higher brainstem and that the motor cortex is merely a platform at which the impulses arrive. Whichever view is accurate, the impulses course from the motor cortex down the *pyramidal* (corticospinal) *tract* to the muscles.

## Spoonerisms: Evidence for Planning

There is considerable evidence suggesting that speakers hold a complete phrase in some stage of readiness for speech. Much of this evidence is in the form of commonly produced word reversals and phoneme reversals. Perhaps the most well-known examples of such reversals are *spoonerisms*, named after William A. Spooner, an English clergyman and dean of New College at Oxford University in the early 20th century. He is less famous for his lectures and sermons than for his amusing speech reversals. Instead of saying, "You've missed my history lectures," he would say, "You've hissed my mystery lectures," a classic spoonerism. He is also reputed to have said, "Work is the curse of the drinking class." Such transpositions of words or sounds from the end of the intended phrase to the beginning would not occur unless speakers formulated plans for the generation of utterances. Spoonerisms and other kinds of speech errors thus reveal something of interest about speech production. Table 3.1 lists examples of speech sound errors collected by Victoria Fromkin (1973). Note that reversals of sounds always involve two consonants or two vowels (consonants never change places with vowels); the errors are always consistent with the rules of English ("optimal" may be rendered as "moptimal" but never as "ngoptimal," because [ŋ] in English never initiates a syllable); and most errors involve the first syllable, often the first sound, of a word. Interesting, too, is

**TABLE 3.1**  Segmental Errors in Speech

| Errors | | Examples |
|---|---|---|
| **Consonant Errors** | | |
| Anticipation | A reading list | A leading list |
| | It's a real mystery | It's a meal mystery |
| Perseveration | Pulled a tantrum | Pulled a pantrum |
| | At the beginning of the turn | At the beginning of the burn |
| Reversals (spoonerisms) | Left hemisphere | Heft lemisphere |
| | A two-pen set | A two-sen pet |
| **Vowel Errors** | | |
| Reversals | Feet moving | Fute meeving |
| | Fill the pool | Fool the pill |
| **Other Errors** | | |
| Addition | The optimal number | The moptimal number |
| Movement | Ice cream | Kise ream |
| Deletion | Chrysanthemum plants | Chrysanthemum p ants |
| Consonant clusters split or moved | Speech production | Peach seduction |
| | Damage claim | Clammage dame |

Segmental errors in speech can involve vowels as well as consonants. Some typical types of substitution of sounds are shown. Such errors provide evidence that the discrete phonetic segments posited by linguistic theory exist in the mental grammar of the speaker. (Reprinted with permission from Fromkin, V. A., Slips of the Tongue. *Sci. Am. 229,* 1973, 114.)

## CLINICAL NOTE

It is impossible to overestimate the importance of the normal functioning of the CNS to speech and language. If any component of the CNS that is relevant to speech or language is damaged, the result will almost certainly be a disruption of the communication process. For example, damage or dysfunction at the cortical level can result in *spasticity*, often observed among victims of *cerebral palsy*. Muscles contract but fail to relax. Damage in the higher brainstem can result in the unintended addition of uncontrolled movements to voluntary acts (*athetosis*, another common symptom of cerebral palsy), or in the hypokinesis or rigidity common in Parkinson's disease. Global damage or oxygen deprivation can result in *mental retardation*, which limits, among other things, the development of language ability in proportion to the degree of the damage. More discrete CNS disorders can produce a variety of learning disabilities, such as attention deficit disorder, problems reading (*dyslexia*), inability to attach meaning to the sound patterns of speech (*auditory agnosia*), various and complex disorders in language (*developmental aphasia*), or problems not only with language but also with communication and human relationships in general (*autism*).

Injury to or dysfunction of the cerebellum can affect the coordination and strength of the movements of the organs of speech. The cerebellum, posterior to the brainstem and below the cerebrum, has long been known to regulate the timing of the components of complex skilled movements. In addition, the cerebellum receives information about the position and movement of structures from sensors in muscles and joints and has many connections with the spinal cord as well as with the cerebrum. Cerebellar disorder underlies ataxic dysarthria, a disorder marked by errors of articulation, and by distortions of prosody and phonation.

the observation that the stress and intonation of the phrase or sentence remain constant in the face of word changes. In one of Fromkin's examples of word reversals, "Seymour sliced the knife with the salami," the pitch rise and increased intensity that would have occurred in "knife" in the intended sentence occurred instead in the second syllable of the word "salami" in the version of the sentence in which the words were transposed. These errors suggest the existence, in the CNS, of neurophysiologic mechanisms for planning speech production before motor commands are sent to the muscles. It is clear that, as a rule, speakers do not simply call forth one word at a time when they produce sentences.

## PNS Control of Speaking

More is known about the activity of the cranial and spinal nerves that form the PNS than is known about the more complex activity of the brain. The circuitry of the PNS has been mapped. We know that certain motor neurons activate certain muscles and that particular sensory neurons conduct information from certain kinds of sense receptors. The interactions, coordination, and use of this circuitry, however, are not well known. The coordination of various motor neurons for a particular act, for example, is not completely understood, nor is the role of sensory information in the control of movement. We understand that someone intends to do something and we understand the more peripheral actions that result (nerve activity, muscle contractions, movements), but we do not yet understand how intentions are transformed into actions. That is, we cannot explain the method of coordination and control, especially for complicated actions such as speaking or playing a sport. These actions require rapid adjustments to constantly changing internal and external conditions.

What do we know about the role of the PNS in the control of speech? Cranial nerves emerge from the base of the brain, and many of them activate groups of muscles important to speech production. The muscles innervated by cranial nerves lie in the head and the neck. Also within this area are receptors (for hearing, touch, and sense of position and movement of the articulators) that presumably are used when children are learning to speak. Information is carried from these receptors along sensory fibers among the cranial nerves.

Spinal nerves are also active in speech. Those that emerge from the ventral (front) side of the vertebral column activate muscles used in the control of respiration for speech. These nerves come primarily from the cervical (neck), thoracic (chest), and abdominal sections of the vertebral column and serve the muscles of inhalation and exhalation. In contrast, receptors sensitive to muscle activity in these areas are served by sensory fibers that enter the dorsal (back) side of the vertebral column quite close to the surface of the body. That is why you may temporarily lose the sense of feeling or touch in your hand if you were to carry an unduly heavy backpack pressing on a dorsal root of sensory fibers serving that hand. Appendix A contains a list of the peripheral nerves that are most important for the production of speech. These will be discussed as the muscles and receptors that they serve are introduced.

## The Motor Unit

The interface between the nervous system and the muscular system is called the motor unit. A motor unit consists of a single motor neuron and the striated (voluntary) muscle fibers that the neuron serves. Typically, each motor neuron activates several muscle fibers. When the neuron stimulates the muscle fibers, a small electrical signal called an *action potential* produces a mechanical twitch. This signal can be amplified and recorded using a technique known as electromyography (EMG) (see Chapter 14). When we say that we are contracting a particular muscle, we are actually firing many motor units simultaneously.

The action potentials from motor units produced at low levels of muscle contraction are small in amplitude compared with those of the motor units recruited later at higher levels of contraction. The electrical signal given off when a muscle contracts is an interference pattern that is the sum of the activity from the individual motor units involved, just as an acoustic interference pattern is the sum of the particular frequencies and phase differences of its component tones (see Chapter 2). Figure 3.13 illustrates the summation of many motor units to form an interference pattern recorded by EMG.

The firing of motor units produces muscle activity but not necessarily movement.

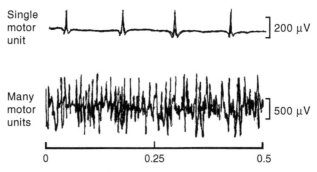

**FIGURE 3.13** Interference pattern in the lower part of the figure reflects the summed activity of many motor units. Both single motor units and complex muscle activity may be recorded by electromyography.

You can tense the muscles of your index finger, both the flexor and the extensor, producing an EMG signal from both, but the finger does not move because agonist–antagonist activity is balanced. The movements that produce speech, however, are the result of the coordination of many muscles whose activity is the result of the firing of many motor units.

In summary, the nervous system activates many groups of muscles that are coordinated so as to produce movements of structures in the abdomen, thorax, larynx, and vocal tract, resulting in audible air pressure changes. To power the whole system, then, we need a supply of air to flow through the vocal tract.

## RESPIRATION

### Modification of Airstream for Speech Sounds

The production of all speech sounds is the result of modification of the airflow from the lungs. The speaker must produce a stream of exhaled air and then modify it in ways that make it audible to a listener.

The number of ways that humans do this to produce the sounds of the world's many languages is impressively large, especially since the speech mechanism comprises a limited set of component parts and a limited set of processes for modifying the airstream. A speaker has only a few movable parts with which to create sounds: the vocal folds, tongue, jaw, lips, and soft palate. Likewise, there are only a few cavities that serve as resonators: the mouth, pharynx, and nasal cavities being the primary ones. Yet speakers of the world produce speech sounds in a multitude of ways. They phonate during the production of some sounds but not others. They create a large variety of vocal tract shapes to vary resonance. They generate aperiodic sounds of various durations such as hisses, clicks, and small explosions of air. They grunt, murmur, and vary loudness. A few sounds are produced on air intake rather than outflow, and in some languages, sounds that are otherwise identical are made distinctive by a change in relative pitch.

English has approximately 40 phonemes, listed in Appendix B. They are all created by making exhaled air audible. The two primary methods used for making the airflow audible are phonation and the production of consonant noises. Phonation is the creation of a nearly periodic sound wave by the rapid opening and closing of the *glottis* (the space between the vocal folds). The continuous flow of air from the lungs is thus chopped into a discontinuous series of tiny audible puffs of air. The aperiodic sound source that may accompany consonant production is created by positioning articulators so that they form occlusions or constrictions in the vocal tract. As the flow of air is released from the occlusions or channeled through the constrictions, aperiodic sounds are created, most frequently in the mouth, or *oral cavity*. Some English phonemes require both periodic and aperiodic sources of sound. Both the sounds of phonation and the sounds of consonant noise are resonated in the *vocal tract*.

Try to produce some examples of these types of sounds. First, say the vowel "ah" ([ɑ]), a phonated sound. All English vowels are classified as phonated (voiced) sounds. The vocal folds are set into vibration, producing the source of the sound, which gets its characteristic [ɑ] quality from the acoustic resonance, provided in this case by a large oral cavity and a relatively small pharyngeal cavity. Next produce the sounds [s] and [t]. These sounds exemplify two different kinds of consonant noise. The source of these sounds is not at the vocal folds but in the oral cavity. The [s] noise is produced by forcing the airstream through a narrow constriction. The airflow is stopped completely for [t] by raising the apex of the tongue to the alveolar ridge while the velum is raised to prevent air from escaping through the nasal cavity. When the apex of the tongue is lowered, airflow will be released, producing a transient burst of noise. As in the case of [ɑ],

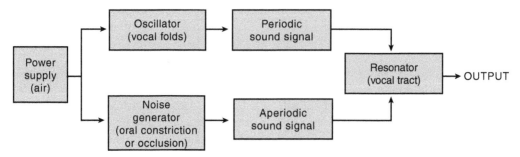

**FIGURE 3.14** Block diagram of speech production. Air is converted into a periodic or aperiodic acoustic signal that is modified by the vocal tract.

the sounds produced by the airflow obstructions for [s] and [t] are resonated in the vocal tract. Finally, produce the sound [z], which combines the periodic source of phonation with the aperiodic source generated in the same way as that for [s]. To hear the difference between a purely period source and simultaneous periodic and aperiodic sources, prolong [s] and after a second or so start to phonate. The result will be [z]. See if you can take a deep breath and continuously alternate between the production of [s] and [z].

The speech production mechanism is often described as the product of one or more sound sources (periodic, aperiodic, or both) and a variable filter or resonator. This

*source–filter* view of speech production, discussed more fully in Chapter 5, is shown in Figure 3.14.

## Negative-Pressure Breathing

To prepare to exhale for the production of speech sounds, a speaker must inhale a sufficient amount of air. Under normal circumstances, air is taken into the lungs in much the same way it is taken into an accordion or bellows (Fig. 3.15). Press the keys as hard as you will on an accordion, and no sound will emerge unless you first increase the volume of its air reservoir by pulling the ends of the accordion away from each other

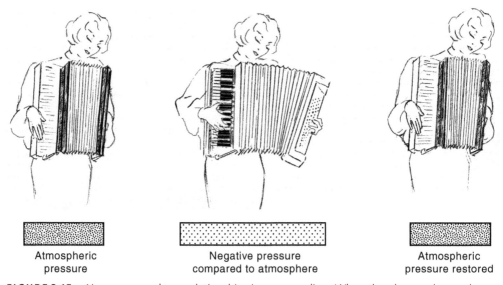

Atmospheric pressure    Negative pressure compared to atmosphere    Atmospheric pressure restored

**FIGURE 3.15** Air pressure–volume relationships in an accordion. When the player enlarges the accordion, pressure falls. Air then enters through an inlet valve to equalize pressure.

and then begin to push them toward each other. The enlargement reduces the pressure inside the air reservoir relative to the external air pressure in accordance with Boyle's law. Robert Boyle, a 17th-century British physicist, discovered that volume and pressure are inversely related. Therefore, increasing the volume of an enclosed space decreases the air pressure within it. The air reservoir of an accordion, however, is not a completely enclosed space because it has an inlet for outside air. Because unequal pressures always equalize themselves if given the chance, air is drawn into the accordion's reservoir through the inlet. To produce musical tones you must reverse the process by pushing the ends of the accordion together. This decreases the volume of the air reservoir. Once again the inverse relationship between volume and pressure described by Boyle's law comes into play. In this case, the decrease in volume momentarily increases the internal air pressure, which causes the air to rush out of the instrument, setting its reeds into vibration and producing musical tones.

The flow of air into and out of the air reservoir of an accordion is analogous to what occurs in the lungs as we breathe: we expand our chest and lungs, causing air to flow in to equalize the negative pressure or partial vacuum; then we contract our thorax and lungs, causing air to flow out to equalize the positive pressure created by the contraction. It is by changing the volume that we change the pressure.

During inhalation, air passes through the oral cavity or nose, the pharynx, the larynx, and then into the lungs via the trachea, bronchi, and bronchioles, the passageways increasingly branching and diminishing in size, until the air reaches the small sacs (alveoli) that compose the major part of the lungs. There the exchange of oxygen for carbon dioxide from the blood, which is essential for life, takes place.

## The Respiratory Mechanism

A surplus of carbon dioxide and a need for oxygen is automatically signaled in the

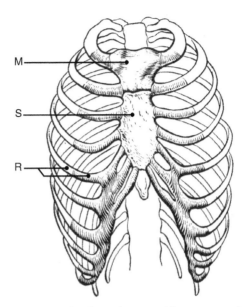

**FIGURE 3.16**  Thoracic cage with osseous and cartilaginous shaded portions. M, manubrium; S, sternum; R, rib. (Adapted with permission from Basmajian, J. V., *Primary Anatomy*, 6th ed. Baltimore: Williams & Wilkins, 1970.)

medulla oblongata, the reflex seat for respiration in the brainstem. The medulla, in turn, initiates nerve impulses from the brain and the spinal cord to various muscles in the thorax or rib cage. The thorax (Fig. 3.16) is bounded by the vertebrae in the back and the sternum, or breastbone, in the front. Completing the thorax are 12 pairs of ribs, which form a skeletal framework from the sternum and manubrium in the front to the vertebrae in the back. The ribs are osseous (bony) except for the section of each rib that connects with the sternum. These sections are made of cartilage. The lower ribs share cartilaginous attachments to the sternum, and the lowest two ribs are attached only to the vertebral column at the back. These are the so-called floating ribs.

This barrel-shaped cavity, the thorax, has as its floor a dome-shaped sheet of muscle called the *diaphragm* (Fig. 3.17), which also serves as the ceiling for the abdominal cavity. The lungs rest on the diaphragm, and because they are spongy, elastic masses of air cells that lack muscles and because they

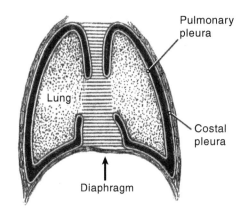

**FIGURE 3.17** Schematic coronal section of thorax showing costal and pulmonary pleurae.

adhere to the deep (interior) surface of the rib cage and to the diaphragm, their size and shape change as the rib cage expands and contracts. The rib cage is lined with a membrane called the *costal* (rib) *pleura*, or *parietal pleura*. This membrane folds back on itself to form, in effect, a second membrane, called the *pulmonary pleura* (or sometimes the *visceral pleura*) that covers the lungs. These two membranes, the costal and pulmonary pleurae, adhere to one another and, at the same time, can slide across one another almost without friction because of a viscous fluid between them. (Similarly, liquid between two thin plates of glass enables the plates to move across each other, while the surface tension of the fluid holds them together.) This pleural linkage between the lungs, diaphragm, and ribs enables the lungs to expand and contract as the thoracic cage changes volume. When the dome-shaped diaphragm flattens, increasing the size of the thorax, lung volume increases; when the diaphragm rises, decreasing the size of the thorax, lung capacity decreases. In a similar manner, when the thorax expands (by rib elevation) or contracts (by rib depression), the lungs also expand and contract.

## Inspiration

### *For Quiet Breathing*

For quiet inspiration (inhalation), the medulla automatically sends neuronal impulses via

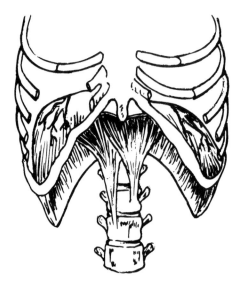

**FIGURE 3.18** Anterior view of the diaphragm.

the spinal cord to the pertinent thoracic muscles. Several nerves emerge from the spinal cord at the level of the neck (*cervical nerves*) and join to form a nerve bundle known as the *phrenic nerve*. The phrenic nerve innervates the diaphragm, the dome-shaped sheet of muscle fibers that separates the thoracic and abdominal cavities (Fig. 3.18). When nervous stimulation is sufficient to cause a contraction of the diaphragm, the muscle fibers shorten, pulling the central part down toward the level of the diaphragm's edges, which are attached to the lower ribs. The effect is to flatten the diaphragm to some extent. Because the diaphragm forms the floor of the thoracic cavity, thoracic volume increases vertically as the floor lowers. One can often observe the abdomen protruding during inspiration because of the downward pressure of the diaphragm on the organs within the abdomen. The flattening of the diaphragm also exerts an outward force on the lower ribs to which it is attached. This causes the rib cage to expand laterally and from back to front.

As the diaphragm is lowering, nerves emerging from the spinal cord at the level of the chest (*thoracic nerves*) transmit impulses to the muscles that run between the ribs. Eleven sets of these intercostal muscles

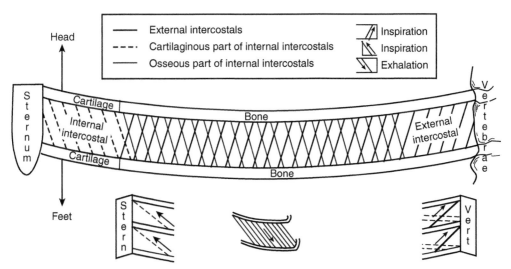

**FIGURE 3.19**  Wraparound representation of the functions of the external and internal intercostal muscles as suggested by Fredericka Bell-Berti.

(inter = between; costal = ribs) connect the osseous portion of the ribs. There are two layers of intercostal muscles, one superficial to the other (Fig. 3.19). The *external intercostal muscles* connect the osseous portion of the ribs but do not connect the cartilaginous sections near the sternum. They lie superficial to the *internal intercostal muscles*, which connect both the cartilaginous and osseous portions of the ribs except where the ribs are attached to the vertebrae at the rear of the thoracic cage. The muscle fibers of the external and internal intercostal muscles course in opposite directions. The external fibers course obliquely from the vertebrae down and out as they extend toward the sternum, whereas the internal fibers course obliquely in the opposite direction from the sternum down and out, as they extend toward the vertebrae.

During inspiration, the external intercostal muscles and the section of the internal intercostals that lie between the cartilaginous portions of the ribs (the *interchondral part*) contract to elevate the ribs. The vertebrae thus act as fulcrums for the external intercostals, supplying leverage so that when the muscles shorten, the main effect is to lift the ribs below each vertebra. The same effect can be imagined in the front, where the internal intercostal muscles join the interchondral portions of the ribs. The muscle fibers course

down and away from the sternum, which supports the upper part of each muscle, again supplying the leverage necessary to lift the ribs below. This action is aided by the *torque* supplied by the twisting of the cartilages. Elevation of the ribs is thus produced by the joint efforts of the external intercostal muscles and the interchondral parts of the internal intercostal muscles, aided by a slight rotation of the cartilages. The result of these actions is an expansion of the thoracic cavity in both the anterior to posterior dimension and the lateral dimension (Fig. 3.20).

As the volume of the rib cage increases, so does the lung volume, because of the pleural linkage. This reduces the air pressure inside the lungs relative to atmospheric pressure. Consequently, air from the outside flows to the area of lower pressure, within the lungs.

The upper airways serve as the conduit for the inhaled air (Fig. 3.21). In restful breathing, air normally enters the nasal cavities, where it is warmed, moistened, and filtered before it proceeds, successively, through the pharynx, larynx, and trachea (windpipe). The air then passes through the bronchi, bronchioles, and finally into the alveolar sacs of the lungs. Air can also enter the respiratory system via the mouth, but mouth breathing (useful during heavy

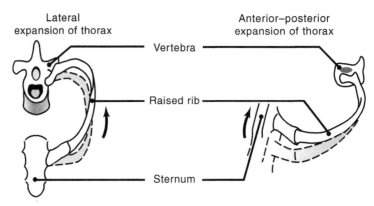

**FIGURE 3.20** Movements of the ribs in inspiration. Inspiration lifts the ribs, increasing the transverse dimension of the chest, and raises the front end of the rib, increasing front-to-back diameter.

exercise to increase the rate and volume of air intake) tends to dry out the oral cavity and the pharynx.

### For Speech Breathing

There are several differences between inspiration during quiet breathing and inspiration for speech. First, the volume of air inspired to produce speech is generally greater than that inspired during quiet breathing, especially if the speaker intends to produce an utterance that is long, loud, or both. To accomplish the inspiration of a greater volume of air, the diaphragm and intercostal muscles can be augmented by any of several muscles

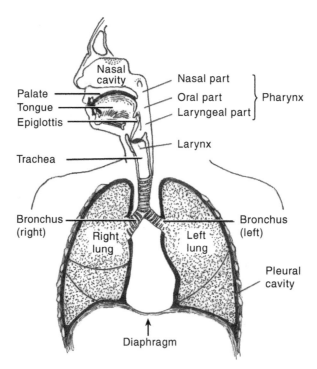

**FIGURE 3.21** Airways of the respiratory system.

capable of sternum and rib elevation: the *sternocleidomastoid*, the *scalenus*, the *subclavius*, and the *pectoralis major* and *pectoralis minor* muscles in front, the *serratus anterior* muscle at the sides, and the *levatores costarum* muscles, *serratus posterior superior* muscle, and *latissimus dorsi* muscle at the back.

A second difference is in the degree of automaticity. We breathe in and out, day and night, conscious and unconscious, and the process is under reflexive control, with the rate and depth of volume change dependent on need. However, we can assume more voluntary control over our breathing. When we are reading a poem or singing a song, we are often conscious of inspiring a larger volume of air in order to be able to complete a long phrase without interruption.

Third, inspiration for speech comprises less of the total respiratory cycle than during quiet breathing. Time your breaths during rest and during the reading of a paragraph; you may not find a significant difference in breaths per minute, which may range from 12 to 20, but the ratio between inspiration time and expiration time will differ markedly. During quiet breathing, inspiration takes up roughly 40% of the respiratory cycle and expiration, 60%. In contrast, inspiration for speech may take up about 10% of the respiratory cycle and expiration, 90% (Fig. 3.22), although these percentages will vary somewhat, depending on the demands of any specific situation.

## Expiration

When the glottis is open for inspiration, air from the outside enters the lungs; when the inspiratory muscle effort is complete (depending on the pressure needs of the task ahead), there is a moment of equalized pressure. The pressure in the lungs is equal to the atmospheric pressure. At a relatively high thoracic volume, however, a large inspiratory force is required to maintain the volume. If one were to relax the inspiratory muscles, the air would suddenly rush out because of the lung–rib recoil. Try it yourself. Inhale deeply by enlarging your rib cage and lung volume. Then, while holding the volume constant, hold your breath but open the glottis. If the glottis is open, pressure above and below must be equal. If you let the inspiratory muscles relax, the air will rush out because of three passive forces: the elastic recoil of the lungs and the rib cage (the expanded elastic tissues of the lungs contracting to their natural shape in response to the lowering of the ribs), the force of the untwisting of the cartilages next to the sternum (*detorque*), and gravity, which may aid in lowering the rib cage. These three passive forces suffice to decrease the volume of the rib cage and lungs. According to Boyle's law, the decrease in volume generates an increase of the pressure within, causing air to flow out. In Figure 3.23, we can see how the pressure–volume relationships for inspiration and expiration contrast with each other. For inspiration, an increase in thoracic volume causes a decrease in pressure. For expiration, a decrease in thoracic volume causes an increase in pressure.

In quiet expiration, the exchange of air is small (approximately 0.5 liter [L]). With deeper breaths, such as those that accompany exercise, the volume of air exchanged increases. The amount of air exchanged during ins and outs of quiet respiration is called *quiet tidal volume*. At rest, people take 12 to 20 breaths per minute, and the inspiration phase is only slightly shorter in duration than the expiration phase. If one were to make a maximum inspiration followed by a maximum

Quiet Breathing

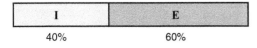

Breathing for Speech

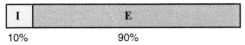

**FIGURE 3.22** Comparison of the inspiratory (*I*) and expiratory (*E*) proportions of the respiratory cycle for quiet breathing and speech.

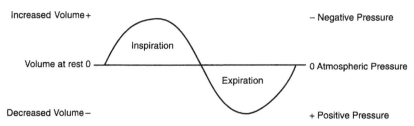

**FIGURE 3.23**  Changes of lung volume and pressure during inspiration and expiration.

expiration, the volume of air inhaled or exhaled would be one's *vital capacity* (VC). A person's VC is related to sex, size, age, health factors, and breathing habits. As an average, human VC is approximately 5 L (somewhat more than 5 quarts), but large male mountain climbers surely have a larger VC than many people. The 0.5 L exchanged during quiet breathing is only 10% of the exchange one is capable of, and as there is an additional 2 L of residual air that one cannot expel, the tidal volume of 0.5 L is only about 7% of total lung volume. Lung volumes and some of the standard terminology used to describe them are given in Figure 3.24.

### For Sustained Phonation

The passive expiratory forces of elasticity, detorque, and gravity are not sufficient by themselves to support singing or speaking. Expiration during phonation differs from that during quiet breathing, and expiration during speech differs from both.

To maintain a constant subglottal pressure so that a note can be sung at a constant intensity, the passive recoil force of the rib cage–lung coupling is used as a background force that is supplemented by actively balancing the muscle contractions of the inspiratory and expiratory muscles. If a singer permitted passive expiratory forces to act unopposed, the lungs would collapse suddenly and the note could not be sustained. The purpose of the balance between the active inspiratory and expiratory forces (muscle contractions) is to control the outflow by slowing it. Rahn et al. (1946) first presented a pressure–volume diagram of the human chest showing the springlike action of the respiratory

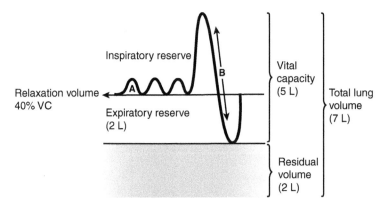

**FIGURE 3.24**  Inspiration and expiration during quiet, or tidal, breathing (*a*) and in maximum exhalation and inhalation (*b*). Standard terminology for various parts of the total lung capacity is indicated. Values for vital capacity (VC), residual volume, and total lung volume are approximate

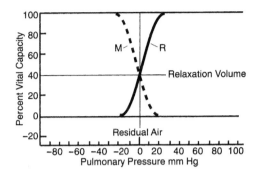

**FIGURE 3.25**  A simplified version of Rahn's pressure–volume diagram. *R* represents the pressure generated when the subject relaxes at various lung volumes. Relaxation volume occurs at about 40% VC; here the elastic forces of the ribs and lungs are balanced. *M* represents the muscle forces needed at various lung volumes to balance the pressure supplied by passive forces.

system. It shows how pressures vary at different lung volumes (Fig. 3.25). Lung volumes are plotted on the ordinate (*y* axis) in terms of the percentage of VC. The relaxation pressure curve (*R*) is plotted by asking people to adjust to a certain lung volume and then open the glottis and relax. At high lung volumes, people exhale during relaxation, whereas at low lung volumes, they inhale. Pulmonary pressure (on the abscissa) is measured and recorded for each lung volume. At high lung volumes, a positive pressure is recorded during relaxation; at low lung volumes, a negative pressure. The S-shaped curve that results is an index of average pressures supplied by the *passive* (nonmuscular) inspiration and expiration forces.

The end of an expiration in restful breathing is marked by a relaxed state in which the tension between the rib cage and the lungs is balanced. This happens at about 40% of VC, the *relaxation volume* or *resting expiratory level* (REL). At volumes above REL, a force is created, mostly from the elasticity of the lungs, which is expiratory. Conversely, at low lung volumes, the relaxation pressure of the lungs and rib cage recoil forces is inspiratory. For example, if you exhale all of

the air you can and open your glottis, you create a large force to assist in inspiration. The relaxation pressure curve in Figure 3.25 thus represents the effects of the forces of lung elasticity and rib cage elasticity, including torque and gravity, that determine how we must use our muscles to make the required changes in lung volume.

The pressure–volume relationships are altered somewhat when a person is lying down, because the abdominal contents press on the diaphragm and increase lung pressure.

Mead, Bouhuys, and Proctor (1968) depict the modifications to this background of recoil force when singers attempt to sustain a tone of low but constant intensity. Maintaining a subglottal pressure of 7 cm $H_2O$ (air pressure is traditionally measured by how far a column of water or mercury would be moved), the vocalist sustains the active muscle force of the inspiratory muscles (during expiration) for the first half of the tone to check the recoil force and eventually increases the active muscle force of the expiratory muscles (Fig. 3.26). For the first part of the tone, the vocalist continues to activate the external intercostal muscles and the interchondral part of the internal intercostal muscles, only gradually reducing the contractions so that the rib cage and lungs decrease in volume smoothly. These muscles serve to break the recoil forces. Thus, inspiratory muscles are used during expiration. As lung volume approaches the state in which the natural output pressure is 7 cm $H_2O$, the expiratory muscles increase activity to maintain the required subglottal pressure at decreasing lung volumes. Mead makes the point that muscle activity must constantly change to sustain a constant subglottal pressure as lung volume changes.

### For Speech

It is important to note that individual muscle activity for conversational speech is not sequenced in an all-or-none fashion. That is, as the research of Hixon and his colleagues

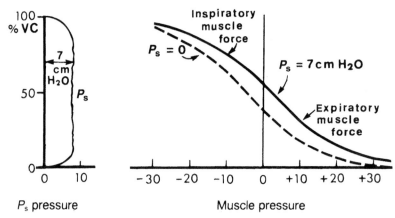

**FIGURE 3.26** Forces required to maintain a constant subglottal pressure ($P_s$) for a sustained tone at varying lung volumes. The *broken line* indicates the inspiratory and expiratory muscle forces needed to balance the recoil forces for zero subglottal pressure. By convention, inspiratory muscle forces are given a minus sign and expiratory muscle forces, a plus sign. The *solid line* indicates the inspiratory or expiratory muscle forces required to produce a constant subglottal pressure of 7 cm $H_2O$.

has shown, both the inspiratory and expiratory muscles are at least minimally active during both phases of respiration for speech. For example, even though the external intercostal muscles are primarily responsible for elevating the rib cage during inspiration and for breaking the descent of the rib cage during the phase of expiration before relaxation pressure is achieved, the internal intercostal muscles are active at the same time. The position of the chest wall, then, at any moment, is the result of combined muscular effort of the agonist–antagonist opposition of the "inspiratory" and "expiratory" muscles. As Weismer (1985) has pointed out, the simultaneous activity of both sets of muscles eliminates a potential hiatus in muscle activity (as relaxation pressure is attained) that would otherwise exist if the expiratory muscles were inactive until the relaxation of the inspiratory muscles had lowered the rib cage to its resting position.

The simultaneous activity of the respiratory muscles also provides a better explanation of how the respiratory mechanism supplies the increases in air pressure that are needed to raise the fundamental frequency ($f_o$) and amplitude of vocal fold vibration

that are needed to signal stressed syllables. During speech, $f_o$ and intensity are constantly changing because some words and syllables are given greater emphasis (stress) than others. For example, during one expiration, a speaker might say, "The **qual**ity of **mer**cy is not **strained** but **drop**peth as the **gent**le **rain** from **heav**en upon the **place** be**neath**," stressing the words or syllables in bold print. Research suggests that the extra subglottal pressure required for the stressed syllables is supplied by contraction of the internal intercostal muscles. If so, we would expect those expiratory muscles to be active at any point in the utterance at which a stressed syllable occurred, even at times long before the rib cage has reached its rest position. The activity of the abdominal muscles (Fig. 3.27) might also increase to supply the added expiratory force needed for stressed syllables that are spoken after the rib cage has contracted beyond its resting position.

The increases in $f_o$, intensity, and duration that commonly underlie the production of stressed syllables may well be a function of a speaker's unconscious attempt to increase intensity and, hence, loudness. The intensity

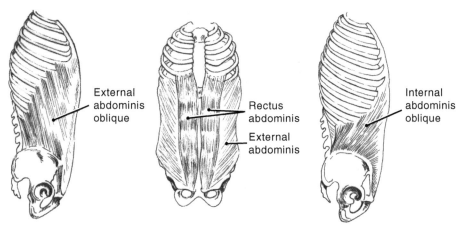

**FIGURE 3.27** Two lateral views and one frontal view of the abdominal muscles used in respiration for speech.

$(I)$ of the voice is primarily controlled by subglottal pressure $(P_s)$ that increases as a function of the third or fourth power of the subglottal air pressure.

$$I = P_s^3 \text{ or } P_s^4$$

As this formula indicates, a small change in pressure generates a large change in intensity. If you double the subglottal pressure, the intensity increases by 8 to 16 times ($2^3 = 8$; $2^4 = 16$), a 9- to 12-dB increase in sound intensity. It seems likely that momentary increases in intensity, generated by pulses of activity in the internal intercostals and the abdominal muscles, are associated with greater stress on syllables. The increase in intensity most often causes a rise in fundamental frequency $(f_o)$ and thus raises the perceived pitch of the stressed syllable. The rise in pitch is often the most important perceptual cue to syllable stress. Finally, the extra effort required to produce the stressed syllable may also be related to its greater duration.

Hixon, Mead, and Goldman (1991) have provided evidence from observations of abdominal movements during speech indicating that the abdominal wall stiffens for both inspiration and expiration during running speech. As in the case of the intercostal muscles, there is an advantage to having the abdominal muscles contract during both inspiration and expiration. Contraction of the abdominal muscles compresses the visceral organs, which, in turn, push up against the bottom of the diaphragm, maintaining it in a high position that will provide the greatest possible inspirational effort as it flattens when it comes time for the speaker to take a breath. There is another advantage to using the abdominal muscles during expiration to maintain a high posture for the diaphragm: Because the diaphragm is attached to the lower ribs (Fig. 3.18), as it flattens during inspiration, it not only extends the vertical dimension of the thorax but also enlarges the lateral and anterior–posterior dimensions of the inferior portion of the rib cage, and so aids in generating the negative pleural pressure needed for inspiration.

The range of durations of phrase groups during conversational speech requires, as we have mentioned, variations in the amount of air inspired (Fig. 3.28). In saying, "I'm nobody. Who are you? Are you nobody too?" a speaker may use one expiration or perhaps two. The location of a break for a breath is partially determined by the text; Emily Dickinson would surely not have wanted us to interrupt her phrase by taking a breath after "Who." Variations in expiratory duration depend on what and how much is spoken and can result in relatively long durations of the expiration. A speaker who wants to finish

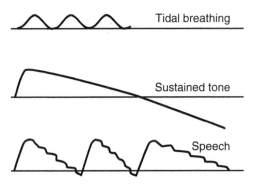

**FIGURE 3.28** Lung volume as a function of time for various respiratory conditions at 40% VC.

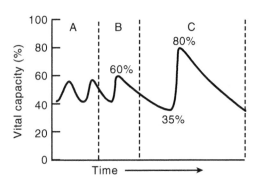

**FIGURE 3.29** Lung volume changes during tidal breathing (*a*), conversational speech (*b*), and loud speech (*c*). (Adapted with permission from Hixon, T. J., Respiratory Function in Speech. In *Normal Aspects of Speech, Hearing, and Language*. F. D. Minifie, T. J. Hixon, and F. Williams (Eds.). Englewood Cliffs, NJ: Prentice-Hall, 1973, p. 115.)

a long phrase without interruption often continues to contract expiratory muscles, using some of the expiratory reserve volume, even at the expense of comfort.

We must mention a final difference between quiet breathing and breathing for speech: the volume of air expended. During restful breathing, we use only 10% of our VC. For example, we may inhale up to 50% of VC and then exhale to 40%. Hixon (1973) reports that in conversational speech, we typically inspire up to roughly 60% of VC

and do not take another breath until we have reached an appropriate stopping place near an REL of about 35% VC. Therefore, we use only about 25% of our VC for conversational speech. During loud speech, we use 45% of VC, the expiratory phase going from perhaps 80% to 35% of VC (Fig. 3.29). It would seem that, barring some respiratory ailment,

---

### $C$LINICAL NOTE

Poor control over the respiratory system can have a number of clinical consequences. In voice disorders, exhaled air is often wasted because of inefficient use of energy rather than because the speaker has not inspired a sufficient volume of air. The irregularities seen in the respiratory patterns of speakers with severe hearing loss are related to anomalies of vocal fold and vocal tract modifications of the airstream. Respiratory irregularities are often seen, too, in the patterns produced by speakers with motor disorders (e.g., cerebral palsy). Irregularities also appear as a lack of coordination between abdominal and thoracic respiratory systems, evidenced during the disfluent utterances of some speakers who stutter. Again, although inefficient use of airflow is often a more serious problem than insufficient airflow, a speaker with motor dysfunction may overcontract the internal intercostal muscles when inhaling. Although the speaker does finally inhale, the antagonistic muscle behavior, of course, reduces the volume of air inspired. In addition, one can observe in relatively inefficient breathers a tendency to expend a great deal of muscular energy lifting the sternum and upper rib cage, a process sometimes called clavicular breathing, when with the same energy applied to different muscles, a speaker could lift the lower ribs and produce a greater thoracic expansion.

the problems of respiration common to some speech pathologies are not a matter of needing more air energy, because only the middle quarter of VC is usually used at conversational levels, but more likely are problems in control and modification of the airstream.

This chapter has been devoted to a discussion of the neurologic and respiratory mechanisms that underlie the production of speech. In the next chapter, we will turn our attention to phonation, the principal source of acoustic energy in the vocal tract.

# REFERENCES AND SUGGESTED READING

## General Works on Speech Production

Barlow, S. M., *Handbook of Clinical Speech Physiology*. San Diego: Singular, 1999.

Dickson, D. R., and Maue-Dickson, W., *Anatomical and Physiological Bases of Speech*. Boston: Little, Brown and Co., 1982.

Harris, K. S., Physiological Aspects of Articulatory Behavior. In *Current Trends in Linguistics*, Vol. 12, No. 4, T. A. Sebeok (Ed.). The Hague: Mouton, 1974, pp. 2281–2302.

Kahane, D. R., and Folkins, J. F., *Atlas of Speech and Hearing Anatomy*. Columbus, OH: Charles E. Merrill, 1984.

Kent, R. D., Atal, B. S., and Miller, J. L. (Eds.), *Papers in Speech Communication: Speech Production*. Woodbury, NY: Acoustical Society of America, 1991.

Lieberman, P., and Blumstein, S. E., *Speech Physiology, Speech Perception, and Acoustic Phonetics: An Introduction*. New York: Cambridge University Press, 1988.

Minifie, F., Hixon, T. J., and Williams, F. (Eds.), *Normal Aspects of Speech, Hearing, and Language*. Englewood Cliffs, NJ: Prentice-Hall Inc., 1972.

Perkell, J. S., *Physiology of Speech Production: Results and Implications of a Quantitative Cineradiographic Study*. Cambridge, MA: MIT Press, 1969.

Seikel, J. A., Drumright, D. G., and Seikel, P., *Essentials of Anatomy and Physiology for Communication Disorders*. Clifton Park, NY: Thomson Delmar Learning, 2004.

Zemlin, W. R., *Speech and Hearing Science: Anatomy and Physiology*, 4th ed. Boston: Allyn & Bacon, 1998.

## Neurophysiology

Broca, P., Remarques Sur La Siège De La Faculté Du Langage Articulé, Suivies D'une Observation D'aphémie (Perte De La Parole). *Bull. Soc. Anatom. Paris. VI. 36*, 1861, 330–357.

Fiez, J. A., Neuroimaging Studies of Speech: An Overview of Techniques and Methodological Approaches. *J. Commun. Disord. 34*, 2001, 445–454.

Fromkin, V. A., Slips of the Tongue. *Sci. Am. 229*, 1973, 110–116.

Lassen, A. R., Ingvar, D. H., and Skinhoj, E., Brain Function and Blood Flow. *Sci. Am. 239*, 1978, 62–71.

Lynch, J. C., The Cerebral Cortex. In *Fundamental Neuroscience*, 2nd ed. D. E. Haines (Ed.). Edinburgh: Churchill Livingstone, 2002, pp. 505–520.

MacKay, D. G., Spoonerisms: The Structure of Errors in the Serial Order of Speech. *Neuropsychologia 8*, 1970, 323–350.

Milner, B., Branch, C., and Rasmussen, T., Observations on Cerebral Dominance. In *Psychology Readings: Language*. R. C. Oldfield and J. C. Marshall (Eds.). Baltimore: Penguin Books, 1968, pp. 366–378. (Later figures given in present text from oral presentation by Milner at ASHA meeting, Las Vegas, 1974.)

Nolte, J., *The Human Brain: An Introduction to Its Functional Anatomy*. Philadelphia: Mosby, 2002.

Penfield, W., and Roberts, L., *Speech and Brain-Mechanisms*. Princeton, NJ: Princeton University Press, 1959.

Wada, J., and Rasmussen, T., Intracarotid Injection of Sodium Amytal for the Lateralization of Cerebral Speech Dominance: Experiments and Clinical Observations. *J. Neurosurg. 17*, 1960, 266–282.

Webster, D. B., *Neuroscience of Communication*, 2nd ed. San Diego: Singular, 1999.

Wernicke, C., *Der Aphasische Symptomencomplex*. Breslau, Poland: Max Cohn & Weigert, 1874.

## Respiration

Campbell, E., The Respiratory Muscles. *Ann. N.Y. Acad. Sci. 155,* 1968, 135–140.

Davies, A., and Moore, C., *The Respiratory System.* Edinburgh, UK: Churchill Livingstone, 2003.

Feldman, J., and McCrimmon, D., Neural Control of Breathing. In *Fundamental Neuroscience.* Zigmond, M., Bloom, F., Landis, S., Roberts J., and Squire, L. (Eds.). New York: Academic Press, 1999, pp. 1063–1090.

Hixon, T. J., Respiratory Function in Speech. In *Normal Aspects of Speech, Hearing, and Language.* F. D. Minifie, T. J. Hixon, and F. Williams (Eds.). Englewood Cliffs, NJ: Prentice-Hall Inc., 1973.

Hixon, T. J., Goldman, M. D., and Mead, J., Kinematics of the Chest Wall During Speech Productions: Volume Displacements of the Rib Cage, Abdomen, and Lung. *J. Speech Hear. Res. 16,* 1973, 78–115.

Hixon, T. J., Mead, J., and Goldman, M. D., Dynamics of the Chest Wall during Speech Production: Function of the Thorax, Rib Cage, Diaphragm, and Abdomen. *J. Speech Hear. Res. 19,* 1976, 297–356. Reprinted in Hixon, T. J. *Respiratory Function in Speech and Song.* San Diego, CA: Singular Publishing Group, 1991, 135–197. Also reprinted in Kent et al., 1991 (q.v.), 297–356.

Hixon, T. J., and Weismer, G., Perspectives on the Edinburgh Study of Speech Breathing. *J. Speech Hear. Res. 38,* 1995, 42–60.

Jürgens, U., Neural Pathways Underlying Vocal Control. *Neurosci. Biobehav. Rev. 26,* 2002, 235–258.

Lofqvist, A., Aerodynamic Measurements for Vocal Function. In *Neurological Disorders of the Larynx.* A. Bletzer, C. Sasaki, S. Falin, M. Brill, and K. S. Harris (Eds.). New York: Thieme, 1992.

Lumb, A., Control of Breathing. In *Nunn's Applied Respiratory Physiology.* A. Lumb (Ed.). Boston: Butterworth Heinemann, 2000, pp. 82–112.

Mead, J., Bouhuys, A., and Proctor, D. F., Mechanisms Generating Subglottic Pressure. *Ann. N.Y. Acad. Sci. 155,* 1968, 177–181.

Petersen, E. S., The Control of Breathing Pattern. In *The Control of Breathing in Man.* B. J. Whipp (Ed.). Manchester, U.K.: Manchester University Press, 1987, pp. 1–28.

Rahn, H., Otis, A. B., Chadwick, L. E., and Fenn, W. O., The Pressure-Volume Diagram of the Thorax and Lung. *Am. J. Physiol. 146,* 1946, 161–178.

Stetson, R., *Motor Phonetics: A Study of Speech Movements in Action.* Amsterdam, The Netherlands: North-Holland, 1951. Revised by S. Kelso and K. Munhall, San Diego: Singular Publishing Group, 1988.

Weismer, G., Speech Breathing: Contemporary Views and Findings. In *Speech Science.* R. G. Daniloff (Ed.). San Diego, CA: College-Hill Press, 1985, pp. 47–72.

Whalen, D., and Kinsella-Shaw, J., Exploring the Relationship of Inspiration Duration to Utterance Duration. *Phonetica. 54,* 1997, 138–152.

Winkworth, A. L., Davis, P. J., Adams, R. D., and Ellis, E., Breathing Patterns During Spontaneous Speech. *J. Speech Hear. Res. 38,* 1995, 124–144.

# The Raw Materials—Phonation

# 4

*Wherefore, let thy voice*
*Rise like a fountain*

—Alfred, Lord Tennyson, "Morte d'Arthur"

## PHONATION

### Conversion of Air Pressure to Sound

The power supply for speech is the exhaled air from the lungs, but it is actions of the upper airways that convert this supply to audible vibrations for speech. As we have mentioned earlier, speakers use two methods of transforming the air into speech sounds. The first method involves using the air pressure to set the elastic vocal folds in the larynx into vibration, producing a periodic sound wave (one with a repeated pattern). The second method involves allowing air to pass through the larynx into the upper vocal tract (the space extending from the vocal folds to the lips or the nostrils), where various modifications of the airstream result in noises: bursts, hisses, or sequences of such aperiodic sound waves (with no repeated pattern). These two

methods can be combined to produce sounds that require simultaneous periodic and aperiodic sources of sound. The first method, that of setting the vocal folds into vibration, is termed *phonation*, and it is this mode of sound production that will consider now.

### Myoelastic Aerodynamic Theory of Phonation

The vocal folds are shelflike elastic protuberances of tendon, muscles, and mucous membrane that lie behind the Adam's apple, or thyroid cartilage, and run anteroposteriorly. Their tension and elasticity can be varied; they can be made thicker or thinner, shorter or longer; they can be widely separated, brought together, or put into intermediate positions; and they can be elevated or depressed in relation to the cavities above. In running speech, all of these adjustments occur at very rapid rates. The continuous changes of vocal fold position and shape are the result of an evolutionary change in the vocal folds from a simple sphincter or valve-like mechanism, found in lower forms of life, to the complex structure of the human larynx, in which the muscles controlling the folds are divided into several groups with specific functions, allowing a wide range of adjustments.

When the vocal folds are brought together and are vibrating, they are in the *phonatory mode*. Before considering the laryngeal structures and their functions in phonation, you can gain an immediate understanding of the physiology of vocal fold vibration by producing the labial vibration known as the "Bronx cheer" or "raspberry." To produce a Bronx cheer you first need to place your tongue between your lips, pushing the lower lip slightly forward with the tip of your tongue. Make an airtight seal between the upper lip and the superior surface of the tongue. Then, exhale relatively forcibly. This will set your lower lip into audible vibration. The sound is that of air escaping in rapid bursts, not the sound of the motions of the lower lip or the tongue. It is apparent that the lip movements are caused by the air pressure that blows the lower lip away from the tongue. This is a passive process: Although the lips and tongue must be brought together by muscle activity, the lip muscles do not produce the lip movements that generate the sound. The muscles must, of course, produce just the right amount of contact between the tongue and the lips for vibration to occur. If you try to produce the Bronx cheer with your lips slightly apart, or tightly pursed, you will meet with failure. Although the Bronx cheer is quite easily observed, until relatively recently there was no general agreement that the vocal folds worked in somewhat the same way.

In the middle of the 18th century, it was generally thought that vocal folds vibrated like strings, directly producing vibrations in air. Even as recently as 1950, Husson, a proponent of the neurochronaxic theory of vo-cal fold vibration, proposed that the vocal folds vibrated as a consequence of individual nerve impulses (generated at the fundamental frequency [$f_0$] rate) sent to the vocalis muscle, rather than as a consequence of the force of exhaled air on the vocal folds. The currently accepted theory of phonation, however, is essentially that proposed by both Helmholtz and Müller in the 19th century and amplified by van den Berg in a series of papers in the 1950s: the *myoelastic aerodynamic theory* of phonation. The key word is aerodynamic. The vocal folds are activated by the airstream from the lungs rather than by nerve impulses. "Myoelastic" refers to the ways in which the muscles (myo-) control the elasticity and tension on the vocal folds so that they can be set into vibration and so that changes can be made in their frequency of vibration.

The number of times the vocal folds are blown apart and come together per second is their fundamental frequency of vibration, that is, the $f_0$ of phonation. Men's voices have an average $f_0$ of approximately 125 Hz. Women are more apt to phonate with an $f_0$ greater than 200 Hz. The $f_0$ of children is higher than 300 Hz. Vocal fold size is one determinant of $f_0$. The greater the length and vibrating mass of the vocal folds, the lower the $f_0$. On average, men have longer and more massive vocal folds than women. Men's vocal fold lengths typically range from 17 to 24 mm, whereas the lengths of women's vocal folds range between 13 and 17 mm. Given a pair of vocal folds of a particular length and mass, however, a person can increase the frequency of vibration appreciably by lengthening and tensing the folds, which decreases their effective mass and increases their elasticity. Note that mass and tension are more important than length in determining $f_0$: Lengthening the folds might be expected to lower $f_0$ but does not, because making them longer makes them less massive and more tense, causing $f_0$ to rise. Usually, the vocal folds may be stretched by 3 or 4 mm. Singers are trained to have a range of two octaves, each octave being a doubling of frequency. A bass voice can go as low as about 80 Hz and a lyric soprano, higher than 1 kHz. Muscular activity is thus important in the control of phonation: Muscles bring the folds together so that they can vibrate, and muscles regulate their thickness and tension to alter the $f_0$.

The essential point of the myoelastic theory, however, is that the determinants of the vibratory cycle are aerodynamic. Air pressure from the lungs blows the vocal folds apart and so opens the glottis during each vibration. The folds come together again during each vibration because of (1) the maintenance of the instructions to the muscles to keep the vocal folds adducted during phonation, (2) the inherent elasticity of the folds, and (3) the sudden drop in air pressure below the folds as the vocal folds are forced apart allowing the air flow to streams through the open glottis.

More recent theorizing about vocal fold vibration has led to the development of the cover-body theory (also called the "two-mass model"). This theory attempts to explain how the unique structure of the vocal folds accounts for the wide range of frequencies, amplitudes, and vocal qualities that a human can produce while phonating. The structure of the vocal folds, described in great detail by Hirano and others (1985), consists of a relatively pliable "cover," formed partly of mucous membrane, that overlies a relatively stiff "body" composed mainly of muscle fibers.

The vibration of the cover ranges from very similar to very dissimilar to that of the body. The degree of similarity or difference, which determines many of the acoustic characteristics of phonation, depends on the activity of the intrinsic laryngeal muscles.

Whatever the theory, an explanation of the details of phonation requires anatomic knowledge of the larynx. Only the anatomy essential to a basic understanding of vocal fold function for speech will be presented below.

## Framework of the Larynx

In addition to its use for speech, the larynx is used (1) to control the flow of air into and out of the lungs providing oxygen to the body and eliminating carbon dioxide; (2) to prevent food, water, and other substances from entering the lungs; (3) to aid in swallowing; and (4) to enable a buildup of pressure within the thorax for such functions as coughing, vomiting, defecating, and lifting heavy objects.

The larynx lies below the *hyoid bone* at the top of the *trachea* (Fig. 4.1). The hyoid bone is suspended under the jaw and can best be felt by tilting the head back slightly. A small horseshoe-shaped bone, it is distinguished from the laryngeal and tracheal cartilages by its rigidity. The trachea, a series of horseshoe-shaped cartilages with the open part at the back, can be felt at the anterior

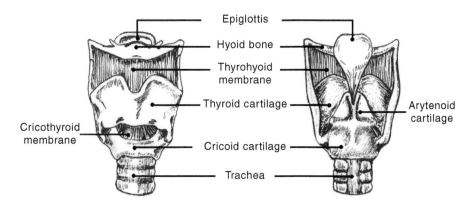

**FIGURE 4.1**   Anterior (*left*) and posterior (*right*) views of the larynx.

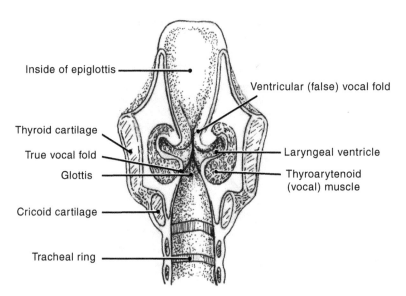

Inside of epiglottis

Ventricular (false) vocal fold

Thyroid cartilage

True vocal fold

Glottis

Laryngeal ventricle

Thyroarytenoid
(vocal) muscle

Cricoid cartilage

Tracheal ring

**FIGURE 4.2** Frontal section of the larynx. Notice the constrictions formed by the ventricular folds and the true vocal folds.

base of the neck. The laryngeal framework lies anterior to the lower pharynx, from which the esophagus branches off posteriorly before descending to the stomach. Food and liquids, therefore, must pass over the entrance to the lungs to gain access to the entrance to the stomach, a seemingly inefficient arrangement, which is the price paid for the evolutionary adaptation of the larynx as a sound source for speech. During swallowing, a leaf-shaped cartilage, the *epiglottis*, covers the entrance to the larynx. In other animals, the larynx is positioned high in the throat and can be coupled to the nasal airways, in which case food and liquids pass from the mouth around the sides of the larynx and straight into the esophagus, with no danger of entering the trachea.

The larynx is a tube composed of cartilages bound together by ligaments and connecting membranes and covered by mucous membrane. The enclosed area forms an hourglass space (Fig. 4.2) with a vestibule above two sets of folds, the *ventricular folds*, or "false vocal folds," and the "true vocal folds" used for phonation. The ventricular folds form a second constriction just above the true vocal folds. The vertical space

between the two sets of folds is called the *laryngeal ventricle*, and the space between the true vocal folds is called the *glottis*. Below the vocal folds the space widens again within the cartilaginous framework of the trachea.

The cartilages that enclose the laryngeal space and support the muscles that regulate changes in it are the *thyroid, cricoid,* and *arytenoid cartilages*. The cricoid cartilage (Fig. 4.3, *c* and *d*), so named because it is shaped like a signet ring (Greek *krikos* = ring; oid = like), is a specially adapted tracheal ring. The top ring of the trachea is distinctive because of the large plate (lamina) that forms its posterior surface (Fig. 4.3*c*), in contrast to the other tracheal rings, which are open at the back. The narrow front and sides of the cartilage form the arch, and the broad lamina at the back forms the signetlike part of the ring, which faces posteriorly.

Although the vocal folds are not attached to the cricoid cartilage, the cricoid articulates with three cartilages that do support the vocal folds: the thyroid cartilage and two arytenoid cartilages. The arytenoid cartilages (Fig. 4.3, *a* and *b*) are roughly pyramidal, and they articulate with the cricoid cartilage at concave depressions on their inferior

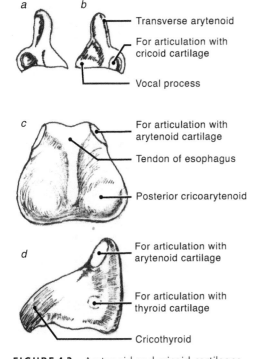

Transverse arytenoid

For articulation with cricoid cartilage

Vocal process

For articulation with arytenoid cartilage

Tendon of esophagus

Posterior cricoarytenoid

For articulation with arytenoid cartilage

For articulation with thyroid cartilage

Cricothyroid

**FIGURE 4.3** Arytenoid and cricoid cartilages. *a.* Left arytenoid cartilage, medial aspect. *b.* Right arytenoid cartilage, medial aspect. *c.* Cricoid cartilage, posterior aspect. *d.* Cricoid cartilage, left lateral aspect.

surfaces that fit over convex facets on the top surfaces of the cricoid lamina. A small projection at the base of each arytenoid cartilage (the vocal process) extends anteriorly and is the point of attachment for the vocal ligament. The vocal ligament and the *thyroarytenoid muscle* that lie lateral to it are stretched between the vocal process of the arytenoid cartilages in the back and the deep angle of the thyroid cartilage in the front (Fig. 4.4).

These structures (the vocal processes of the arytenoid cartilage, the vocal ligaments, the thyroarytenoid muscle, and the mucous membrane lining the inner surface on both sides of the glottis) form the true vocal folds. The vocal process, which projects into the posterior third of the folds, forms the *cartilaginous* portion of the glottis. The anterior two thirds of the folds are the *membranous* portions of the glottis. The patterns of vibration of the cartilaginous and membranous portions of the glottis differ from each other.

The extension at the lateral base of each arytenoid cartilage is called the muscular process because three muscles important for the positioning of the vocal folds are attached to it (Fig. 4.4). The muscular process extends posteriorly and somewhat laterally.

The largest cartilage of the larynx, the thyroid cartilage, so named because it is like a shield (Greek *thyreos* = large shield), lies anterior to the arytenoid cartilages, which its sides enclose, and superior to the cricoid cartilage, the top laminal crest of which it also encloses. The two laminae or plates of the thyroid cartilage meet anteriorly and from an

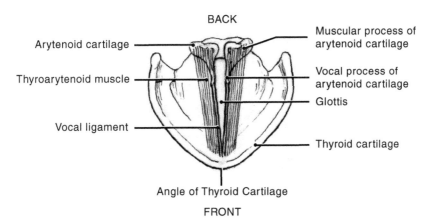

BACK

Arytenoid cartilage

Muscular process of arytenoid cartilage

Thyroarytenoid muscle

Vocal process of arytenoid cartilage

Glottis

Vocal ligament

Thyroid cartilage

Angle of Thyroid Cartilage

FRONT

**FIGURE 4.4** Superior view of larynx showing the relations among the thyroid, cricoid, and arytenoid cartilages and the thyroarytenoid muscle.

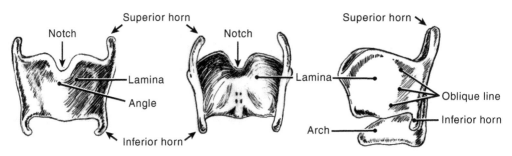

**FIGURE 4.5** Left to right, anterior, posterior, and lateral views of the thyroid cartilage. Lateral view includes the cricoid cartilage.

angle that is more acute in men (about 90°) than in women (about 120°), hence the common term "Adam's apple" instead of "Eve's apple." There is a notch (Fig. 4.5) where the laminae separate above the angle; you can usually locate it by feeling along the midline of your neck with your index finger. The plates are widely separated in the back and extend into two superior horns that project toward the hyoid bone above. The two smaller inferior horns articulate with the cricoid cartilage below by fitting into a round facet on each side of the cricoid lamina (Fig. 4.3*d*).

The cartilages of the larynx can move in relation to one another to a limited degree. The thyroid and cricoid cartilages can rock back and forth on each other. We will describe these motions later in the discussion of pitch change. The arytenoids can rotate and rock on the cricoid cartilage and can also slide a bit toward one another. The muscles attached to the muscular process of the arytenoid cartilages control these movements, as described in the following discussion of vocal fold adjustments.

## Vocal Fold Adjustments During Speech

The vocal folds at rest are separated (abducted), creating a V-shaped glottal space with its apex behind the thyroid cartilage and its widest separation at the back, where the folds attach to the vocal process of the arytenoid cartilages (Fig. 4.4). During running speech, the vocal folds are separated for voiceless speech sounds, such as the consonants /s/ and /t/, and are brought together (adducted) for voiced sounds, such as the vowels and diphthongs /u/, /i/, and /aɪ/ in the words "two" /tu/, "tea" /ti/, and "tie" /taɪ/. They are less firmly brought together for voiced consonants such as /z/ and /v/, for which phonation is needed in addition to large air pressures in the oral cavity (Fig. 4.6).

### Voiceless Consonants

The simplest adjustment of the vocal folds during speech is the one made for voiceless consonants. The folds abduct to allow the passage of sufficient air from the lungs to create noises in the oral cavity. Voiceless consonants are often interspersed in the speech stream singly or in clusters, demanding rapid glottal opening to interrupt phonation. The job is done by a pair of large triangular muscles attached by tendons to the top of the muscular process of each arytenoid cartilage (Fig. 4.7); the muscle fibers fan out as they course back and down to attach to the dorsal plates of the cricoid cartilage. Named for their position and attachments, the *posterior cricoarytenoid muscles*, on contraction, rotate the arytenoid cartilages, abducting the vocal processes, and thus the vocal folds. Innervation to these and almost all of the other intrinsic muscles of the larynx is supplied by the *recurrent nerve*, a branch of the vagus, the tenth cranial nerve. The posterior cricoarytenoid is the only muscle that acts to abduct the vocal folds.

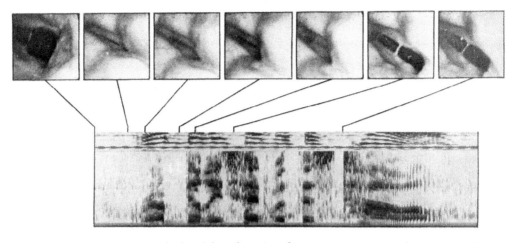

rʌ b bɪ l i z hɛdwɪθɚ ɪ s t    a    w!

**FIGURE 4.6** Glottis viewed from above with a fiberoptic bundle at various times in the production of a sentence. The posterior part of the glottal chink is at the lower right in each view. Note the open glottis in the first frame for inspiration, the relatively closed glottis in the third and fifth frame for a vowel, and the relatively open glottis in the sixth frame for a voiced fricative consonant. (The structure apparently connecting the folds in the rightmost views is a bead of mucus.) (Reprinted with permission from Sawashima, M., Abramson, A. S., Cooper, F. S., and Lisker, L., Observing Laryngeal Adjustments during Running Speech by Use of a Fiberoptics System. *Phonetica 22,* 1970, 193–201.)

## Phonated Speech Sounds

Widely separated vocal folds cannot be set into vibration, so to produce the phonated sounds of speech, the normally separated folds must be adducted or nearly so. To adduct or approximate the vocal folds, the arytenoid cartilages must be brought closer together, with their vocal processes rocked inward toward one another. A strong band of muscular fibers runs horizontally across the posterior surfaces of the arytenoid cartilages. This muscle, the *transverse interarytenoid muscle,* is overlaid by some muscular fibers in the shape of an X called the *oblique interarytenoid muscles* (Fig. 4.8). Together, termed the *interarytenoid (IA) muscle,* they adduct the arytenoid cartilages and the vocal folds. The IA muscle is thought to be the primary adductor of the vocal folds. The *lateral cricoarytenoid (LCA) muscles* also aid in adduction of the vocal folds by rocking the muscular process of the arytenoids forward and down, pressing the vocal processes together (Fig. 4.9). The simultaneous contraction of the IA and

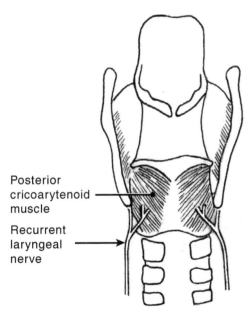

Posterior
cricoarytenoid
muscle

Recurrent
laryngeal
nerve

**FIGURE 4.7** Posterior view of the posterior cricoarytenoid muscle. Innervation is via the recurrent branch of the vagus nerve (cranial nerve X).

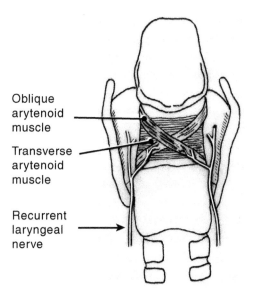

Oblique arytenoid muscle

Transverse arytenoid muscle

Recurrent laryngeal nerve

**FIGURE 4.8**　Posterior view of the transverse and oblique arytenoid muscles. Together these muscles constitute the interarytenoid muscle.

LCA can produce the stronger adduction of the folds that is usually used for vowel production. For speech sounds requiring phonation along with an uninterrupted flow of air

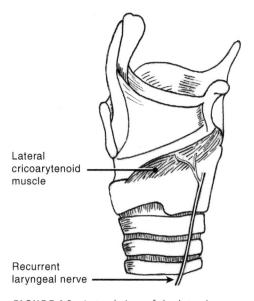

Lateral cricoarytenoid muscle

Recurrent laryngeal nerve

**FIGURE 4.9**　Lateral view of the lateral cricoarytenoid muscle with the left side of the thyroid cartilage removed.

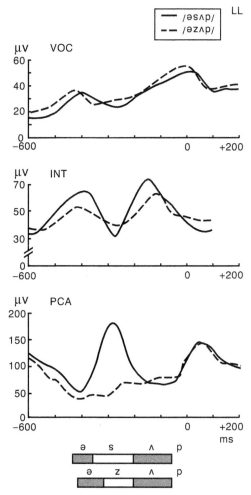

**FIGURE 4.10**　Superimposed electromyography curves for voiced (z; *broken line*) and voiceless (s; *solid line*) fricatives in nonsense syllables. Although vocalis muscle (VOC) activity is similar for both, for /s/, interarytenoid (INT) activity is reduced when posterior cricoarytenoid (PCA) activity is greatly increased. (Modified with permission from Hirose, H., and Gay, T., The Activity of the Intrinsic Laryngeal Muscles in Voicing Control. *Phonetica, 25,* 1972, 140–164.)

for a sound source above the glottis, the vocal folds are often less completely adducted. Hirose and Gay (1972) (Fig. 4.10) differentiated the functions of laryngeal muscles by measuring the electrical activity generated as these muscles contract. The recording method (electromyography), as we have already noted, is explained in Chapter 14.

The vocal folds themselves are composed of (1) the vocal ligaments, which are the thickened edges of the *conus elasticus* membrane rising from the cricoid cartilage, (2) the muscles that are attached to the ligaments, the internal part of the *thyroarytenoid muscles,* commonly called the *vocalis muscles,* and (3) the mucous membrane that covers them. The vocal ligaments and the vocalis muscles, which form the body of the vocal folds, emerge from the projection of the arytenoid cartilage known as the vocal process. The posterior portions of the vocal folds are thus stiffer than the anterior portions because of the presence of the arytenoid cartilage. The folds become increasingly flexible in their anterior, membranous portions. When relaxed, the vocal folds are relatively thick, vibrating in an undulating manner as the mucous membrane moves somewhat independently like flabby skin on a waving arm. The lateral fibers of the thyroarytenoid muscle extend to the muscular process of the arytenoid cartilage, some of them wrapping around the arytenoid, where they commingle with the IA muscles. More research is needed to differentiate the roles of the medial and lateral fibers of the thyroarytenoid muscles in phonation, but in general the medial (vocalis) fibers are thought to tense the folds.

The muscle activity needed to adduct and tense the vocal folds simply readies them for vibration but does not cause the vibration itself. For the Bronx cheer, you had to put your tongue and lips together, and that required muscular effort, but the sound itself was produced by aerodynamic forces acting on the elastic body of the lower lip. The two aerodynamic forces that produce vibration of the vocal folds are the *subglottal air pressure* ($P_s$) applied to the lower part of the folds, forcing them apart, and the negative pressure that occurs as air passes between the folds (the *Bernoulli effect*). These positive and negative pressures set the vocal folds into vibration because of the elasticity of the folds.

## Subglottal Air Pressure

Consider first that once the elevated subglottal air pressure reaches what is called the *phonation threshold pressure,* the glottis is forced to open as the vocal folds separate. During each opening of the glottis, a tiny puff of air escapes, cut off sharply by the abruptly closing glottis. Because the folds vibrate rapidly (usually more than 100 times per second), one puff follows another in rapid succession. This chain of air puffs sets up an audible pressure wave at the glottis. A necessary condition for phonation is that the air pressure below the folds must exceed the pressure above the folds. If the pressure above the folds increases so that the pressure difference across the glottis necessary for phonation is lost, phonation ceases. You can test this by trying to prolong the closure period of a voiced stop consonant such as a [b]. You can phonate during the [b] closure only for a short time because the labial and velopharyngeal closures for [b] block the flow of air out of the vocal tract and so cause the supraglottal air pressure to increase until it equals the subglottal air pressure. Because there is no longer more pressure below the folds than above them, phonation is not possible. For speech at conversational level, a subglottal air pressure in the range of 7 to 10 cm $H_2O$ (centimeters of water pressure) is sufficient to produce phonation at approximately 60-dB intensity.

The effect of subglottal air pressure sufficient to separate a pair of vocal folds can be seen in Figure 4.11. This figure shows schematic diagrams made from a movie of a larynx during phonation. The glottis begins to open as the bottom portions of the vocal folds separate. The separation then proceeds upward to the top of the folds. As the top of the vocal folds separates, the bottom portions begin to approximate. The approximation of the folds then continues upward until the glottis is closed from top to bottom and the next cycle of vibration is ready to begin. Thus, there is a vertical phase difference, creating a wavelike motion of the

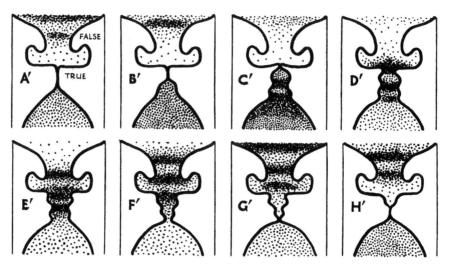

**FIGURE 4.11**   Cross sections of the vocal folds during vibration. The folds open and close from bottom to top. (Reprinted with permission from Vennard, W., *Singing: The Mechanism and the Technic*. New York: Carl Fischer, 1967.)

folds, the normal movement during vibration for chest voice. If the speaker speaks or sings in a high falsetto voice, however, the vertical phase difference is lost and each of the taut folds moves as a unit. Regardless of the mode of vibration, the closing phase of each cycle is the result of the tendency of the elastic folds to move back to their adducted position (the adductor muscles remain active during all phases of the phonatory cycle) and of the second aerodynamic phenomenon important to phonation, the pressure drop explained by the Bernoulli effect.

## The Bernoulli Effect

Daniel Bernoulli, an 18th-century mathematician and physician, developed the kinetic theory of gases and liquids, part of which is known as the Bernoulli effect or principle. The Bernoulli effect is based on the observation that when a gas or liquid flows through a constricted passage, the velocity (speed in a given direction) increases. The increase in velocity causes a decrease of pressure within the stream of gas or liquid relative to pressure exerted by the walls of the passage. In other words, the inward pressure perpendicular to the airflow is greater

than the outward pressure. Figure 4.12 illustrates the increase in velocity within a narrow portion of a passage and the resulting decrease in pressure against the lateral walls. If the walls are sufficiently pliable, the reduction in outward pressure moves them toward each other. Translated to the larynx, the Bernoulli effect results in the vocal folds

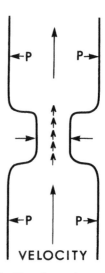

**FIGURE 4.12**   Flow through a constricted passage. In the constriction, velocity is greater, but pressure on the inner sides of the constriction is correspondingly reduced.

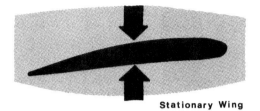

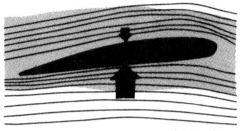

Stationary Wing

Moving Wing

**FIGURE 4.13** Aerodynamic forces on an airplane wing.

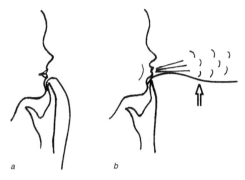

*a* *b*

**FIGURE 4.14** The Bernoulli principle. (*a*) No airflow. (*b*) When blowing increases airflow on the upper side of the paper, pressure is lower on the top than on the bottom, and the sheet rises.

being drawn toward each other: The narrow space created at the moment they are blown apart causes the air pressure within the glottis to decrease.

The conventional airplane wing is designed to take advantage of the Bernoulli effect to elevate an aircraft. The wing is streamlined on the top surface (Fig. 4.13), permitting a higher velocity of air current than that passing beneath. The higher velocity results in a drop in pressure against the top surface, which creates a difference between the pressures under and over the wings, elevating the plane. You can elevate a piece of paper, using the same principle, by holding one end of it under your lips and blowing air across the top (Fig. 4.14).

We experience the Bernoulli phenomenon constantly. When a draft of air flows through a narrow corridor, the doors opening into rooms off the hall slam shut, because the pressure on the hall side of the doors is lower than that on the room side. If you have ever been in a lightweight car cruising alongside a heavy truck on a highway and felt your car being sucked alarmingly close to the truck, it is because the faster airstream created between your car and the

truck has lowered the pressure against the truck side of your car relative to the other side.

## Vocal Fold Vibration

As we have seen, each cycle of vocal fold vibration is caused first by the subglottal air pressure that has built up sufficiently to separate the folds and by the Bernoulli effect, which accounts for a sudden drop in pressure against the inner sides of each fold that sucks them together again as the air rushes through the glottis at an increased velocity. The whole process is made possible by the fact that the folds themselves are elastic. Their elasticity not only permits them to be blown apart for each cycle, but the elastic recoil force (the force that restores any elastic body to its resting place) works along with the Bernoulli effect to close the glottis for each cycle of vibration.

The vocal folds move in a fairly periodic way. During sustained vowels, for example, the folds open and close in a repeated pattern of movement. This action produces a barrage of airbursts that sets up an audible pressure wave (sound) at the glottis. The pressure wave of sound is also periodic: the pattern repeats itself. Like all sound sources that vibrate in a complex periodic fashion, the vocal folds generate a harmonic series (see Chapter 2) consisting of an $f_o$ and many whole number multiples of that $f_o$. The $f_o$ is the number of glottal cycles (openings and closings) per second.

The human voice is a low-frequency sound compared with most of the sounds of the world, including those made by other sound sources above the larynx. Because it contains many harmonics, the voice is also a complex sound. We never hear the unmodified sound of vocal fold vibration, however, because by the time it has reached the lips of the speaker, it has been changed by the rest of the vocal tract. If we were to place a microphone just above the vocal folds, we might record a sound that has a spectrum resembling those shown in Figure 4.15, consisting of the $f_o$ (the frequency of the vibration itself), a second harmonic (two times the $f_o$), a third harmonic (three times the $f_o$),

and so forth. It is characteristic of the human voice that the higher harmonics have less intensity than the lower harmonics, so that although the voice contains many high-frequency components, there is more energy in the low frequencies. The intensity falls off at about 12 dB per octave (each doubling of the frequency).

Low-pitched and high-pitched voices sound different in part because the spacing of their harmonics is different. Figure 4.15 shows the difference. Notice the closer spacing of the harmonics in the adult male's voice, which has an $f_o$ of 150 Hz. Because the harmonics are whole number multiples of the $f_o$, they are separated by 150 Hz. In contrast, a child phonating with an $f_o$ of 300 Hz would generate harmonics that are separated by 300 Hz. Analogously, an individual adjusting the $f_o$ of his or her vocal

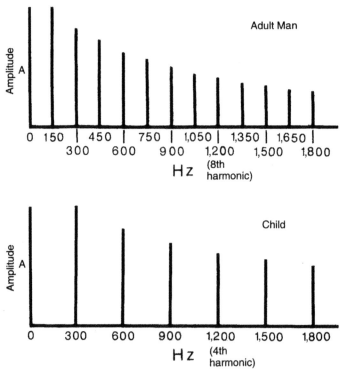

**FIGURE 4.15** Spectra of sounds resulting from vocal fold vibration. The spectra represent different fundamental and harmonic frequencies of vibration, which account for the difference in the harmonic spacing.

fold vibrations changes the harmonic spacing similarly: The higher the $f_o$, the greater harmonic spacing; the lower the $f_o$, the less the space (frequency difference) between the harmonics. Notice that both spectra in the figure, the adult male's and the child's, have a similar shape because the amplitudes of the harmonics decrease as their frequencies increase.

## Fundamental Frequency

The human voice is composed of many frequencies; it is a complex tone. A listener's perception of a speaker's pitch depends mostly on the lowest (fundamental) frequency in the speaker's voice. The $f_o$ is constantly changing, as we know when we listen for the intonation patterns of sentences.

## *C*LINICAL NOTE

Although it is true that some voice disorders involve interactions between the respiratory and phonatory systems, many are caused by abnormalities of phonation. For instance, paralysis of one or both vocal folds can cause *spasmodic dysphonia* (also called *spastic dysphonia*). The inability to phonate at all, breaks in normal phonatory output, and "strangled" voice quality are all symptoms of this disorder. Normal phonation may, of course, be rendered impossible for those patients in whom all or part of the larynx, including the vocal folds, has been surgically removed because of cancer. Speakers who have undergone such surgery must learn to vibrate other tissues and muscle masses, such as scar tissue or the cricopharyngeus muscle, to provide a source of sound for speech. Some alaryngeal speakers have to resort to an artificial sound source, an electrolarynx, that they hold to the outside of the neck. This produces a "voice" with a mechanical quality.

Less catastrophic disorders are commonly found among speakers. For instance, a *breathy voice*, still occasionally popular with some movie stars and celebrities who wished to convey "sexiness," is the result of failing to adduct the vocal folds sufficiently, particularly in the cartilaginous portions of the glottis. They are close enough to vibrate, but the sound of continuously released air accompanies the sound wave set up by the air pressure volleys. A *hoarse voice* is caused by irregularities in the folds. When the vocal folds are irritated or swollen, as they may be during a cold with accompanying laryngitis, the voice becomes hoarse. Hoarseness can also be indicative of vocal abuse. One cause of vocal abuse may be the application of too much tension to the muscles of the larynx, causing *contact ulcers*, lesions produced by the arytenoid cartilages banging against one another. Another cause of abuse is overusing the voice, causing nodules to develop along the edges of the vocal folds. Vocal nodules may also be caused by overuse of *glottal attack*, for which the vocal folds are tightly, rather than lightly, adducted before phonation. A very high subglottal pressure is thus needed to blow the vocal folds apart. Hirose and Gay (1972) have shown that glottal attack is accompanied by an early onset of activity in the lateral cricoarytenoid muscles (Fig. 4.16), which compress the center of the vocal folds. This early compression provides the time needed for the pressure buildup required to initiate phonation.

Abnormal laryngeal behavior has also been implicated in stuttering. Some people who stutter contract the adductor and abductor muscles of the larynx simultaneously, rather than reciprocally. This causes the glottis to be "frozen" in either an open or a closed state. Thus, for example, if it becomes necessary to produce an unphonated sound followed by a phonated sound (e.g., in the word "so"), the speaker may still be contracting his posterior cricoarytenoid muscle (abductor) at the same time as his interarytenoid muscles (adductors). Until the conflict is resolved, the glottis cannot close and phonation cannot begin. The time needed to resolve the conflict may account for the blocks and perseverations that mark episodes of stuttering.

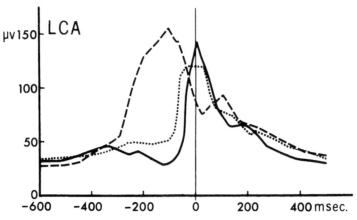

**FIGURE 4.16** Contrasting muscle activity patterns in the lateral cricoarytenoid (LCA) muscle for various forms of vocal attack. The onset of the vowel is marked as 0. Activity is earliest for glottal attack (*broken line*), later for normal voiced attack (*dotted line*), and latest for voiceless aspirate attack (*solid line*). The measure of muscle activity is obtained by smoothing muscle interference patterns. (See Fig. 3.13 and the discussion of Fig. 14.3.) (Reprinted with permission from Hirose, H., and Gay, T., *Folia Phoniatrica* (*Basel*). Basel: S. Karger AG, 1973.)

The question "Are you sure?" is likely to have a rising intonation pattern, whereas the statement "I'm sure" usually has a falling intonation pattern. The speaker produces these different intonation patterns by varying the $f_o$ of vocal fold vibration.

According to the myoelastic aerodynamic theory of phonation, frequency of vocal fold vibration is determined primarily by the elasticity, tension, and mass of the vocal folds. More massive folds (longer and thicker) vibrate naturally at lower frequencies than shorter and thinner folds. Vocal folds vibrate faster when they are tense than when they are slack. The most efficient way to make a given set of vocal folds more tense and less massive (thinner) is to stretch them.

Before discussing the physiology of the vocal fold adjustments that regulate fundamental frequency and thus pitch changes, we must clarify the relationship between vocal fold length and mass and fundamental frequency. Imagine that we were to measure the length and mass of the vocal folds of two people, an adult man and an adult woman, during restful breathing. In most instances, we would find that the adult man, who has larger and more massive vocal folds, would produce a lower average $f_o$ than the adult woman who has shorter and less massive vocal folds. A child, whose vocal folds are even shorter and less massive, will produce a higher $f_o$ than an adult woman. There are various values given for the average fundamental frequency of an adult man, but most of them are in the neighborhood of 125 Hz. The values given for adult women are about 100 Hz higher. The average $f_o$ for children (300 Hz and higher) is more variable because children's vocal fold mass and length are continually changing as they grow. Differences in the basic length and mass of the vocal folds also explain why one adult man is a baritone and another is a tenor and why one adult woman is an alto and another is a soprano.

But, because the $f_o$ produced by any speaker is constantly changing during the production of running speech, the average values are rarely attained. For instance, if an adult woman with an average $f_o$ of 225 Hz uttered a sentence, we might discover that there was only a brief moment—a few milliseconds—during which the average $f_o$ was produced. The rest of the sentence would exhibit fundamental frequencies both higher and lower than the average. Indeed, it would be the pattern of $f_0$ changes that was linguistically significant and not the specific $f_0$ values at any given moment. That is why we must now explore the mechanisms for changing $f_0$ and, to the listener's ears, pitch.

Vocal fold lengthening by a particular speaker will stretch and thin the effective vibrating portion of the folds, adding tension and thereby producing a higher fundamental frequency. In other words, the decrease in mass and the increase in tension override the effect of the increase in length, and so $f_0$ rises. The paired muscles responsible for stretching the vocal folds and thereby controlling $f_0$ change are the *cricothyroid muscles*.

Because each vocal fold lies between the thyroid cartilage and an arytenoid cartilage, the way to stretch the folds is to increase the distance between these cartilages. The cricothyroid muscles can do just that. Because they are attached to the side of the cricoid ring and rise, some fibers almost vertical and others at an oblique angle to the thyroid cartilage (Fig. 4.17), their contraction pulls the two cartilages toward one another by lifting the anterior arch of the cricoid cartilage toward the thyroid cartilage. The closing of the space between the cricoid arch and

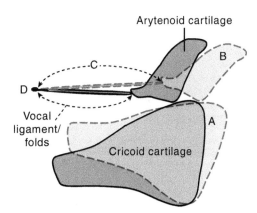

FIGURE 4.18 Effect of cricothyroid muscle contraction on vocal fold length, mass, and tension. *Broken lines* indicate the positions of the cricoid (*A*) and arytenoid (*B*) cartilages and the lengthened, thinned, and tensed vocal folds (*C*) after the contraction of the cricothyroid muscle. *D* is the point of attachment of the vocal folds to the thyroid cartilage.

the front of the thyroid has been likened to the closing of the visor on the helmet of a suit of armor. Figure 4.17 shows the location of one of the cricothyroid muscles on the left side of the larynx. The effect that their contraction has in elevating the front of the cricoid cartilage is to tip the posterior plate of the cricoid backward (Fig. 4.18). The arytenoid cartilages ride on the cricoid cartilage, and the vocal folds, anchored anteriorly to the thyroid cartilage, are therefore stretched, thinned, and made more elastic. The innervation of the cricothyroid muscle is from the superior laryngeal nerve (vagus, or tenth cranial nerve). The cricothyroid is the only intrinsic laryngeal muscle innervated in this way; all the other intrinsic laryngeal muscles are innervated by the recurrent nerve (another branch of the vagus nerve).

The addition of longitudinal tension to the vocal folds increases the $f_0$ at which they vibrate, at least for much of the frequency range used in speech. For extreme frequencies, other mechanisms are thought to be instrumental in pitch control. At high frequencies, such as for falsetto voice, the cricothyroid muscle further increases tension, although no further lengthening is

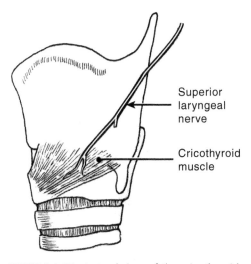

FIGURE 4.17 Lateral view of the cricothyroid muscle, innervated by the superior laryngeal branch of the vagus nerve (cranial nerve X).

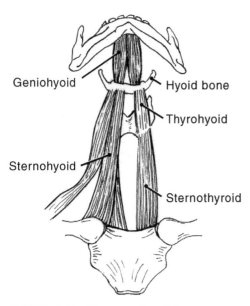

**FIGURE 4.19** Strap muscles of the neck—anterior view from below.

Geniohyoid

Hyoid bone

Thyrohyoid

Sternohyoid

Sternothyroid

possible. The vocal folds are pulled extremely taut and forgo their usual wavelike motion. The vocal ligaments vibrate more like strings.

At extremely low frequencies, the strap muscles of the neck, particularly the *sternohyoid muscle* (Fig. 4.19), participate in lowering the $f_0$. You may have noticed that the larynx rises slightly in the neck for high frequencies or, more noticeably, lowers in the neck for low frequencies. The muscles above the hyoid bone (*suprahyoid muscles*) elevate the larynx; the muscles below the hyoid bone (*infrahyoid muscles*) lower the larynx. Raising the larynx may increase tension in the conus elasticus, a membrane that emerges from the cricoid cartilage and rises to the vocal folds, where its thickened border becomes the vocal ligament. Lowering the larynx presumably decreases the tension on the conus elasticus. Increased tension in the conus elasticus as a result of laryngeal elevation and decreased tension in the case of laryngeal lowering therefore affects the fundamental rate of vibration of the vocal folds.

Tension in the vocal folds can also be increased by contraction of the thyroarytenoid muscles themselves, especially in the fibers of

the vibrating portions known as the "vocalis muscles." The vocalis muscles (the medial fibers of the thyroarytenoid) are antagonistic to the cricothyroid muscles, because they shorten rather than lengthen the folds, but both sets of muscles can increase tension in the folds to raise $f_0$. It is possible that the vocalis muscles tune the vocal folds to make the cricothyroid lengthening more effective.

It seems, then, that $f_0$ is primarily affected by applying more or less longitudinal tension to the vocal folds via the cricothyroid muscles. Secondary effects result from (1) applying more or less vertical tension to the folds by elevating or depressing the larynx using the strap muscles of the neck and (2) varying subglottal pressure (see the following paragraphs).

## Relation Between Frequency and Intensity

We have seen that by increasing the subglottal air pressure while keeping other factors

LOWER FREQUENCY, LOWER INTENSITY

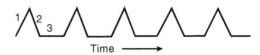

Time

HIGHER INTENSITY, HIGHER FREQUENCY

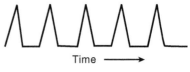

Time

Increased P$_s$

**FIGURE 4.20** Schematic diagram of the movement of the vocal folds during phonation. At high subglottal pressure ($P_s$, *bottom*), the folds remain closed for a greater proportion of the vibratory cycle (30% to 50%) and close more rapidly. Frequency tends to increase along with intensity. Compare with lower subglottal pressure (*top*): *1*, abducting; *2*, adducting; *3*, adducted. Folds remain open for 50% to 75% of the cycle and close slowly.

constant, we can increase vocal intensity. However, if subglottal pressure is increased without muscular adjustments of the vocal folds, the $f_o$ as well as the intensity increases. If someone is phonating a steady tone and is (gently) punched in the stomach, the tone not only gets louder but also increases in pitch. The pitch rise may occur because of reflexive tensing of the vocal folds or because the increased subglottal air pressure causes the vocal folds to adduct more quickly as a result of the heightened Bernoulli effect. In contrast, when one is speaking at the end of a breath, the $f_o$ drops naturally along with the intensity by about 2 to 7 Hz. A singer or a speaker can, however, reverse this affinity. A singer who wants to increase intensity but maintain the $f_o$ must lower the resistance to the airflow at the vocal folds, ei-

ther by relaxing the cricothyroid muscle a bit or by decreasing the internal vocal fold tension by relaxing the thyroarytenoid muscle. Similarly, when asking "Are you sure?" to signal the question with a rising $f_o$, the speaker must work against the natural fall in frequency at the end of a breath group by increasing cricothyroid activity, stretching the folds, and at the same time increasing internal intercostal muscle activity to give added stress to the word "sure."

Increased vocal intensity results from greater resistance by the vocal folds to the increased airflow. The vocal folds are blown further apart, releasing a larger puff of air that sets up a sound pressure wave of greater amplitude. The vocal folds not only move farther apart for each vibratory cycle of increased intensity but also stay adducted for

**TABLE 4.1** Summary of Events During Phonation

| Peripheral Nerves | Muscles | Movements | Air Pressure | Air Movement |
|---|---|---|---|---|
| Cranial nerve X (vagus): recurrent branch | PCA | Open vocal folds before thorax enlargement | | → Air enters via larynx to lungs |
| | → IA → | Adduction of vocal folds | | |
| | → LCA → | Medial compression of vocal folds | $P_s$ builds | |
| | → Voc. → | Intrinsic tension | Pressure drops across glottis, $P_s > P_{supra}$ | |
| Cranial nerve X (vagus): external branch of superior laryngeal nerve | → CT → | Longitudinal tension | Resistance offered to $P_s$ by vocal fold tension | |
| | | Vocal folds → blown open | Subglottal air pressure overcomes vocal fold resistance | → Released puff of air |
| | | Folds sucked ← together | Negative pressure vs. lateral edges of folds as velocity of air increases (Bernoulli effect) | → Airstream cut off |
| | | Vocal folds part ← | $P_s$ builds again | → Another puff of air released |

PCA, posterior cricoarytenoid muscle; IA, interarytenoid muscle; LCA, lateral cricoarytenoid muscle; Voc. vocalis muscle; CT, cricothyroid muscle; $P_s$, subglottal pressure; $P_{supra}$, supraglottal pressure.

a larger part of each cycle. In Figure 4.20 the changes in the vocal fold movement are schematized and presented with the resulting change in waveform.

Table 4.1 summarizes the chain of events in vocal fold vibration from neural impulses to the resulting change in air pressure and airflow. Arrows pointing to the right indicate muscular adjustments, whereas arrows pointing to the left indicate aerodynamic forces.

## Toward Speech Sounds

Thus far, we have described the processes of respiration and phonation. We have seen that phonation is a dynamic process, varying as it does during running speech in intensity, frequency, and quality. Phonation must be coordinated with respiration. The motor commands to the larynx must be appropriately related to those of the respiratory system. For instance, to take a breath for speech, the glottis must open quickly before the thorax expands, and when the vocal folds adduct for phonation, the action must be simultaneous with expiration. But the output of the phonatory system does not, by itself, produce the rapidly varying acoustic stream that carries the phonetic segments of speech. To understand the production of speech sounds fully, we must extend our discussion beyond the sources of sound (respiration and phonation) to include the filtering action of the vocal tract above the larynx.

## REFERENCES AND SUGGESTED READING

### General Works on Speech and Voice Production

Baken, R. J., An Overview of Laryngeal Function for Voice Production. In *Vocal Health and Pedagogy*. R. T. Sataloff, (Ed.). San Diego: Singular Press, 1998, pp. 27–45.

Berhrman, A., *Speech and Voice Science*. San Diego: Plural Publishing, 2007.

Daniloff, R., Schuckers, G., and Feth, L., *The Physiology of Speech and Hearing*. Englewood Cliffs, NJ: Prentice-Hall Inc., 1980.

Dickson, D. R., and Maue-Dickson, W., *Anatomical and Physiological Bases of Speech*. Boston: Little, Brown and Co., 1982.

Ferrand, C. T., *Speech Science,* 2nd ed. Boston: Allyn and Bacon, 2007.

Fujimura, O., Body-Cover Theory of the Vocal Fold and Its Phonetic Implications. In *Vocal Fold Physiology*. K. Stevens and M. Hirano, (Eds.). Tokyo: University of Tokyo Press, 1981, pp. 271–281.

Hixon, T. J., Weismer, G, and Hoit, J. D., *Preclinical Speech Science*. San Diego: Plural Publishing, 2008.

Kahane, D. R., and Folkins, J. F., *Atlas of Speech and Hearing Anatomy*. Columbus, OH: Charles E. Merrill, 1984.

Kent, R. D., Atal, B. S., and Miller, J. L., (Eds.), *Papers in Speech Communication: Speech Production*. Woodbury, NY: Acoustical Society of America, 1991.

Lieberman, P., and Blumstein, S. E., *Speech Physiology, Speech Perception, and Acoustic Phonetics: An Introduction*. New York: Cambridge University Press, 1988.

Ludlow, C. L., Central Nervous System Control of the Laryngeal Muscles in Humans. *Respir. Physiol. Neurobiol. 147,* 2005, 205–222.

Perkell, J. S., *Physiology of Speech Production: Results and Implications of a Quantitative Cineradiographic Study*. Cambridge, MA: MIT Press, 1969.

Titze, I., *Principles of Voice Production*. Englewood Cliffs, NJ: Prentice-Hall, 1994.

Zemlin, W. R., *Speech and Hearing Science: Anatomy and Physiology,* 4th ed. Boston: Allyn & Bacon, 1998.

### Phonation

Atkinson, J. E., Correlation Analysis of the Physiological Factors Controlling Fundamental Voice Frequency. *J. Acoust. Soc. Am. 63,* 1978, 211–222.

Faaborg-Andersen, K., Electromyographic Investigation of Intrinsic Laryngeal Muscles in Humans. *Acta. Physiol. Scand. 41,* Suppl. 140, 1957, 1–148.

Faaborg-Andersen, K., Yanagihara, N., and von Leden, H., Vocal Pitch and Intensity

Regulation: A Comparative Study of Electrical Activity in the Cricothyroid Muscle and the Airflow Rate. *Arch. Otolaryngol. 85,* 1967, 448–454.

Gay, T., Hirose, H., Strome, M., and Sawashima, M., Electromyography of the Intrinsic Laryngeal Muscles During Phonation. *Ann. Otol. Rhinol. Laryngol. 81,* 1972, 401–409.

Hirano, M., and Kakita, Y., Cover-Body Theory of Vocal Fold Vibration. In *Speech Science.* R. G. Daniloff, (Ed.). San Diego, CA: College-Hill Press, 1985, pp. 1–46.

Hirose, H., and Gay, T., The Activity of the Intrinsic Laryngeal Muscles in Voicing Control. *Phonetica 25,* 1972, 140–164.

Honda, K., Laryngeal and Extra-Laryngeal Mechanism of $F_0$ Control. In *Producing Speech: Contemporary Issues.* F. Bell-Berti and L. J. Raphael, (Eds.). New York: American Institute of Physics, 1995, pp. 215–245.

Hunter, E. J., Titze, I. R., and Alipour, F., A Three-Dimensional Model of Vocal Fold Abduction/Adduction. *J. Acoust. Soc. Amer. 115,* 2004, 1747–1759.

Husson, R., *Étude des Phénomenes Physiologiques et Acoustiques Fondamentaux de la Voix Chantée* [Thesis]. University of Paris, 1950.

Ishizaka, K., and Flanagan, J. L., Synthesis of Voiced Sounds from a Two-Mass Model of the Vocal Cords. *Bell Syst. Tech. J. 51,* 1972, 1233–1268. Reprinted in Kent et al., 1991 (q.v.), 183–218.

Ludlow, C. L., and Hart, M. O. (Eds.), Proceedings of the Conference on the Assessment of Vocal Pathology, *ASHA Reports, 11,* 1981.

Müller, J., *The Physiology of the Senses, Voice, and Muscular Motion with the Mental Faculties* (Translated by W. Baly). London: Walton & Maberly, 1848.

Plant, R., and Hillel, A., Direct Measurement of Onset and Offset Phonation Threshold Pressure in Normal Subjects. *J. Acoust. Soc. Amer. 116,* 2004, 3640–3646.

Sawashima, M., and Hirose, H., Laryngeal Gestures in Speech Production. In *The Production of Speech.* P. MacNeilage, (Ed.). New York: Springer-Verlag, 1983, pp. 11–38.

Titze, I. R., On the Mechanics of Vocal-Fold Vibration. *J. Acoust. Soc. Am. 60,* 1976, 1366–1380.

Titze, I. R., On the relation between subglottal pressure and fundamental frequency in phonation. *J. Acoust. Soc. Amer. 85,* 1989, 901–906.

Titze, I. R., Jiang, J., and Drucker, D., Preliminaries to the Body-Cover Theory of Pitch Control. *J. Voice. 1,* 1988, 314–319.

van den Berg, I., Myoelastic-Aerodynamic Theory of Voice Production. *J. Speech Hear. Res. 1,* 1958, 227–244.

Von Helmholtz, H., *Die Lehre der Tonempfindungen als physiologische Grundlage für die Theorie der Musik.* Braunschweig, Germany: F. Vieweg & Sohn, 1863.

# The Articulation and Acoustics of Vowels

# 5

*Take care of the sense, and the sounds will take care of themselves.*
–The Duchess, *Alice's Adventures in Wonderland*, Chapter 9, by Lewis Carroll
(Charles Ludwidge Dodgson)

In the last chapter, we saw that the exhaled airstream can be used to provide two types of sound source. It can be segmented into separate puffs by the vibrating vocal folds to provide the periodic sound of phonation or it can pass through the open glottis to provide energy for the production of aperiodic sound above the larynx. In either case, whether the source is at the glottis or in the mouth, the sound is filtered by the resonant frequencies of the vocal tract. Those resonant frequencies are determined by the sizes and shapes of the various spaces in the vocal tract; those sizes and shapes, in turn, are determined by the movements and positions of the articulators, including the tongue, soft, palate, lips, and jaw. In this context, resonance refers to the acoustic response of air molecules within the oral, nasal, and pharyngeal cavities to some source of sound that will set them into vibration.

We will see that the movements of the articulators are necessary both for producing sound sources in the vocal tract itself and for altering the acoustic resonance characteristics of the vocal tract according to the various requirements for different speech sounds. Although this chapter is concerned mainly with vowels, you will notice that consonants are occasionally mentioned below. This is because the principles of resonance and articulation that are discussed here are also relevant to consonant sounds that are the subject of the following chapter.

## THE VOCAL TRACT: VARIABLE RESONATOR AND SOUND SOURCE

### Resonating Cavities

The resonating cavities of the vocal tract include all of the air passages above the larynx

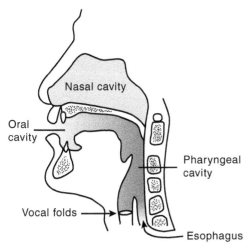

**FIGURE 5.1** A section of the head showing the major cavities of the vocal tract.

from the glottis to the lips (Fig. 5.1). The large resonating cavities are the pharyngeal cavity, the oral cavity, and—when the velum is lowered, opening the velopharyngeal port—the nasal cavity. The air spaces between the lips, between the teeth and the cheeks (buccal cavities), and within the larynx and the trachea are smaller resonators within the vocal tract. As we saw in Chapter 2, an air-filled tube resonates at certain frequencies depending on (1) whether it is open at one or both ends, (2) its length, (3) its shape, and (4) the size of its openings.

Musical instruments have resonators to amplify and filter sound. Stringed instruments are designed with resonating chambers graded in size to impart specific qualities to the sounds they produce. The large resonating chamber of the double bass emphasizes the low frequencies of a complex sound, whereas the smaller resonating chamber of a violin emphasizes the high frequencies. The size and shape of the resonating chamber of a stringed instrument usually cannot be changed. In contrast, the shapes and sizes of the human vocal resonators can be varied by moving and positioning the articulators. For example, tongue elevation enlarges the area of the pharyngeal resonating cavity, whereas tongue fronting decreases the area of the front (oral) resonating cavity. Conversely, tongue depression reduces the area of the pharyngeal resonating cavity, and tongue retraction enlarges the area of the front (oral) resonating cavity. Lip protrusion lengthens both the oral resonating cavity and the entire vocal tract; larynx lowering lengthens both the pharyngeal cavity and the entire vocal tract.

In general, the larger a vocal tract is, or the larger a particular resonating cavity is, the lower the frequencies to which it will respond; the smaller a vocal tract or a resonating cavity is, the higher the frequencies to which it will respond. The resonating cavities we have described here (and the vocal tract as a whole) serve as variable resonators for both vowels and consonants. Our concern in this chapter is to describe how the vocal tract and the resonating cavities it comprises function to produce vowel sounds.

## Sound Sources for Vowels

English vowels are classified as phonated or voiced sounds. This is because the sound source for vowels is almost always the vibrations of the vocal folds. Whispered (unphonated) speech is the exception, not the rule. For most of the speech we produce and hear, phonation supplies the acoustic input to the resonating cavities that modify the glottal waveform in various ways to produce individual vowels.

It is important, however, to note that although vowels may be *classified* as voiced sounds, an aperiodic source, such as that produced while whispering, will resonate in much the same way in the vocal tract as the periodic source supplied by phonation. Bringing the vocal folds close enough to make the airstream passing between them become turbulent (but not close enough to set the folds into vibration) will generate the aperiodicity that characterizes a whisper. Thus, it is possible to produce any given vowel, /i/ for instance, either in a phonated or a whispered version.

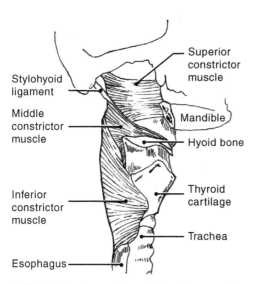

**FIGURE 5.2** Lateral view of the pharyngeal constrictor muscles.

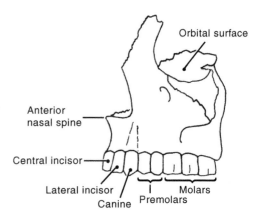

**FIGURE 5.3** The maxilla, with teeth indicated.

## LANDMARKS OF THE VOCAL TRACT

### Pharynx

The posterior part of the vocal tract is formed by a tube of muscles known as the pharynx. The muscles are divided into three groups according to their position (Fig. 5.2). The inferior constrictor muscles are at the level of the larynx; the middle constrictor muscles start high in the back and course down to the level of the hyoid bone, and the superior constrictor muscles form the back of the pharynx from the level of the palate to the mandible. Contraction of the constrictor muscles narrows the pharyngeal cavity, and relaxation of the muscles widens it. The nasal, oral, and laryngeal cavities open into the pharyngeal cavity. The parts of the pharynx adjacent to each cavity are called the nasopharynx, oropharynx, and laryngopharynx, respectively.

### Oral Cavity

The oral cavity is bounded in front and along the sides by the teeth set into the upper jaw, or *maxilla* (Fig. 5.3), and the lower jaw, or *mandible* (Fig. 5.4). The most important teeth

for speech are the *incisors*, the flat-edged biting teeth in the front of the mouth. There are two central and two lateral incisors in each jaw. The tip of the tongue is braced behind the lower incisors during the production of many vowels, especially those produced in the front of the oral cavity, such as /i/ and /e/. The incisors are also used, in conjunction with the lower lip and the tongue, to create constrictions for many consonant sounds, such as /f/, /θ/, and /s/. The roof of the oral cavity consists of the *hard palate* (Fig. 5.5) and the soft palate, or *velum*. The anterior two thirds of the hard palate is formed by the palatine process of the maxilla, and the other third is formed by part of the palatine bone. An important landmark on the hard palate is the superior *alveolar ridge*. With the tip of your tongue, you can feel the rough surface of the alveolar ridge protruding behind the upper teeth. More English speech

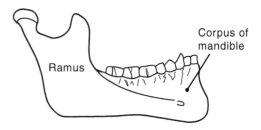

**FIGURE 5.4** The mandible. Two major sections are the ramus and corpus of the mandible.

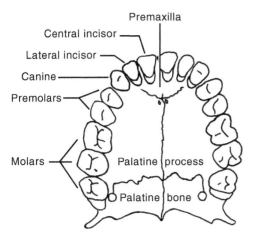

Premaxilla
Central incisor
Lateral incisor
Canine
Premolars
Molars
Palatine process
Palatine bone

**FIGURE 5.5**  The hard palate, consisting of the premaxilla and palatine processes of the maxillary bone and the palatine bone. The bones are fused along the lines indicated. The irregular ridges along the anterior portion of the premaxilla, called rugae, are the locus of maximum constriction for many speech sounds.

sounds are articulated at or near the alveolar ridge than at any other place of articulation. The major point of constriction for many vowels is formed by arching the tongue high in the oral cavity slightly posterior to the alveolar ridge. Alveolar consonant sounds, for which the constriction of the vocal tract involves contact between some portion of the tongue and the alveolar ridge, include /t,d,n,s,z,r,l/. The area just behind the alveolar ridge (the *alveolar-palatal* or *postalveolar* area) is the place of articulation for the affricate sounds /ʧ/ and /ʤ/.

## Velum

The greater part of the velum, or soft palate, consists of a broad muscle that enters it laterally from the temporal bones behind and above on each side. This muscle, the *levator palatini* muscle, is appropriately named, because its function is to elevate or lower the soft palate, thus closing the entrance to the nasal cavities above (see Fig. 6.3.) The levator palatini muscle has often been likened to a sling running beneath the velum. Contraction of the levator palatini muscle can cause

the soft palate to move up and back until it makes contact with the posterior wall of the pharynx. This action (*velopharyngeal closure*) occurs to some degree for all of the vowel sounds in English, and for all consonants except for the three nasal sounds /m/, /n/, and /ŋ/, which require nasal resonance. For these nasal sounds, the velopharyngeal port is opened by relaxation of the levator palatini muscles. The most posterior portion of the velum is the uvula, a fleshy appendage that hangs down into the pharynx. You can see your uvula in a mirror if you open your mouth and depress your tongue while saying /ɑ/.

## The Tongue: Extrinsic Musculature

The floor of the oral cavity is largely formed by the muscle mass of the tongue. The bulk of the tongue can be moved in three directions: up and back, down and back, and up and forward. These movements within the oral cavity and the pharynx are caused by contraction of the extrinsic muscles of the tongue, which have attachments to structures outside of the tongue itself (Fig. 5.6).

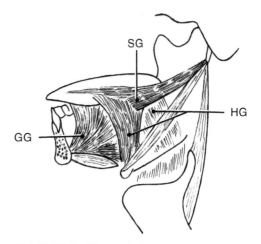

SG
HG
GG

**FIGURE 5.6**  The extrinsic tongue musculature in lateral view. The styloglossus muscle (SG) elevates and backs the tongue, the hyoglossus muscle (HG) depresses the tongue, and the genioglossus muscle (GG) fronts and elevates the tongue.

The *styloglossus* muscle is attached to the styloid process of each temporal bone. The muscle fibers run down and forward, inserting into the sides of the tongue. Contraction of the styloglossus muscle pulls the tongue back and up. This movement is important for the production of vowel sounds such as /u/ as in "Sue."

The *hyoglossus* muscle is attached to the hyoid bone. Its fibers run in a thin sheet up into the lateral base of the tongue. Hyoglossus contraction results in tongue depression and backing. The sounds /ɑ/ and /a/ have low tongue positions that are achieved in part because of the contraction of the hyoglossus muscle.

The *genioglossus* muscle is attached to the inside of the mandible at the superior mental spine. The muscle fibers radiate up and back to insert throughout the length of the tongue, down to and including the hyoid bone. Contraction of the genioglossus muscle draws the hyoid bone and the tongue root forward and results in a forward and upward movement of the tongue body that is important for the articulation of vowels such as /i/ and /e/.

The fourth and the last of the extrinsic muscles of the tongue, the *palatoglossus* muscle, is described below (Chapter 6) in the discussion of the velopharyngeal mechanism.

## The Tongue: Intrinsic Musculature

Unlike the extrinsic tongue muscles, with their attachments to external structures, the intrinsic tongue muscles are contained entirely within the tongue body. Whereas the extrinsic muscles determine the gross position of the tongue body, the intrinsic muscles of the tongue determine the shape of its surface (Fig. 5.7).

The *superior longitudinal* muscle consists of many muscle fibers coursing from the back of the tongue to the tip, just below the superior surface of the tongue. Contraction of the superior longitudinal muscle curls the tongue tip up, as in the articulation of the vowel /ɝ/ and some allophones of the consonants /l/ and /r/.

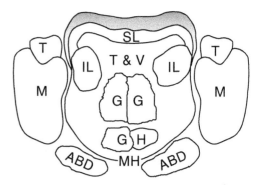

**FIGURE 5.7**   The tongue in frontal section. Intrinsic muscles are indicated by * in the following list. *SL, superior longitudinal muscles; *T and V, transverse and vertical muscles; *IL, inferior longitudinal muscles; GG, genioglossus muscles; GH, geniohyoid muscles; MH, mylohyoid muscles; ABD, anterior belly of the digastric muscles; T, teeth; M, mandible.

The *inferior longitudinal* muscles, also running from the root to the tip of the tongue, along the underside of the tongue, act to depress the tongue tip, as in the articulation of the vowel /i/.

The major portion of the tongue mass lies between the superior and inferior longitudinal muscles. Muscle fibers coursing from top to bottom of the mass (*vertical muscles*) interweave with muscle fibers coursing from the middle of the tongue out to the sides (*transverse muscles*). Together the intrinsic muscles shape the tongue, especially its tip, into a variety of configurations, many of which contribute to vowel production.

## The Lips

Many facial muscles intermingle with the fibers of the major lip muscle, the orbicularis oris, which encircles the lips (Fig. 5.8). Contraction of the orbicularis oris is necessary to round and protrude the lips for the production of such vowels as /u/ and /o/. Orbicularis oris contraction is also needed for the complete labial closure of consonant sounds such as /p/, /b/, and /m/.

Other facial muscles, such as the *risorius* (Fig. 5.8), may be active in adjusting the

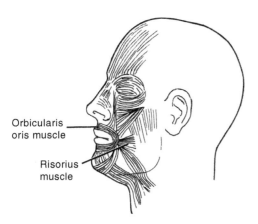

**FIGURE 5.8** The facial muscles, indicating the position of the orbicularis oris and the risorius muscles.

corners of the mouth to aid in the sort of lip spreading that many speakers use when articulating vowels such as /i/ in "we." The fibers of the facial muscles vary considerably in the way they are distributed from one individual to another.

## ACOUSTIC THEORY OF VOWEL PRODUCTION

The acoustic theory of vowel production is the product of research carried out over a considerable period in many countries. From the 1940s to the 1960s, researchers in Japan, Sweden, and the United States gave the theory the basic form it has today. Gunnar Fant's *Acoustic Theory of Speech Production,* published in 1960, related a source–filter account of vowel production to the resonances shown on sound spectrograms. Fant used a model, developed by Stevens and House, that varied three parameters (the location of the main tongue constriction, the amount of lip protrusion, and vocal tract cross-sectional area) to predict the frequencies of vocal tract resonances.

### Resonance of a Tube Open at One End

During vowel production, the vocal tract approximates a tube of uniform diameter open at one end (the lips) and closed at the other (the glottis, during vocal fold adduction).

The lowest natural frequency at which such a tube resonates will have a wavelength ($\lambda$) four times the length of the tube. The wavelength of a tube that is 17 cm long (the length of an average adult male's vocal tract) will thus be $4 \times 17$ cm, or 68 cm. The lowest resonant frequency at which the air within such a tube naturally vibrates equals the velocity of sound in air divided by the wavelength ($f$ = velocity divided by wavelength). Because the velocity of sound is 34,400 cm/s, the formula for the lowest resonant frequency ($R_1$) of a 17-cm tube open at one end is

$$R_1 = c/\lambda = 34{,}400 \text{ cm per sec}/68 \text{ cm}$$
$$= 506 \text{ Hz}$$

where $c$ is a constant, because in a given medium and at a given temperature, sound travels at a constant velocity. Therefore, the lowest resonant frequency of such a tube is approximately 500 Hz.

The tube also resonates at odd multiples of that frequency. Why odd multiples? Because the even multiples are not effective resonant frequencies. Figure 5.9 illustrates both the compatibility of the odd multiples and the incompatibility of the even multiples with the 500-Hz resonance of the tube. The combination of $R_1$ (500 Hz) with its even multiples ($R_2$, 1,000 Hz; $R_4$, 2,000 Hz; $R_6$, 3,000 Hz) results in opposing, neutralizing forces at the zero crossing, the point where the waveforms of $R_1$ and its even-numbered multiples cross the $x$-axis. In contrast, when $R_1$ is combined with each of its odd multiples ($R_3$, 1,500 Hz; $R_5$, 2,500 Hz), both waves are moving in the same direction at the zero crossing and so reinforce each other.

### Resonance of Male Vocal Tract

Tubes, then, when energized, resonate naturally at certain frequencies that depend on the length and configuration of the tube. A human vocal tract is similar to the sort of acoustic resonator we have been describing. There are, of course, some differences:

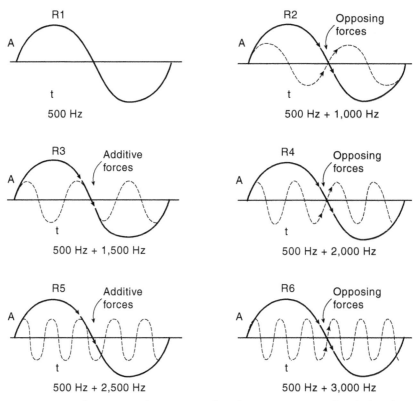

**FIGURE 5.9** The resonant frequencies of a tube open at one end and closed at the other. The even harmonics are not effective resonant frequencies because they are canceled at the entrance to the tube (opposing forces), whereas the odd harmonics are compatible (additive forces).

Unlike the rigid tube, the vocal tract has soft, absorbent walls. Furthermore, unlike the tube, its cross-sectional area is not uniform; it varies from one location to another along its length. Finally, the vocal tract contains a bend of approximately 90° where the oral cavity meets the pharynx. Nonetheless, the similarity between the rigid, straight tube and the soft-walled tube with its right-angle bend and variable cross-sectional area is close enough for our discussion.

Chiba and Kajiyama (1941) illustrated the resonances of a tube open at one end and closed at the other, and they related these resonances to those occurring in a vocal tract that is fairly uniform in cross section (Fig. 5.10).

Resonance occurs in such a tube when the velocity of the air molecules at the open end is at a maximum. Accordingly, the tube in Figure 5.10 contains a plot of air molecule velocity. The first (lowest frequency) resonance $(R_1)$ of such a tube or tract is shown at the top of the figure. It is a frequency whose wavelength is four times the length of the tube, and we can see that when one fourth of the wave is within the tube, the velocity of air molecules will reach a maximum at the open end of the tube, or in the case of the human resonator, at the lips. At the closed end of the tube (equivalent to the glottis in a vocal tract), the velocity is at a minimum but the pressure is high. This is because the molecules are crowded together, with little room to move because of the "dead end" formed by the closed end of the tube by the vocal folds. The second frequency at which resonance occurs, shown in the middle of Figure 5.10

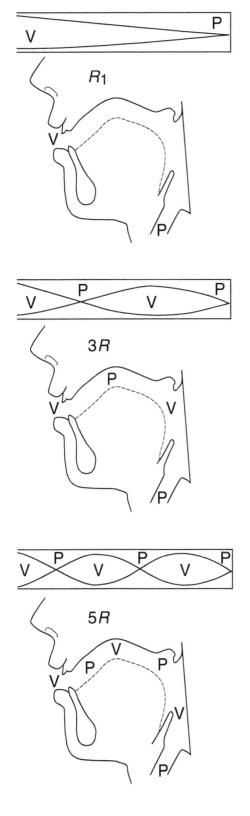

$(3R)$, is three times the lowest resonant frequency, because when three fourths of the wave is in the tube, the velocity of the air molecule again reaches a maximum at the lips. For $3R$ there are two points of maximum velocity and two points of maximum pressure within the vocal tract. The third resonance $(5R)$, shown at the bottom of the figure, is a frequency with a wavelength shorter than the tube or vocal tract. It is five times the lowest resonance, so five fourths of the wave fits into the length of the tube. The velocity is maximum at three places, again including the lips (the open end of the tube), and there are three locations of maximum pressure in the oral cavity.

The points of maximum velocity and pressure are important because resonances change in frequency when the vocal tract is constricted near a point of maximum velocity or maximum pressure. Remember that points of maximum pressure correspond to points of minimum velocity and vice versa. Figure 5.11, a plot of variation in pressure (as opposed to the plot of velocity in Fig. 5.10), illustrates the inverse relationship between pressure and velocity. In general, constrictions at points of maximum velocity lower resonant frequency, and constrictions at points of maximum pressure raise the resonant frequency.

Vocal tract resonances $(R_1, R_2, R_3, \ldots)$ are called *formants*. The lowest resonant frequency, or first formant $(F_1 = R_1)$, is most responsive to changes in mouth opening. Speech sounds requiring small mouth openings have low-frequency first formants. Conversely, open-mouth sounds are characterized by relatively high-frequency first formants. (The first formant at its highest frequency value is still the lowest resonance

**FIGURE 5.10** The resonances of the vocal tract. V, points of maximum velocity; P, points of maximum pressure; R, resonances. (Adapted with permission from Chiba, T., and Kajiyama, M., *The Vowel: Its Nature and Structure.* Tokyo: Kaiseikan, 1941.)

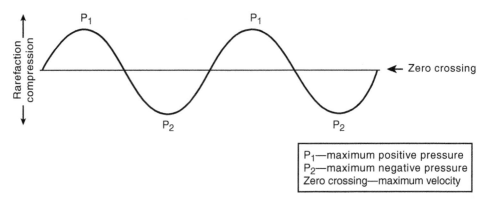

P₁—maximum positive pressure
P₂—maximum negative pressure
Zero crossing—maximum velocity

**FIGURE 5.11**  The inverse relationship between pressure and velocity for a sine wave. Pressure is greatest at points $P_1$ and $P_2$ for positive and negative values. Velocity is greatest at zero crossings and at a minimum at $P_1$ and $P_2$.

of the tract.) The second formant ($F_2 = R_3$) is most responsive to changes in the size of the oral cavity. Tongue backing or lip rounding may lower the frequency of this formant, as these constrictions occur in areas of high velocity, but any tongue or jaw activity that narrows the region in the oral cavity where the pressure is relatively high causes an increase in the frequency of $F_2$. The third formant ($F_3 = 5R$) is responsive to front versus back constriction.

## SOURCE AND FILTER

Let us return to our consideration of an unconstricted vocal tract. Imagine a sound produced at the vocal folds passing through the air-filled cavities of a tract that resonates at frequencies of 500, 1,500, and 2,500 Hz, about the same resonant frequencies as the 17-cm tube discussed in the previous section. To understand the basis for this output, it is useful to view the speech production mechanism as a combination of a source (e.g., vocal fold vibrations) and a filter (resonant responses of the supraglottal vocal tract—the resonating cavities above the larynx).

Figure 5.12 contrasts the waveforms of a vowel sound at its source and at the lips. The source waveform could be recorded directly by suspending a miniature microphone just above the vocal folds as the speaker phonated while producing the vowel. At first glance, it looks as if the vowel has more high-frequency energy than the waveform of its glottal source. The exact nature of the changes undergone in transfer can better be appreciated by contrasting the Fourier spectra. A Fourier analysis (see Chapter 2) is an analysis of a complex wave into its component frequencies.

The spectrum of the sound source (the sound produced at the vocal folds) can be seen to consist of a fundamental frequency ($f_0$; corresponding to the frequency of vocal fold vibration) and many multiples, or harmonics, of the fundamental frequency (Fig. 5.13). These harmonics tend to diminish in intensity as they increase in frequency. If we could hear it, the sound of phonation would resemble a buzz, not a speech sound. The middle spectrum is a plot of the resonant

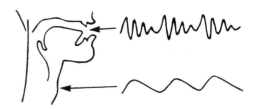

**FIGURE 5.12**  A sound wave at the lips and at the glottis. The waveform changes during passage through the vocal tract. The tract has acted as a filter.

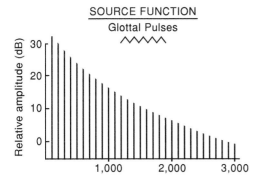

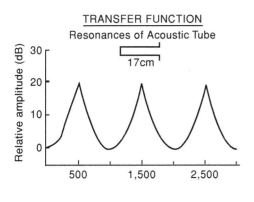

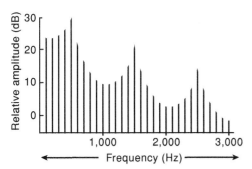

**FIGURE 5.13** *Top*: The spectrum of the glottal source. *Bottom*: The spectrum of the source after filtering by a transfer function corresponding to a neutral vocal tract, with a radiation effect added. *Center*: The transfer function.

frequencies of a neutrally shaped vocal tract, computed, as we have seen above, to be approximately 500, 1,500, and 2,500 Hz. These are the frequencies at which the air in a tract of that shape and length would vibrate maximally in response to another complex sound. When the sound source represented by the first spectrum is transmitted through the filter of a vocal tract that resonates at the frequencies indicated in the second spectrum, the resulting sound is a product of the two. Specifically, the glottal source with its many harmonics (the *source function*) is filtered according to the frequency response of the vocal tract filter (the *transfer function*). The harmonics of the glottal sound wave that are at or near the spectral peaks of the transfer function of the vocal tract are resonated, and those distant from the resonant frequencies of the tract lose energy and are thus greatly attenuated. The sound that emerges at the end of the tract (the lips) has the same harmonics as the sound at the source (the glottis), but the amplitudes of the harmonics have been modified, altering the quality of the sound.

The frequencies mentioned above, 500, 1,500, and 2,500 Hz, are appropriate only for a neutrally shaped average male vocal tract and are not the resonant frequencies for a vocal tract that is longer, shorter, or different in configuration (i.e., not neutrally shaped). A speaker can move lips, tongue, and jaw, creating many vocal tract sizes and shapes. Any change of vocal tract configuration alters the frequencies at which the cavities resonate. Unlike the neutral tubelike configuration of the vocal tract when a speaker says "uh" [ʌ] or the [ə] in the second syllable of "sofa," most of the vocal tract shapes assumed for speech sounds are much more constricted in certain parts of the tube than in other parts. This alters the cavity sizes, so they resonate to frequencies that are different from those of the neutrally shaped vocal tract. The odd multiples of the lowest resonance that occurred for the tubular tract of uniform shape are lowered or raised in frequency because of the locations of the constrictions and changes in the volumes of the cavities. The resonant frequencies thus no longer display the simple 1:3:5 ratio.

The vocal tract is thus a variable resonator, and as its shape changes because of changes in articulator placement, the formants change in frequency, producing a variety of sounds. A convincing demonstration of the effect of the vocal tract as a variable resonator is to phonate at a constant pitch while articulating a continuous sequence of vowels. The sound source produced by the vocal folds remains constant; the only changes are in the shapes of the resonator caused by the changing articulation. Simply by changing the vocal tract shape, you can make all of the vowel sounds. This is true, as we have mentioned above, even if you whisper, that is, use an aperiodic sound source. The filter of the system, the vocal tract, will resonate in much the same way it does when the source 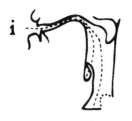 is periodic (phonated), and so the equivalent vowels are produced.

can assume a fixed vocal tract shape and produce the same vowel repeatedly with widely different fundamental frequencies and harmonics. Singing the vowel [i] up the scale, you are conscious of maintaining the appropriate vocal tract shape for [i] for each note, although the fundamental frequency of the sound source is changing, causing the spacing between the harmonics to change also (see Figs. 4.15 and 5.17). Despite these differences, the resonances of the vocal tract  remain virtually the same.

Analogously, as we have seen above, if the source ($f_o$) remains constant, the shape of the vocal tract can independently change, causing a change in the resonant frequencies and, thus, in the vowel that is produced.

### Vowels: /i/, /ɑ/, and /u/

To better understand the production of the vowels we hear, let us consider the sounds /i/, /ɑ/, and /u/. These vowels represent extremes in articulation and thus in the shaping of the vocal tract that filters the glottal source of sound (amplifying some harmonics and attenuating others) to produce different vowel sounds. That is, any vowel sound that emerges from the lips is a product of vocal fold vibration (the source function) and the resonances of a particular vocal tract shape and length (the filter or transfer function) plus an effect of sound radiation at the lips. The source function and the filter are largely independent of each other. For example, you

### High Front Unrounded Vowel

The sound /i/ in "see" is distinctive because of the high-frequency energy from the resonances in the oral cavity. To resonate at such high frequencies, the oral cavity must be made small. That is why the speaker fronts the tongue toward the alveolar ridge. A tracing from a radiograph (Fig. 5.14) of the vocal tract of a speaker saying [i] shows that the tongue mass fills most of the oral cavity, leaving a small volume of air to vibrate in the space anterior to the constriction formed by the tongue. The pharynx, in contrast, enlarges because the posterior part of the tongue has been raised, that is, lifted out of the pharyngeal space.

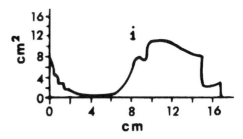

**FIGURE 5.14**  *Left*: Lateral view of the tongue for the vowel [i]. *Right*: The cross section of the vocal tract for [i]. The abscissa indicates distance from the lips. (Adapted with permission from Fant, G., *Acoustic Theory of Speech Production*. The Hague, The Netherlands: Mouton, 1970.)

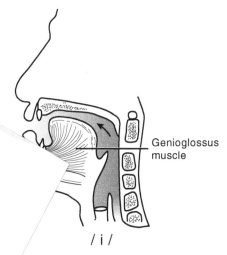

/ i /

**FIGURE 5.15**  The genioglossus muscle pulls the tongue up and forward for the vowel [i].

The right side of Figure 5.14 shows Fant's measurements of the cross-sectional area in square centimeters at various distances from the lips. These calculations were made by using lateral radiographic measures to estimate three-dimensional cross sections of the vocal tract. The vocal tract is narrowly constricted at 4 and 6 cm back from the lips and widens considerably at 10 and 12 cm back from the lips. The muscle that is the primary agent for this adjustment of tongue fronting and elevation is the genioglossus muscle (Fig. 5.15), innervated by the hy-

poglossal (twelfth cranial) nerve. Because the tongue is high and fronted and there is no lip protrusion, /i/ is classified as a high front unrounded vowel.

The left side of Figure 5.16 shows a possible output spectrum for the articulation of /i/. Note that the fundamental frequency of the source is 150 Hz. The transfer function of the vocal tract configuration for /i/ is superimposed on the spectrum. If we had used this transfer function with a sound source having an $f_0$ of 300 Hz, the harmonic structure of the vowel would be different: the harmonics of an $f_0$ of 300 Hz are spaced more widely than those of an $f_0$ of 150 Hz. But because the articulation and therefore the transfer function remain the same, the resonant (formant) frequencies would remain unchanged. Figure 5.17 demonstrates this principle for three sources with fundamental frequencies of 100, 150, and 200 Hz. When each source serves as the input to a vocal tract that is shaped to produce the vowel /i/, the output spectra have peaks of resonance at the same frequencies. A different speaker, of course, with a different-size vocal tract and slightly different articulatory habits, would produce different formant frequencies, but the pattern of one very low formant ($F_1$) and two relatively high formants ($F_2$, $F_3$) would remain the same as long as the articulation conforms

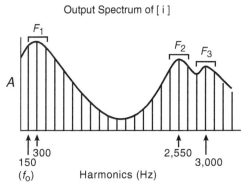

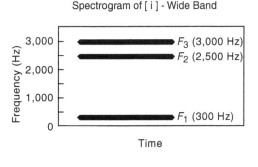

**FIGURE 5.16**  *Right*: Schematic spectrogram of the vowel [i] as in the word "beat." *Left*: A spectrum of the same sound. $F_1$, $F_2$, and $F_3$ represent the vocal tract resonances. The spectrogram shows frequency ($f$) changes in time. The spectrum shows the amplitude ($A$) of the component frequencies or harmonics. The center frequency of the formants does not always match the frequency of an individual harmonic.

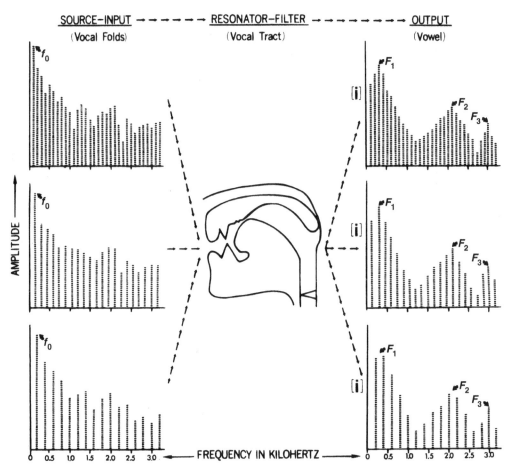

**FIGURE 5.17** Input–output spectra for a single resonator–filter: the vocal tract shaped to produce the vowel /i/. The frequencies of the resonance peaks of the output spectra are identical.

to the pattern for /i/ that we have described. A typical formant pattern for this vowel is $F_1$, 270 Hz; $F_2$, 2,290 Hz; and $F_3$, 3,010 Hz (Table 5.1).

A comparison of the output spectrum in Figure 5.16 with the spectrum for the neutral vowel (Fig. 5.13) shows that for /i/, $F_1$ is lower because the high-velocity area between the lips is narrowed, whereas $F_2$ and $F_3$ are both higher in frequency because the shortened oral cavity resonates at higher frequencies.

Therefore, the output of the vocal tract is primarily determined by the transfer function of the resonating cavities and thus ultimately by the articulators that shape those cavities. In the output (the sound that emerges at the lips), the harmonics closest to the resonances of the tract are resonated, and those furthest from the resonances lose energy in transmission. The schematic rendering of a sound spectrogram of [i] on the right side of Figure 5.16 depicts the formants of the vocal tract as broad bands of energy. Formants are numbered from low to high frequency: The first formant, $F_1$, is around 300 Hz, $F_2$ is at 2,500 Hz, and $F_3$ is at 3,000 Hz.

The frequency of a formant is measured at the center of the band of energy. This frequency may or may not correspond to the frequency of one of the harmonics. In the example given in Figure 5.16, the $F_2$ frequency is 2,500 Hz, but the harmonic with the

**TABLE 5.1**  Averages of Formant and Fundamental Frequencies (in Hertz) of Vowels Spoken by 33 Men, 28 Women, and 15 Children

|        | /i/ | | | /I/ | | | /ɛ/ | | |
|--------|-----|-----|-----|-----|-----|-----|-----|-----|-----|
|        | **M** | **W** | **Ch** | **M** | **W** | **Ch** | **M** | **W** | **Ch** |
| $F_1$  | 270 | 310 | 370 | 390 | 430 | 530 | 530 | 610 | 690 |
| $F_2$  | 2,290 | 2,790 | 3,200 | 1,990 | 2,480 | 2,730 | 1,840 | 2,330 | 2,610 |
| $F_3$  | 3,010 | 3,310 | 3,730 | 2,550 | 3,070 | 3,600 | 2,480 | 2,990 | 3,570 |
| $f_0$  | 136 | 235 | 272 | 135 | 232 | 269 | 130 | 223 | 260 |

|        | /æ/ | | | /ɑ/ | | | /ɔ/ | | |
|--------|-----|-----|-----|-----|-----|-----|-----|-----|-----|
|        | **M** | **W** | **Ch** | **M** | **W** | **Ch** | **M** | **W** | **Ch** |
| $F_1$  | 660 | 860 | 1,010 | 730 | 850 | 1,030 | 570 | 590 | 680 |
| $F_2$  | 1,720 | 2,050 | 2,320 | 1,090 | 1,220 | 1,370 | 840 | 920 | 1,060 |
| $F_3$  | 2,410 | 2,850 | 3,320 | 2,440 | 2,810 | 3,170 | 2,410 | 2,710 | 3,180 |
| $f_0$  | 127 | 210 | 251 | 124 | 212 | 256 | 129 | 216 | 263 |

|        | /U/ | | | /u/ | | | /ʌ/ | | |
|--------|-----|-----|-----|-----|-----|-----|-----|-----|-----|
|        | **M** | **W** | **Ch** | **M** | **W** | **Ch** | **M** | **W** | **Ch** |
| $F_1$  | 440 | 470 | 560 | 300 | 370 | 430 | 640 | 760 | 850 |
| $F_2$  | 1,020 | 1,160 | 1,410 | 870 | 950 | 1,170 | 1,190 | 1,400 | 1,590 |
| $F_3$  | 2,240 | 2,680 | 3,310 | 2,240 | 2,670 | 3,260 | 2,390 | 2,780 | 3,360 |
| $f_0$  | 137 | 232 | 276 | 141 | 231 | 274 | 130 | 221 | 261 |

|        | /ɝ/ | | |
|--------|-----|-----|-----|
|        | **M** | **W** | **Ch** |
| $F_1$  | 490 | 500 | 560 |
| $F_2$  | 1,350 | 1,640 | 1,820 |
| $F_3$  | 1,690 | 1,960 | 2,160 |
| $f_0$  | 133 | 218 | 261 |

M, man; W, woman; Ch, child; $F_1$, $F_2$, $F_3$, first, second, third formants; $f_0$, fundamental frequency.

Adapted with permission from Peterson, G. E., and Barney, H. L., Control Methods Used in a Study of the Vowels. *J. Acoust. Soc. Am. 24*, 1952, 183.

greatest amplitude in this formant is at 2,550 Hz for a source with a 150-Hz $f_0$ and would be 2,400 Hz for a source with an $f_0$ of 300 Hz.

As we have mentioned, an alternative method of displaying vowel formants is shown at the right of Figure 5.16, a schematic rendering of a wideband spectrogram. It differs from the output spectrum at the left of the figure in several ways, most importantly in that time is a parameter of the display: the output spectrum is an instantaneous representation of the resonant charac-teristics of the vowel, whereas the spectro-gram depicts the peaks of resonance as they change over time. Because we are assuming a static vocal tract shape, the formants in this spectrogram do not change in frequency. In normal speech, however, the articulators are in virtually continuous motion, and so the cavity shapes and the formants contin-uously change. Thus, it is much easier to display those changes in a wideband spec-trographic representation than it would be if we had to refer to a sequence of many out-put spectra made at different times during the

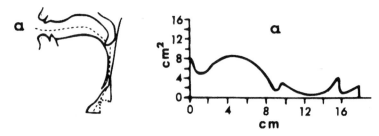

**FIGURE 5.18** Lateral view of the vocal tract and vocal tract area function for /ɑ/. (Adapted with permission from Fant, G., *Acoustic Theory of Speech Production.* The Hague, The Netherlands: Mouton, 1960.)

production of an utterance. (See Chapter 13 for a detailed discussion of spectrograms and spectra.)

Another way the wideband spectrogram differs from the output spectrum is that it provides no specific information about the frequencies of the individual harmonics that compose the resonance peaks of the vocal tract. You cannot tell from looking at the schematic wideband spectrogram in Figure 5.16 which harmonic frequencies make up the formants or, for that matter, how many harmonics fall within the bandwidth of each formant. Such information, however, is irrelevant if the point of interest is the center frequencies of the formants (resonance peaks), because they are determined by the articulation of the vowel and will remain essentially unchanged whether the frequencies of the fundamental and harmonics were higher or lower, or even whether they changed during the articulation of the vowel. In fact, as we mentioned earlier, for the same articulatory or vocal tract configuration, the center formant frequencies will be little different even when the vocal tract is resonating to an aperiodic source, as in the whispered vowels, which contain no harmonics.

## Low Back Vowel

The oral cavity is larger and the pharyngeal cavity smaller for the vowel /ɑ/ than for /i/. The size of the oral cavity for /ɑ/ may be increased in two ways: lowering the tongue

passively by lowering the jaw or actively by depressing the tongue. It is also possible to combine these two strategies.

Jaw lowering is partially controlled by the anterior belly of the digastric muscle. This paired muscle originates near the posterior surface of the mandibular symphysis and attaches to the body of the hyoid bone near the minor horn. Figures 5.19 and 6.11 show lateral and inferior views, respectively, of the anterior belly of the digastric muscle, which is innervated by motor fibers from the trigeminal (sixth cranial) nerve.

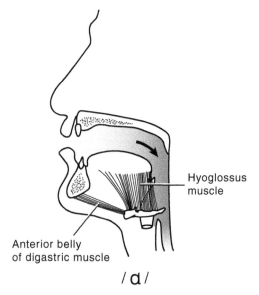

Hyoglossus muscle

Anterior belly of digastric muscle

/ ɑ /

**FIGURE 5.19** For [ɑ], the anterior belly of the digastric muscle is active in jaw opening and/or the hyoglossus muscle is active in depressing the tongue.

Enlargement of the oral cavity by active lowering of the tongue can also be achieved by contraction of the hyoglossus muscle. As Figure 5.19 shows, the fibers of this muscle course down from the tongue and insert into the body and major horn of the hyoid bone. It is innervated by the hypoglossal (twelfth cranial) nerve.

Active or passive lowering of the tongue for /ɑ/ provides the large oral cavity and small pharyngeal cavity volumes that characterize this vowel (Fig. 5.19). As we would expect, the small pharyngeal cavity resonates to higher frequency harmonics in the source, generating a relatively high-frequency first formant, whereas the large oral cavity resonates to low-frequency harmonics in the source and thus generates a relatively low-frequency second formant (Fig. 5.18). Typical frequencies for the first three formants of /ɑ/ are $F_1$, 730 Hz; $F_2$, 1,090 Hz; and $F_3$, 2,440 Hz (Table 5.1). Thus, the articulatory differences between /i/ and /ɑ/ are reflected in the acoustic differences. (Remember that /i/ has a large pharyngeal cavity and low-frequency $F_1$ and a small oral cavity and high-frequency $F_2$.)

## High Back Rounded Vowel

The third articulatory extreme in vowel production is /u/. This vowel is articulated with the dorsum of the tongue raised toward the roof of the mouth near the juncture between the hard palate and the velum. This is accomplished by contracting the styloglossus muscle (Figs. 5.6 and 5.20), which is innervated by the hypoglossal (twelfth cranial) nerve. Many speakers also round and protrude the lips by contracting the orbicularis oris muscle (Fig. 5.20), which is innervated by the facial (seventh cranial) nerve.

The acoustic effect of this positioning of the lips and tongue is threefold: First, the protrusion of the lips increases the overall length of the vocal tract and thus lowers the frequencies of all the formants. Second, the raising of the tongue dorsum pulls the bulk of the tongue out of the pharyngeal cavity,

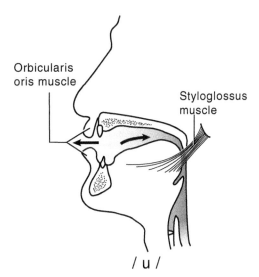

**FIGURE 5.20**  The activity of the orbicularis oris muscle protrudes the lips as the styloglossus muscle elevates the back of the tongue for [u].

enlarging it and allowing it to resonate to the low-frequency harmonics composing the first formant of this vowel. Third, the posterior constriction formed by the raised tongue dorsum and the protrusion of the lips lengthen the oral cavity, allowing it to resonate to the relatively low-frequency harmonics that make up the second formant of /u/ (Fig. 5.21). Typical frequencies for the first three formants of /u/ are $F_1$, 300 Hz; $F_2$, 870 Hz; and $F_3$, 2,240 Hz (Table 5.1).

At normal rates of speech, /u/ is frequently produced with little or no lip protrusion. To achieve the appropriate elongation of both the oral cavity and the vocal tract as a whole, speakers must therefore resort to alternative articulatory strategies. These include a greater degree of tongue retraction than would be used if the lips were protruded. This permits the speaker to attain an oral cavity length that is equivalent to that produced when the lips are rounded and protruded and the tongue is in a more fronted position. Thus, it is possible to generate the second resonant frequency for /u/ by more than one articulatory strategy. Similarly, a vocal tract length equivalent

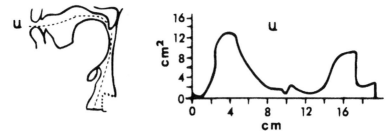

**FIGURE 5.21** Lateral view of the vocal tract and vocal tract area function for [u]. There are two distinct cavities for this vowel. (Adapted with permission from Fant, G., *Acoustic Theory of Speech Production.* The Hague, The Netherlands: Mouton, 1960.)

to that produced by lip protrusion can be attained by lowering the larynx. Again, the desired acoustic effect can be achieved by more than one articulatory configuration. This one-to-many relationship between acoustics and articulation is typical of many speech sounds.

Let us make one final observation before going on to discuss other vowels: The formant frequencies provided for /i/, /ɑ/, and /u/ have been deliberately labeled typical. Absolute frequencies cannot be given because the resonance characteristics of each vocal tract differ to some extent from those of every other. This variability is a function of three kinds of differences among speakers. First, as we noted earlier, the overall size of vocal tracts differs among speakers. Second, the relative size of parts of the vocal tract may differ. For example, the pharynx is generally smaller relative to the oral cavity in women than in men.

Third, a particular sound may be articulated differently by different speakers because of their dialects or idiolects or even by the same speaker as the context changes. The differences account, in part, for our ability to recognize individual speakers on the basis of differences between the qualities of equivalent sounds, aside from the differences between voice (source) characteristics. We shall see in later chapters that these differences raise interesting and difficult questions about how to explain the fact that listeners can perceive different acoustic signals as linguistically equivalent entities.

## The Relationship Between Acoustics and Articulation

The sounds we have been discussing, /i/, /ɑ/, and /u/, occupy a special place in traditional articulatory-based descriptions of most languages. The earliest of these articulatory descriptions, now well over 100 years old, were based almost entirely on the impressionistic, introspective evidence of phoneticians who viewed vowel articulation primarily as functions of tongue shape and tongue position. Lip posture, because it was so easily observable, also formed one of the bases for description.

With the introduction of more objective techniques for describing articulation, the importance of the tongue root and jaw position became known, and the development of acoustic analysis led investigators to explore the relationships among articulation, the dimensions of the resonating cavities, and the acoustic features of speech, especially with regard to formant frequencies. Research into these relationships has led to general agreement that the frequencies of formants cannot be attributed solely to a particular resonating cavity within the vocal tract. That is, the formants are understood as the acoustic response of the vocal tract as a whole to the components of the source.

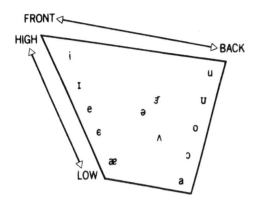

RELATIVE TONGUE POSITIONS FOR VOWELS

**FIGURE 5.22** The traditional vowel quadrilateral. The location of each phonetic symbol represents the position of the high point of the tongue within the part of the oral cavity in which vowel constrictions are formed.

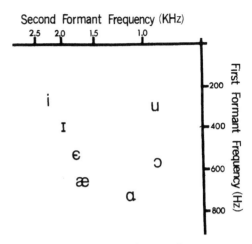

**FIGURE 5.23** Average formant frequencies of 33 adult male speakers of English. (Data from Peterson, G. E., and Barney H. L., Control Methods Used in a Study of the Vowels. *J. Acoust. Soc. Am. 24*, 1952, 183.)

Nonetheless, in practice, speech scientists have found it impossible to ignore the well-established correlations (implied in our discussion of /i/, /ɑ/, and /u/) among (1) the frequencies of the first two formants, (2) the dimensions of the oral and pharyngeal cavities, and (3) the traditional description of the tongue, the jaw, and the lip position in vowel articulation. Let us now be explicit about the basis of these correlations.

Figure 5.22 depicts the traditional vowel quadrilateral (sometimes called the vowel triangle, although it has four sides). The basic parameters of this quadrilateral are tongue height (high to low) and tongue advancement (front to back). The quadrilateral is thus a schematic representation of the portion of the oral cavity within which the high point of the tongue moves while forming constrictions during vowel articulation. The relative position of any phonetic symbol in the quadrilateral is taken to represent the position of the highest point on the superior surface of the tongue in the articulation of the vowel it represents. Despite some discrepancies between the locations of these symbols and the high point of the tongue as viewed in radiographic studies, the description given in

the vowel quadrilateral generally conforms to the known facts, and it is particularly relevant to the measured frequencies of vowel formants.

The correlation between the articulatory parameters of the vowel quadrilateral and the acoustic output of the vocal tract will be obvious if we inspect Figure 5.23, a plot of the average first and second formant frequencies of 33 men taken from Table 5.1. The basic similarity between this formant frequency plot and the arrangement of the vowel symbols in the vowel quadrilateral is clear, and it is not merely coincidental.

To fully explain the basis of the similarity, we must describe how the positioning of the articulators affects the size and shape of the oral and pharyngeal resonating cavities. Figure 5.24 displays the interrelationships among (1) articulator activity and placement, (2) the resulting resonance cavity sizes, and (3) the formant frequencies generated for a number of English vowels. The frequency of $F_1$ is closely correlated with (1) the area of the lower portion of the pharyngeal cavity and (2) the degree of mouth opening at the lips. The frequency of $F_2$ is correlated with the length of the front (oral) cavity.

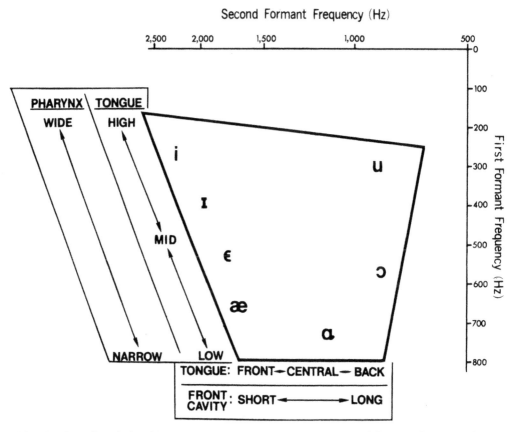

**FIGURE 5.24** The relationships among tongue position, cavity size, and formant frequency for some English vowels.

Consider the first formant. As the tongue moves from a high to a low position, the pharyngeal cavity decreases in volume (Fig. 5.25). The basic reason for the decrease in volume is the incompressibility of the tongue: as it descends into the smaller area within the mandible, the tongue root is forced back into the pharyngeal cavity. Conversely, as the tongue body rises, the tongue root is pulled out of the pharyngeal cavity. This means that vowels with higher tongue positions have larger pharyngeal cavities that will resonate to lower frequencies in the source. Vowels with lower tongue positions will have smaller pharyngeal cavities that will resonate to higher frequencies in the source. The correlation between lip opening and $F_1$ frequency can be inferred from the articulation, as the higher vowels are characterized by raised jaw positions and smaller lip apertures, whereas the lower vowels display low jaw positions and larger lip apertures.

The second formant frequencies of the vowels correlate in a straightforward way with the length of the oral resonating cavity. In the front vowel series in the traditional vowel quadrilateral (Figs. 5.22 and 5.25), each vowel has a slightly more retracted tongue position than the one above it. For the back series, each vowel has a slightly more retracted tongue position than the one below it. If we assume that the location of the vowels within the quadrilateral is essentially correct, then as we articulate the vowels on the perimeter of the quadrilateral from /i/ down to /æ/, across the bottom to /ɑ/ and then up to /u/, we are repeatedly retracting the high point of the tongue. Because the

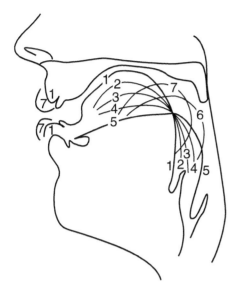

**FIGURE 5.25** The vocal tract shape, for the vowels in the words (1) "heed," (2) "hid," (3) "head," (4) "had," (5) "father," (6) "good," and (7) "food." (Reprinted with permission from Ladefoged, P., *A Course in Phonetics.* Fort Worth: Harcourt Brace Jovanovich, 1975.)

high point of the tongue marks the posterior limit of the front or the oral resonating cavity, that cavity grows longer throughout this series of vowels. Lip rounding may supplement the retraction of the tongue by elongating the oral cavity for many of the back vowels. Thus, the short oral cavity associated with the advanced tongue positions of

the front vowels such as /i/ and /I/ resonates to high frequencies in the source. The longer the oral cavity becomes as the tongue is retracted (and the lips protruded), the lower the frequencies in the source that will be resonated.

Acoustically, the critical dimension is front cavity length, not tongue position or lip protrusion. We remarked earlier that back, "lip-rounded" vowels are not always articulated with maximum rounding (protrusion). We can see now that reduced degrees of lip rounding can be compensated for by increased degrees of tongue retraction to yield a front resonating cavity of the appropriate length for a given vowel.

The effect of these articulatory and acoustic relationships on the formant frequencies of the vowels on the perimeter of the vowel quadrilateral can be seen in Figures 5.26 to 5.28: (1) A generally consistent lowering of $F_2$ as the front (oral) resonating cavity is enlarged because of tongue retraction (and lip protrusion) and (2) a general raising of $F_1$ from /i/ through /ɑ/ as the pharyngeal cavity size is decreased (because of tongue lowering) and the lip aperture is increased (because of jaw lowering), and a lowering of $F_1$ from /ɑ/ through /u/ as the pharyngeal cavity size is increased (as the tongue rises) and the lip aperture is diminished (as the jaw rises) (Fig. 5.25).

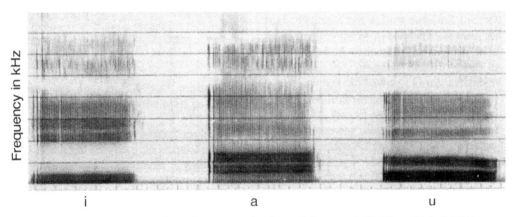

**FIGURE 5.26** Spectrogram of steady-state productions of the vowels [i], [a], and [u]. A 1-kHz calibration tone is indicated. (Spectrogram courtesy of Kay Elemetrics.)

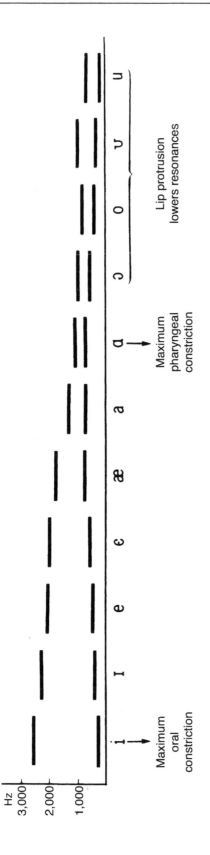

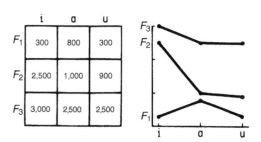

**FIGURE 5.28** Relationships among $F_1$, $F_2$, and $F_3$ for /i/, /ɑ/, and /u/.

These explanations are only a first approximation of causality, and the response of the vocal tract as a whole, rather than of the individual resonating cavities, must be considered to account fully for formant frequencies. This is obvious if we consider the articulation of the vowel /ɑ/, in which the highest point of the tongue is so depressed that it can scarcely be said to divide the vocal tract into front (oral) and back (pharyngeal) cavities. Nonetheless, speech scientists generally infer causality from the correlations presented here and often make such assumptions as "the fronting of the tongue results in a rise in the frequency of $F_2$" and "a fall in the frequency of $F_1$ indicates that the tongue and jaw have been raised." The pervasiveness and usefulness of such assumptions suggest that they are, for the most part, reliable.

In point of fact, the correlations between articulation and acoustics can be more satisfactorily represented in a number of ways. Ladefoged (1975), for example, achieves a closer match between formant frequencies and actual tongue positions and shapes (as depicted in radiographs) by plotting $F_1$ against the difference between $F_2$ and $F_1$ rather than by simply plotting $F_1$ directly against $F_2$. This results in a more physiologically accurate placement of the back vowels

**FIGURE 5.27** Two-formant vowels, synthesized on the Pattern Playback. The symbols indicate the identification of each pattern by listeners. The lettering indicates the vocal tract characteristics of the corresponding vowels.

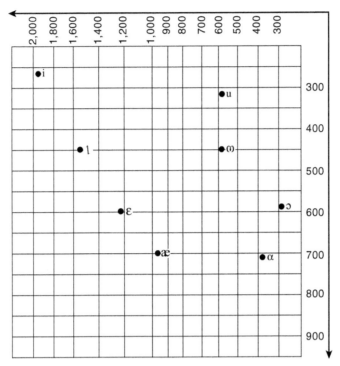

**FIGURE 5.29**  A formant chart showing the frequency of the first formant on the ordinate (vertical axis) plotted against the difference in frequency of the first and second formants on the abscissa (horizontal axis) for eight American English vowels. The symbol "ω" is equivalent to "U." (Modified with permission from Ladefoged, P., *A Course in Phonetics*. Fort Worth: Harcourt Brace Jovanovich, 1975.)

(Fig. 5.29) by showing [ɔ] and [ɑ] to be farther back than [u] and [ʊ].

It may well be that phoneticians have been unconsciously charting the vowels according to their acoustic reality rather than their articulatory reality. It seems clear that the vowel quadrilateral data are more nearly a direct reflection of the acoustic than the articulatory data. As Ladefoged points out, the impressions of vowel height are "more closely determined by the first formant frequency than by the [actual] height of the tongue."

Similarly, impressions of tongue advancement are "more simply expressed by reference to the difference between the first and second formant frequencies than to any measurement of the actual [horizontal] position of the tongue." In addition, Fant has observed that the highest point of the tongue is not as important as the maximum constriction and the length of the tract from the glottis to this point. For example, the highest point of the tongue for /ɑ/ is in the oral cavity, but the point of maximum constriction is in the pharyngeal cavity, closer to the glottis.

## The Relationship Between Acoustics and Vocal Tract Size

There is no set of absolute formant frequency values for any of the vowels. This is because vocal tracts of different size resonate to different frequencies. In a 1952 study, Peterson and Barney measured the formant frequencies of 76 speakers (33 men, 28 women, and 15 children). The subjects were recorded as they produced English vowels in an /hVd/

## $C$LINICAL NOTE

There are several speech disorders that can be related to the deviant articulation and resonance of vowels. Perhaps, the most noticeable of these disorders can be found in the speech of the hearing-impaired, especially children who are congenitally deaf. Lacking the auditory input of other speakers, and being deprived of the auditory feedback from their own speech production, hearing-impaired speakers tend to produce vowels that are not clearly differentiated from each other and which are in many ways dissimilar to those produced by speakers with normal hearing. There is evidence that the tongue and jaw movements of hearing-impaired speakers are constrained compared with those of normal-hearing speakers. This, in turn, causes the vowel formants to be more similar to each other, accounting for the lack of differentiation among the vowels. Other disorders that can be manifest in faulty vowel production are apraxia of speech, the dysarthrias, and cerebral palsy. Foreign accent, although not actually a pathologic condition, is often treated by speech pathologists and is often marked by the use of vowels not typical of English.

Whatever the cause of the difficulty in producing vowels, the effect is often visible in acoustic displays such as wideband spectrograms and wideband amplitude spectra. (See Chapter 13 for a full discussion of these types of acoustic display.) Using the available technology, it is possible for clients to view such displays of their own speech instantaneously and to compare their acoustic output with that of a speaker with normal speech. This sort of feedback is often effective in allowing the client to sense the connections between articulatory movements or positions and the resulting acoustic output. Once the connections are understood, clients can adjust their articulatory or acoustic outputs so that they approximate the models supplied by clinicians.

context. The average formant frequencies for the three groups of speakers are shown in Table 5.1. There are marked differences among the groups for the first three formant frequencies for each vowel. Nonetheless, the relative positions of the vowels in an $F_1$ by $F_2$ formant plot (Fig. 5.30) are remarkably similar. In general, as we would expect, the larger vocal tracts generate lower resonant frequencies than the smaller ones. Thus, the lowest formant frequencies are those of the men and the highest are those of the children, whereas those of the women display intermediate values. The frequency differences, however, do not relate only to the differences in overall vocal tract dimensions, but also to the larger ratio of pharyngeal cavity area to oral cavity area for adult males as compared to women and children.

### Tense and Lax Vowels

Some of the vowels (and diphthongs) in English are of intrinsically greater duration than others. These vowels are usually characterized by tongue movements that deviate more from the so-called neutral position for schwa than do the vowels of intrinsically shorter duration. However, the vowels with the more extreme tongue positions and greater duration are termed *tense* vowels, more because of evidence about their distribution in words than because of their method of production. Tense vowels can appear in open syllables, such as "see," "say," "so," "sue," "saw," "sigh," "cow," and "soy." The vowels with less extreme tongue positions and shorter duration are *lax* vowels. Most lax vowels appear only in closed syllables (syllables that end in consonants), not in open syllables at the ends of words. Examples of English lax vowels are found in the words "sit," "set," "sat," and "soot."

The tense vowels can be divided into two subclasses according to whether the vocal tract is held relatively constant throughout the vowel or there is a distinct change in the vocal tract shape during production.

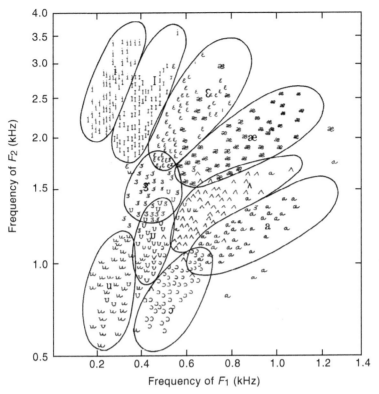

**FIGURE 5.30**  Average formant frequencies for some English vowels spoken by men, women, and children. (Data from Peterson, G. E., and Barney, H. L., Control Methods Used in a Study of the Vowels. *J. Acoust. Soc. Am. 24*, 1952, 183.)

Virtually, all of the "simple" tense vowels are diphthongized to a greater or lesser extent. Vowels such as those in the words "say" and "so" are marked by more extreme diphthongization than those in the words "see" and "sue." Try saying these words to see whether you can distinguish between (1) the changes in vocal tract shape and differences in duration that differentiate the more diphthongized tense vowels from those that are less diphthongized and (2) the tense from the lax vowels in general.

## DIPHTHONG PRODUCTION

A diphthong is a vowel of changing resonance. Common diphthongs are the vocalic portions of the words in the following sentences:

How Joe likes toy trains!
/aʊ/ /oʊ/ /aɪ/ /ɔɪ/ /eɪ/
I don't play cowboy.
/aɪ/ /oʊ/ /eɪ/ /aʊ/ /ɔɪ/

Those "tense" vowels that require a changing vocal tract shape are also considered to be diphthongs. The diphthongs ending with vocal tract shapes appropriate for [ɪ] ([eɪ], [aɪ], and [ɔɪ]) entail tongue movement forward and up from the [e], [a], and [ɔ] positions, and the diphthongs ending with vocal tract shapes appropriate for [ʊ] ([oʊ] and [aʊ]) entail tongue movement back and up, concurrent with lip protrusion. The sounds [ɪi] and [ʊu] as in "see" and "sue," respectively, are often diphthongs too, but the vocal tract and resonance changes are less extensive than in the other diphthongs.

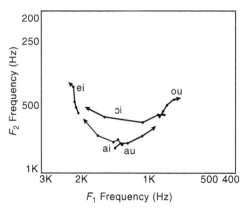

**FIGURE 5.31**  First and second formants for the diphthongs. The first formant frequencies are plotted on the ordinate and the second formant frequencies on the abscissa. *Arrows* indicate the direction of formant movement. (Replotted with permission from data in Holbrook, A., and Fairbanks, G., Diphthong Formants and Their Movements. *J. Speech Hear. Res. 5,* 1962, 38–58.)

Acoustic studies of formant changes in diphthongs have shown $F_1$ and $F_2$ formant shifts characteristic of each diphthong. Holbrook and Fairbanks (1962) measured formant frequencies of diphthongs from spectrograms of 20 male speakers saying "My name is John___" with Hay, High, Hoy, Hoe, Howe, and Hugh as last names. $F_1$ by $F_2$ plots show acoustic overlaps, but when the samples are limited to those closest to the median, patterns are more discrete. Figure 5.31 shows that the longer diphthongs with more extensive changes ([aɪ], [aʊ], and [ɔɪ]) undershoot the final goals [ɪ] and [ʊ] more than the shorter diphthongs ([eɪ] and [oʊ]). The authors noted that [eɪ] extends from [aɪ] in an almost continuous fashion, as does [oʊ] from [aʊ]. Together they form the trough of an inverted triangle.

Muscle use for diphthongs is similar to that for vowels, although contractions sometimes shift gradually from one muscle group to another. For example, to produce [aɪ], the tongue-lowering muscles are gradually replaced by tongue fronting and elevating muscles, such as the genioglossus and geniohyoid muscles.

Peterson and Lehiste (1961) measured the durations of diphthongs, along with other *syllabic nuclei,* and found that the shorter diphthongs [eɪ], [oʊ], and [ɝ] change slowly and continuously, whereas the longer diphthongs [aɪ], [aʊ], and [ɔɪ] evidenced a steady state at the beginning followed by a longer transition, and ended with a shorter off-glide near the terminal target.

## REFERENCES AND SUGGESTED READING

### General Acoustics of Speech

Denes, P. B., and Pinson, E. N., *The Speech Chain,* 2nd ed. New York: W. H. Freeman, 1993.

Fant, G., *Acoustic Theory of Speech Production.* The Hague, The Netherlands: Mouton, 1960.

Fry, D. B. (Ed.), *Acoustic Phonetics: A Course of Basic Readings.* New York: Cambridge University, 1975.

Kent, R. D., and Read, C., *The Acoustic Analysis of Speech.* San Diego: Singular Publishing Group, 1992.

Lehiste, I. (Ed.), *Readings in Acoustic Phonetics.* Cambridge, MA: MIT Press, 1967.

Olive, J. P., Greenwood, A., and Coleman, J., *Acoustics of American English Speech: A Dynamic Approach.* New York: Springer-Verlag, 1993.

Pickett, J. M., *The Acoustics of Speech Communication.* Boston: Allyn & Bacon, 1999.

Potter, R. K., Kopp, G. A., and Green, H. C., *Visible Speech.* New York: Van Nostrand Co., 1947.

Stevens, K. N., *Acoustic Phonetics.* Cambridge, MA: MIT Press, 1998.

### Articulation and Resonance: Vowels and Diphthongs

Bell-Berti, F., *The Velopharyngeal Mechanism: An Electromyographic Study.* Haskins Laboratories Status Report (Suppl.). New Haven, CT: Haskins Laboratories, 1973.

Chiba, T., and Kajiyama, M., *The Vowel: Its Nature and Structure.* Tokyo: Kaiseikan, 1941.

Hillenbrand, J., Getty, L. A., Clark, M. J. and Wheeler, K., Acoustic Characteristics of

American English Vowels. *J. Acoust. Soc. Am. 97*, 1995, 3099–3111.

Holbrook, A., and Fairbanks, G., Diphthong Formants and Their Movements. *J. Speech Hear. Res. 5*, 1962, 38–58.

Kuehn, D. P., and Dalston, R. M., Cleft Palate Studies Related to Velopharyngeal Function. In *Human Communication and Its Disorders*. H. Winitz (Ed.). Norwood, NJ: Ablex, 1988.

Ladefoged, P., *A Course in Phonetics*, 3rd ed. New York: Harcourt Brace Jovanovich, 1993.

Ladefoged, P., *Vowels and Consonants*, 2nd ed. Malden, MA: Blackwell Publishing, 2005.

Lubker, J. F., An Electromyographic-Cinefluorographic Investigation of Velar Function During Normal Speech Production. *Cleft Palate J. 5*, 1968, 1–18.

Moll, K., and Daniloff, R. G., Investigation of the Timing of Velar Movements During Speech. *J. Acoust. Soc. Am. 50*, 1971, 678–684.

Peterson, G. E., and Barney, H. L., Control Methods Used in a Study of the Vowels. *J. Acoust. Soc. Am. 24*, 1952, 175–184.

Peterson, G. E., and Lehiste, I., Duration of Syllable Nuclei in English. *J. Acoust. Soc. Am. 32*, 1960, 693–703.

Peterson, G. E., and Lehiste, I., Transitions, Glides, and Diphthongs. *J. Acoust. Soc. Am. 33*, 1961, 268–277.

Raphael, L. J., and Bell-Berti, F., Tongue Musculature and the Feature of Tension in English Vowels. *Phonetica 32*, 1975, 61–73.

Rayleigh, J. W. S., *Theory of Sound*. London: Macmillan, 1878.

Stevens, K. N., and House, A. S., An Acoustical Theory of Vowel Production and Some of Its Implications. *J. Speech Hear. Res. 4*, 1961, 303–320.

Stevens, K. N., and House, A. S., Development of a Quantitative Description of Vowel Articulation. *J. Acoust. Soc. Am. 27*, 1955, 484–493. Reprinted in Kent et al., 1991 (q.v.), 401–410.

Stone, M. A., Guide to Analyzing Tongue Motion from Ultrasound Images. *Clin. Linguist. Phonet. 19*, 2005, 455–501.

Stone, M., Epstein, M., and Iskarous, K., Functional Segments in Tongue Movement. *Clin. Linguist. Phonet. 18*, 2004, 507–521.

Story, B. A., Parametric Model of the Vocal Tract Area Function for Vowel and Consonant Simulation. *J. Acoust. Soc. Am. 117*, 2005, 3231–3254.

Tuller, B., Harris, K. S., and Gross, B., Electromyographic Study of the Jaw Muscles During Speech. *J. Phonet. 9*, 1981, 175–188.

# The Articulation and Acoustics of Consonants

# 6

> *God have mercy on the sinner*
> *Who must write with . . .*
> *Only consonants and vowels*

–John Crowe Ransom, *Survey of Literature*

## ARTICULATION AND RESONANCE: CONSONANTS

In the previous chapter, we described how the movements and positions of the articulators are instrumental in shaping the resonating cavities of the vocal tract to modify the sound source for vowels. The relationship between articulation and resonance for vowels is quite similar to that for consonants, especially with regard to the resonant consonants, including the nasals (/m/, /n/, and /ŋ/), the glides (/w/ and /j/), and the liquids (/r/ and /l/). There are, however, some differences that should be mentioned. First, the constrictions used to produce the consonants, especially the nonresonant consonants (stops, fricatives, and affricates), are usually more extreme than those for vow-

els. In the case of the stops and affricates, the constrictions formed by the articulators completely block the flow of air for a brief period of time. Second, there are differences between the ways in which the sources of sound are used in the production of consonants, again especially with regard to the stops, fricatives, and affricates. Whereas the vowels are usually produced only with a periodic source of sound, the consonants may use an aperiodic sound source or a combination of periodic and aperiodic sources.

## TYPES OF SOUND SOURCES: CONSONANTS

As we have seen, the speech sounds that we know as vowels and diphthongs are mainly the result of filtering the complex wave produced at the glottis in the resonating cavities of the vocal tract. The same is true of resonant consonants (nasals, glides, and liquids). The various configurations of the vocal tract thus generate different combinations of resonant frequencies for each sound. The characteristic cavity configurations and resulting resonances for each sound are what make them distinct from one another. But the vocal folds can also be used to generate an aperiodic source of sound to be resonated in the cavities of the vocal tract. This is accomplished by partially adducting the folds, bringing them close enough to each other to make the breath stream turbulent as it flows through the glottis, but not so close as to cause the vocal folds to vibrate. The aperiodic energy generated at the glottis is the source for whispered speech and for the consonant [h].

Aperiodic sounds can also be generated at various locations within the supraglottal vocal tract. One way to do this is to block the flow of air completely for a brief period of time and then to release the built-up air pressure suddenly, as in a stop consonant such as /t/. The term plosive is also used for this kind of sound because of the explosive and transient nature of the airburst.

A second way to produce an aperiodic sound is to force the airstream through an articulatory constriction for a relatively extended period of time. As in the case of the partially closed glottis, this will cause the airstream to become turbulent and will result in a continuous source of noise that is longer in duration than the transient noise bursts of the stops. The fricative /ʃ/, as in "shoe," is an example of a sound that uses a continuous noise source.

## Simultaneous Combinations of Different Sound Sources

Speech sound sources can be combined in a variety of ways. The periodic source produced by the vibrating vocal folds and the continuous noise produced by channeling the airflow through a constriction are frequently heard simultaneously during the productions of voiced fricatives such as /v/, /ð/, /z/, /ʒ/ and at the end of the voiced affricate /dʒ/. Similarly, in certain contexts, the periodic source may be simultaneously combined with the transient aperiodic source at the moment of release of the voiced stops /b/, /d/, and /g/ and at the start of the voiced affricate /dʒ/.

## Sequences of Different Sound Sources

In the course of normally produced speech, there are frequent instances in which the periodic and aperiodic sources must alternate to meet the requirements of the sounds being produced. For instance, in the sentence "She saw Pat race by," there are at least nine locations where phonation alternates with an aperiodic source of sound.

Some sounds or contexts require the alternation of transient and continuous aperiodic sound sources. Such sequences are required to produce both affricates, /tʃ/ and /dʒ/. Both the simultaneous and sequential combinations of sound sources in the vocal tract are resonated by the cavities of the supraglottal portion of the tract. Therefore, the supraglottal vocal tract is always a resonator and often a source of sound for speech as well. The sound sources for speech, their combination, and their uses in speech sound production are summarized in Table 6.1.

In our discussion of the consonants, we will begin with those sounds that most resemble the vowels, the resonant consonants or semivowels, and then describe the less resonant sounds that are produced with a more constricted vocal tract (the fricatives, stops, and affricates). For each class of speech sounds, we shall discuss the physiology and articulation of its production and the acoustic results.

**TABLE 6.1**   Speech Sound Sources

| Source | Resonator | Sound | Manner | Examples |
|---|---|---|---|---|
| Vocal folds | Vocal tract | Periodic | Vowels | /i/ /u/ |
| | | | Diphthongs | /ai/ /ou/ |
| | | | Semivowels | /w/ /y/ |
| | | | Nasals | /m/ /ŋ/ |
| Vocal tract | Vocal tract | Aperiodic | Stops | /p/ /k/ |
| | | | Fricatives | /s/ /f/ |
| | | | Affricate | /ʧ/ |
| Vocal folds and vocal tract | Vocal tract | Mixed periodic and aperiodic | Voiced stops | /b/ /g/ |
| | | | Voiced fricatives | /z/ /v/ |
| | | | Voiced affricate | /ʤ/ |

## CONSONANT PRODUCTION

### Resonant Consonants I: The Semivowels

The semivowel vowel consonants are so named because their articulations and acoustic features resemble those of vowels. That is, the articulators used in their production form only minimum constrictions in the vocal tract, and, as a result, they are characterized by formant structures similar to those of vowels and diphthongs. The similarity to diphthongs is evident in spectrograms of the semivowels in which, depending on context, changes in the formant frequency may be quite evident (Figs. 6.1 and 6.2). Glides and liquids, then, are often similar to diphthongs but with transitions that are articulated more quickly and which thus have a shorter acoustic duration.

The semivowels are usually subdivided into two manners of articulation: The *glides*, /w/ and /j/, as in "we" and "you," and the *liquids*, /r/ and /l/, as in "right" and "light." The similarities of these consonants to vowels are relatively easy to hear. For example, if you articulate the glides /w/ and /j/ at the start of "we" and "you" very slowly, the diphthongs [ui] and [iu] can be heard. The vowel-like quality of the liquid consonant /l/ can be heard if you prolong the final sound in a word such as "full," and that of /r/ is evident as you will discover if you isolate and compare the first sound of "run" to the vowel in the word "earth."

Although the vocal tract is relatively open for the semivowels, as it is for vowels and diphthongs, and although the semivowels are characterized acoustically by formants, they are classified as consonants, not as vowels. The reason for this is that the semivowels occur on the periphery of syllables in English, as do other consonants, and not in the centers or *nuclei* of syllables, as do the vowels and diphthongs. For example, "win" /wɪn/, "yoke" /jok/, "rat" /ræt/, and "leap" /lip/ occur as English words, but /twn/, /pjk/, /drt/, and /plp/ do not, because the latter syllables lack appropriate nuclei formed by vowels and diphthongs articulated with an open vocal tract. The semivowels are always located next to vocalic nuclei, both individually, as in the examples above, and in contexts containing consonant clusters: In "spring, "splash," "twin," and "cute," the semivowels are all adjacent to the vowels or diphthongs: /sprɪŋ/, /splæʃ/, /twɪn/, and /kjut/. The glides occur only before (or between) vocalic nuclei, as in "way," "away," "thwart," "yes," "reuse," and "music." The liquids, /r/ and /l/, by contrast, can occur after vocalic nuclei and before consonants as in "car," "card," "pool," and "pooled."

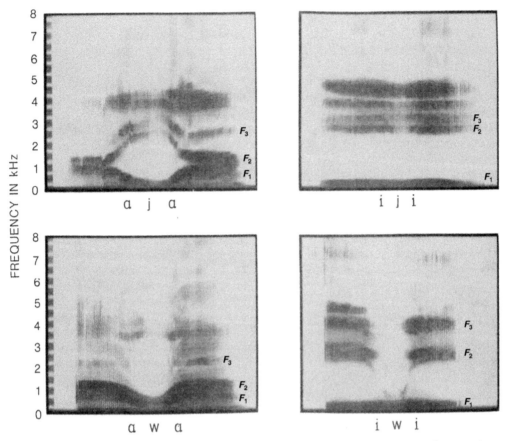

**FIGURE 6.1**  Spectrograms of /ɑjɑ/, /iji/, /ɑwɑ/, and /iwi/. The $F_2$ movement is larger for /ɑjɑ/ than for /iji/, whereas the $F_2$ movement is smaller for /ɑwɑ/ than for /iwi/.

Occasionally, though, liquid semivowels do function as the nuclei of syllables. They share this ability with the nasals, which are also resonant consonants. For example, "ladle" has two nuclei, the diphthong [eɪ] of the first syllable and the [l] of the second syllable. When a consonant serves as a vocalic nucleus in a syllable, a dot is put under the phonetic symbol to indicate that it is functioning as a *syllabic consonant.* Syllabic consonants occur in such words as "waddle" [wɑdl̩], "cotton" [kɑtn̩], and "up or down" [ʌpr̩daʊn], which can be used to express a preference in the cooking of fried eggs.

Let us look at some of the individual characteristics of the resonant consonants, beginning with /j/, a palatal glide. To produce this sound, the tongue blade must ap-

proximate the palate at a position close to that for a high front vowel, and so requires genioglossus muscle activity. During the utterance [ɑjɑ] (Fig. 6.1), the high first formant frequency for first [ɑ] decreases as the tongue rises to the starting position for the /j/ and the pharynx enlarges; the second formant frequency increases because of the tongue fronting and the resultant shortening of the front (oral) resonating cavity. The production of glides requires movement of the tongue and lips to change the vocal tract shape from the starting position (high front tongue position at the start of /j/, similar to that of the vowel /i/) to the next vowel position. It is the sound of the acoustic changes caused by the movements of the articulators that listeners use to recognize glides.

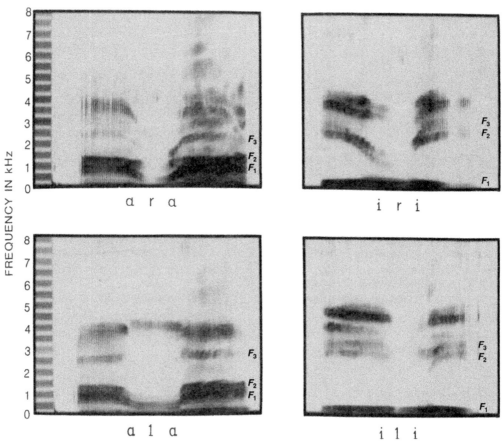

**FIGURE 6.2** Spectrograms of /ɑrɑ/, /iri/, /ɑlɑ/, and /ili/. The $F_3$ movement lowers close to $F_2$ for /r/, whereas it remains high for /l/.

The glide /w/ is analogous to /j/ in its formation. That is, the starting position for /w/ is characterized by a high back tongue position and protruded lips, similar to that of the vowel /u/. The articulators then move rapidly to the position for the following vowel, causing the changes in resonance that allow listeners to recognize /w/. Note that /w/ has two places of articulation: the bilabial protrusion that results from contraction of the orbicularis oris and other lip muscles and the lingua-palatal approximation caused by the contraction of such muscles as the styloglossus, to elevate and retract the tongue.

You can demonstrate the vowel-like nature of the starting positions for the glides by saying the vowel /i/ or the vowel /u/ and then rapidly changing your vocal tract shape to one that is appropriate for some other vowel, /ɑ/ for example. If you make the transition from one vowel to the other continuously and rapidly, you will hear /jɑ/ (if you started with /i/) or /wɑ/ (if you started with /u/).

Because the articulatory configurations for /j/ and /w/ resemble, respectively, /i/ and /u/, the patterns of the formant frequency change are usually predictable as the vocal tract configuration changes to that of the vowel following the glide. The second formant of /i/, you will recall, is higher than that for any other vowel. As a result, $F_2$ will decrease in frequency during the production of /j/. The opposite is true for /w/ for which $F_2$ at onset is very low in frequency, resulting in an increase in $F_2$ frequency when this glide is produced. Because the tongue is very high in the mouth and the pharyngeal cavity is relatively large, $F_1$ is very low (as it is for /i/ and /u/) for both glides. As a result, there is almost always a rise in $F_1$ as the articulators move to the position for the following vowel.

The importance of articulatory movement and changes in resonance in the production (and perception) of the glides can be illustrated by the limiting cases of such syllables as /ji/ (as in "yeast") and /wu/ (as in "woo"). In both cases, the starting and ending vocal tract configurations are similar: for /j/, an /i/-like configuration at syllable onset and the vowel /i/ at offset; for /w/, a /u/-like configuration at syllable onset and the vowel /u/ at offset. Speakers, however, do not simply produce a long /i/ or /u/. Rather, they move the articulators away from the onset configuration and then return them to approximately where they started. This articulatory movement changes the vocal tract resonances and provides the formant frequency changes needed for glide production and perception.

The liquids, /r/ and /l/, are produced in syllable-initial position by raising the tongue toward the alveolar ridge. Differences in the tongue tip configuration and position create the distinctions between the two sounds. For /l/, the tip rests lightly against the alveolar ridge, dividing the airflow into two streams that emerge over the sides of the tongue; hence, it is often called a *lateral* sound. For /r/, the tongue is grooved and the tip does not touch the alveolar ridge, so some of the airflow and acoustic energy emerges centrally, although much of it is laterally emitted, as it is for /l/. The lips are often rounded. Many speakers produce a *retroflex* /r/ by raising the tongue tip toward the alveolar ridge and bending it slightly backward.

Because of the raised tongue tip for the liquids, the superior longitudinal muscle is particularly active in their production. Its antagonist, the inferior longitudinal muscle, may be more active for /r/ than for /l/, especially if the /r/ is retroflexed. The shaping of the tongue dorsum is probably achieved by

the interaction of the vertical and transverse muscles.

The acoustic results of these tongue tip adjustments (Fig. 6.2) are reflected somewhat in the second formant but are particularly obvious in the third formant. For /r/, $F_3$ falls below the $F_3$ frequencies typical of the neighboring vowels, whereas for /l/ it does not depart from them significantly.

There are some noticeable differences between the liquids when they occur in syllable-final as opposed to syllable-initial position. Syllable-initial /l/, as in "leave" and "lip," is articulated with the dorsum of the tongue very low in the mouth. In contrast, syllable-final /l/, as in "full" and "cool," is articulated with the dorsum of the tongue raised somewhat toward the velum. This type of /l/ is associated both with high back vowels and with syllable-final position. It is sometimes called "dark /l/," in contrast to the "light /l/" found in syllable-initial position, especially when it is associated with front vowels.

Similarly, syllable-final /r/ differs from its counterpart in initial position. It often loses its consonantal quality and simply colors whatever vowel it follows. Speakers of some dialects omit the articulatory constriction for [r] at the end of "car," "hear," or "sure" and replace it with vowel lengthening or movement toward a neutral tract shape ([ə]): "hear" becomes /hɪə/ or [hɪ:]. Speakers who do produce /r/-coloring when they articulate syllable-final /r/ do so by elevating the tongue dorsum toward the palate. This causes $F_3$ of the preceding vowel to decrease in frequency, which, as we have seen, is characteristic of other allophones of /r/.

The fact that /r/ and /l/ are so consistently confused in English by native speakers of several Asian languages demonstrates their articulatory and acoustic similarity. Children with developmental speech substitutions often produce the more easily articulated /w/ for the liquids or use /j/ for /l/ and /w/ for /r/. "The little rabbit likes carrots" might be rendered by a young child as [dəwɪtəwæbəjaɪkskæwəts].

## Resonant Consonants II: The Nasals

### *Velopharyngeal Port: Vocal Tract Modifier*

Most of the speech sounds in English are resonated in a two-part tract consisting of the pharyngeal and oral cavities, extending from the vocal folds to the lips. There are three sounds, however, that require added resonance in the nasal cavities: the /m/, /n/, and /ŋ/ as in "mining" ([maInIŋ]). During continuous speech, the entrance to the chambers of the nose must be closed off most of the time because almost all speech sounds are *oral sounds*. It must, in contrast, be open for the three *nasal sounds*. The entrance to the large nasal chambers from the pharyngeal and oral cavities is called the *velopharyngeal port* because it lies between the velum and the walls of the pharynx. It can be closed by elevating and backing the velum until it approximates the posterior pharyngeal wall.

The levator palatini is the muscle primarily responsible for closing the velopharyngeal port. This paired muscle arises from the petrous portion of the temporal bone and from the lower part of the eustachian tube cartilage. It courses down and forward, curving medially from each side to enter the soft palate anterior to the uvula. The fibers from each side intermingle and form the middle of the soft palate (Fig. 6.3). The muscle fibers are positioned like a sling originating at the upper back part of the nasopharynx and running down and forward into the soft palate. The angle of insertion of the levator palatini enables it, on contraction, to elevate and retract the soft palate, closing the entrance to the nasal cavities. Electromyographic investigations by Lubker (1968),

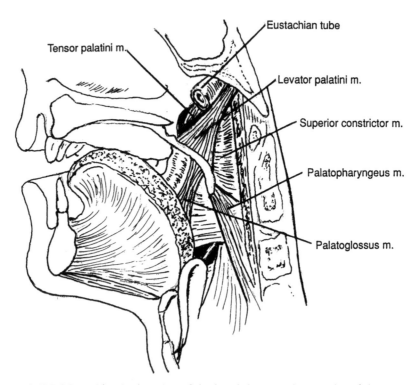

**FIGURE 6.3** Midsagittal section of the head showing the muscles of the pharyngeal port. The palatopharyngeus muscle, not discussed in the text, forms the bulk of the posterior faucial pillar. It is active in reducing pharyngeal size for low vowels and in assisting in velopharyngeal closure.

Fritzell (1969), and Bell-Berti (1973) have demonstrated the importance of levator palatini activity as the prime agent for velopharyngeal closure. Cinefluorographic studies by Moll and others (1971), along with fiberoptic studies by Bell-Berti and her colleagues (1975), have provided data that relate velar movement to muscle activity. (See Chapter 14 for descriptions of research techniques using electromyography [EMG] and fiberoptic imaging.)

Pharyngeal wall movement normally accompanies velopharyngeal closure to form a tighter seal at the port, but it is not clear whether that movement is a consequence of levator palatini activity or contraction of the pharyngeal constrictor muscles.

Innervation of the levator palatini muscles is by the *pharyngeal plexus*, a group of neurons formed from the accessory (eleventh cranial) nerve (which supplies most of the motor innervation), the vagus (tenth cranial) nerve, and the sensory fibers from the glossopharyngeal (ninth cranial) nerve.

The velum, or soft palate, is coupled to the tongue by a muscle confusingly termed the *palatoglossus* muscle in some references and the *glossopalatine* muscle in others. The *anterior faucial pillars*, which one can observe in an open mouth (Fig. 6.4), are made up of the palatoglossus muscle fibers. Because the palatoglossus muscle arises from the transverse muscle fibers within the back of the tongue, ascending to the soft palate on each side to form each anterior faucial pillar, contraction can either lower the palate or elevate the sides and back of the tongue. It is active for some speakers for the tongue elevation required for production of velar consonants /k/ and /g/ and perhaps for lowering the soft palate for /m/, /n/, and /ŋ/.

The uvula possesses its own musculature (the *uvular* muscle) and may add thickness to the velum in closure. The *tensor palatini* muscle does not contribute to velopharyngeal closure, but it is active in opening the eustachian tube leading to the middle ear.

The degree of constriction or closure of the velopharyngeal mechanism varies ac-

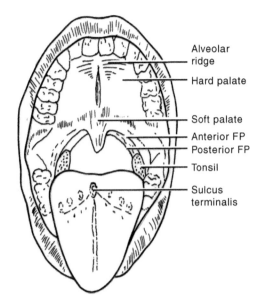

**FIGURE 6.4** Structures of the oral cavity. The uvula can be seen at the rear of the soft palate. FP, faucial pillar.

cording to phonetic context, from the low position typical for nasals to the intermediate positions typical for low vowels to the more nearly closed positions typical for high vowels to the highest positions typical for oral consonants. The high vowels, /i/ and /u/, as in "see" and "Sue," are accompanied by a higher velum than are the low vowels /ɑ/ and /æ/ as in "hot" and "hat." Maximum velar elevation and backing, needed to achieve the tightest seal, occur during the articulation of oral consonants, especially stops and affricates, which require a complete cessation of airflow through the mouth and nose, and fricatives, which require substantial intraoral air pressure (air pressure within the oral cavity). Leakage of air into the nasal cavities could, depending on its degree, make it impossible to produce stops and fricatives acceptably.

In general, then, the levator palatini is least active for nasal consonants and most active in a sequence of a nasal consonant followed by an oral consonant that demands high intraoral pressure. A general rule is that when the velum comes within 2 mm of the pharyngeal wall (producing an open area of about 20 mm$^2$), there is no apparent nasality. A wider opening produces nasal resonance, and speech is definitely perceived as nasal if the velopharyngeal port attains an opening of 5 mm (an area of 50 mm$^2$).

Velar height also plays an important role in adjusting the volume, and thereby the pressure, within the cavities above the larynx. This adjustment is used to facilitate the voiced–voiceless distinction in consonant production. You will recall that to maintain vocal fold vibration, pressure below the vocal folds (subglottal pressure) must exceed the pressure above the vocal folds (supraglottal pressure). This pressure drop across the glottis is difficult to maintain during voiced stops, for the very act of stopping the airstream creates a sudden buildup of supraglottal air pressure that will eventually eliminate the pressure difference across the vocal folds. Raising the velum to its maximum height may create a brief enlargement of the supraglottal volume during voiced stop production, reducing the supraglottal pressure and permitting phonation to continue.

Bell-Berti reports electromyographic findings indicating that speakers vary in their method of enlarging the supraglottal space. Some speakers rely more on elevating the velum, others on relaxing the constrictor muscles or lowering the larynx. This is another example of alternative articulatory strategies leading to the same result, in this case, the maintenance of phonation. The role of the velum in enlarging the supraglottal space will be discussed further, when we consider the production of stop consonants later in this chapter.

### Production of Nasal Consonants

Nasal resonance is mandatory for the production of /m/, /n/, and /ŋ/ in English, so the velum must be low, leaving the entrance to the nasal cavities open. Simultaneously, the oral cavity is occluded in one of three ways. For /m/, the lips are brought together by the orbicularis oris muscles, innervated by the facial (seventh cranial) nerve. The sound from the vocal folds is thus resonated not only in the pharyngeal cavity and in the dead-end of the closed oral cavity but also in the spacious chambers of the nasal cavities. The alveolar nasal /n/, the palatal–velar nasal /ŋ/, and the bilabial nasal /m/ are produced in much the same way except for the differences in the place of the occlusion in the oral cavity. For /n/, the blade or tip of the tongue touches the upper alveolar ridge, with the anterior sides of the tongue touching the upper molars. For /ŋ/, the tongue dorsum touches the posterior part of the hard palate or the anterior part of the soft palate, allowing much less of the oral cavity to resonate as a side branch of the vocal tract. For /m/, oral closure is produced by bringing the lips together. Produce the nasal consonants /m/, /n/, and /ŋ/ in the words "some," "sun," and "sung," one after another, to feel the place of occlusion move back in the mouth from labial to alveolar to palatal–velar. As we shall see, the places of articulation of nasals are essentially the same as those for the stop consonants.

The addition of the nasal branches to the vocal tract creates a larger, longer resonator. We know that the longer the resonator, the lower the frequencies to which it naturally responds. Fujimura (1962) describes the acoustic result of closing the oral cavity while the velum is low as the addition of a characteristic nasal "murmur." This murmur, or formant, lies within the 200- to 300-Hz range for an adult male's tract. It is a bit lower in frequency for [m] than for [n], and lower for [n] than for [ŋ] because the volume of the oral cavity progressively decreases as the location of the articulatory closure moves back in the mouth.

Acoustically, nasal consonants are relatively weak sounds for several reasons. First of all, their articulation creates *antiresonances* within the vocal tract. Antiresonances are, as the term implies, frequency regions in which the amplitudes of the source components are severely attenuated. Although vowels and diphthongs also display antiresonances as troughs between resonance peaks in spectra (Figs. 5.16 and 5.17), their effects are generally much more marked in consonants. This is so because consonants are

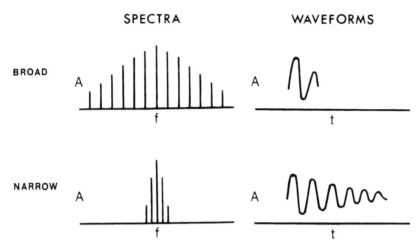

**FIGURE 6.5** Waveforms and spectra of broadly and narrowly tuned resonators. Damping occurs more rapidly for a broadly than a narrowly tuned resonator.

articulated with more severe constrictions and occlusions than vowels. Because all of the nasal consonants are produced with a complete occlusion of the oral cavity, we are not surprised to find antiresonances in their spectra. Resonances and antiresonances can affect each other in a number of ways. For example, if they are close enough in frequency, they can cancel each other. Sometimes a narrow antiresonance in the midst of a broad resonance makes one formant appear to be two when seen in spectrograms.

The elongation of the vocal tract caused by the opening of the velopharyngeal port is another cause of relatively weak intensity of the nasal sounds. The elongated tract results in a broader band of frequency response, and, as you will recall, broadly tuned resonators are more highly damped than narrowly tuned ones (Fig. 6.5). The principal effect, in the case of the nasals, is the creation of antiresonances that cause attenuation of their higher formants relative to those of neighboring vowels.

Antiresonances can also be attributed to the anatomy of the nasal resonator and to the articulation of the nasal consonants. For example, nasals suffer a loss in intensity because sound is absorbed by the soft walls and convolutions within the nasal cavities. The mucous membrane-covered conchae absorb

sound energy like acoustic tiles in a sound-treated room. In addition, because the oral cavity is completely occluded, all of the airflow must be emitted through the nostrils, which do not radiate sound efficiently because of their relatively small openings. Even the hair and the mucous membranes within the nostrils account for a measure of sound attenuation.

The frequency ranges for the antiresonances associated with [m], [n], and [ŋ] vary with the place of articulation and thus with the size of the occluded oral cavity, which acts as an acoustic dead-end. The labial nasal consonant [m] is characterized by an antiresonance lower (in the 500- to 1,500-Hz range) than that for [n] (around 2,000 to 3,000 Hz) or for [ŋ] (above 3,000 Hz). A second antiresonance in the area of 600 Hz for a male tract seems to be consistent regardless of the place of articulation. Figure 6.6 shows the usual formants for [i], which fade for the nasals. Note the added nasal murmur for [m] and [n].

## Nonresonant Consonants I: The Fricatives

The sounds we have been considering thus far, the semivowels and the nasals, are characterized in their articulations by a

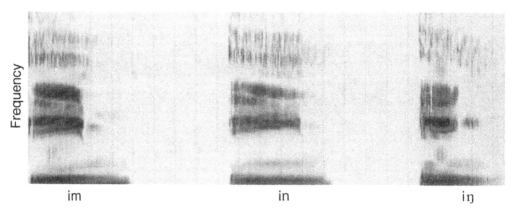

im                          in                          iŋ

**FIGURE 6.6** Spectrogram of [im], [in], and [iŋ]. Formants lose intensity during the nasal. (Digital spectrogram courtesy of Kay Elemetrics.)

relatively free flow of air. Acoustically, they are characterized by formant structure, which is why they are called resonant consonants. We now turn our attention to the nonresonant consonants: the fricatives, stops, and affricates. These sounds are characterized by a much more restricted airflow than the semivowels and nasals. Acoustically, they display little or nothing of the sort of formant structure we have observed in the vowels and resonant consonants.

The obstructions to the airflow in the nonresonant consonants are caused by the articulators forming constrictions and occlusions within the vocal tract that generate aperiodicity (noise) as the airflow passes through them. This aperiodic source of sound is resonated in the tract in much the same way as the periodic source produced by phonation. The most effective resonators for noise sources are those immediately anterior to the constrictions and occlusions that produce them.

The presence of audible noise in the nonresonant consonants accounts for another difference between them and the resonant consonants and vowels. In most languages, including English, resonant consonants and vowels are classified as voiced sounds. Phonologically voiceless vowels, semivowels, and nasals are the exception rather than the rule. There is a practical reason for this: without a periodic source,

many of the resonant sounds would be inaudible at any appreciable distance from a speaker. You can test this by whispering any of the nasals. A voiceless /m/, for instance, is nothing more than an exhalation through the nose.

In the case of the nonresonant consonants, however, noise in the speech signal makes the sounds audible whether or not phonation accompanies their articulation. This creates the possibility of using a single articulation to produce two distinctive speech sounds, one phonated (voiced) and the other unphonated (voiceless). For example, if you articulate the sounds /f/ and /v/ in isolation, you will notice that they share the same labiodental articulation; they are differentiated only by the presence of phonation during the production of /v/ and the absence of phonation during the production of /f/. Pairs of consonant sounds that differ only with regard to their voicing classification are called *cognates*.

The aperiodic source that marks fricatives is created in the vocal tract by sending the breath stream (either phonated or unphonated) through constrictions formed in the tract. The airflow must be strong enough and the constriction narrow enough to make the airflow turbulent, creating frication (noisy random vibrations). The fricative sounds are thus produced by compressing a continuous flow of air through a constriction

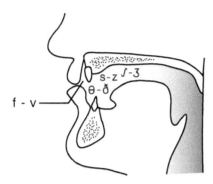

**FIGURE 6.7**  Place of articulation for the fricatives of American English: labiodental, linguadental, alveolar, and palatal (postalveolar).

formed by closely approximating two articulators.

In English, these constrictions are formed at four primary places of articulation: labiodental, linguadental, alveolar, and postalveolar (the front of the hard palate). Figure 6.7 schematizes the four constriction sites. If the glottis is open, the airstream is made audible only at the point of constriction, but if the glottis is closed with the vocal folds vibrating, the result is two sound sources, the periodic sound of phonation and the aperiodic sound of the airstream passing through the constriction.

To develop enough air pressure in the oral cavity to produce noise, the levator palatini muscle must contract, closing the velopharyngeal port sufficiently to avoid a significant flow of air into the nasal cavity. This is an essential aspect of articulation of all nonresonant consonants.

The labiodental fricatives, /f/ (voiceless) and /v/ (voiced), as in "fan" and "van," are formed by bringing the lower lip close to the inferior edges of the upper central incisors. This requires contraction of several muscles in the lower part of the face (especially the inferior orbicularis oris), which are innervated by the facial (seventh cranial) nerve. The linguadental fricatives /θ/ (voiceless) and /ð/ (voiced), as in "*th*igh" and "*th*y," are formed by approximation of the tip of the tongue with the upper incisors. This strategy is not

much different from that used for the labiodentals, but the articulation is accomplished by the muscles of the tongue, with the superior longitudinal muscle, innervated by the hypoglossal (twelfth cranial) nerve, playing a primary role. Because the labiodental and linguadental fricatives are similar in production, they are also similar in their acoustic properties, as we shall see shortly.

The alveolar /s/ and /z/ and the postalveolar /ʃ/ and /ʒ/ fricatives are produced a bit differently, and their distinctive hissing, shushing quality has earned them a subtitle among fricatives: the *sibilants*. Consider the production of [s] (voiceless) and [z] (voiced) as in "Sue" and "zoo." The constriction is formed between the alveolar ridge and the tongue, but speakers vary in which part of the tongue is elevated. Many speakers form the constriction between the tip of the tongue and the alveolar ridge (a *high-point* /s/), whereas others tuck the tip down behind the lower incisors, forming the constriction between the blade of the tongue and the alveolar ridge (a *low-point* /s/).

For [s] and [z], a groove is formed along the tongue midline to channel the airstream. This is accomplished by raising the lateral edges of the tongue to the medial edges of the upper teeth while depressing the center of the tongue. The seal between the edges of the tongue and the teeth is, in any case, essential to prevent the airstream from passing over the sides of the tongue, which would produce a lateral lisp. A second constriction is important to the production of the alveolar fricatives: the opening between the upper and lower incisors must be narrow so that the airstream is directed over the edges of the teeth, creating turbulent airflow behind the teeth. The difficulties in producing /s/ and /z/ for someone who has an open bite or is missing front teeth demonstrate the importance of this second constriction.

The muscle groups implicated in creating the narrow space between the incisors are those of the jaw and tongue. Depending, of course, on the jaw and tongue positions at the onset of motor activity for /s/ or /z/, the jaw

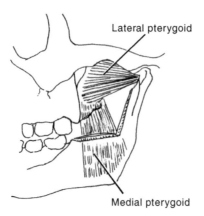

**FIGURE 6.8** The lateral and medial pterygoid muscles in lateral view. The medial pterygoid raises the jaw in speech. The lateral pterygoid has two portions with different functions: the superior part elevates the jaw, and the inferior part lowers the jaw, according to Tuller, Harris, and Gross (1981).

closers, principally the *medial pterygoid* muscle (Fig. 6.8), innervated by the mandibular branch of the trigeminal (fifth cranial) nerve, and tongue elevators (genioglossus and geniohyoid muscles), are more or less active. The pattern of activity within the intrinsic muscles of the tongue also varies with the individual methods of forming the alveolar constriction. Speakers who produce a high-point /s/ or /z/ evidence more activity in the superior longitudinal muscle, whereas those producing low-point sounds show active contraction of the inferior longitudinal muscle.

The articulation of postalveolar /ʃ/ (voiceless) and /ʒ/ (voiced), as in "shoe" and "leisure," although similar in several respects to /s/ and /z/, display some differences. The constriction is made a bit farther back, in the postalveolar area, and the midline groove is considerably shallower than for /s/ and /z/. In addition, the lips may be somewhat rounded and protruded. Lip rounding may also accompany the production of /s/ and /z/ but is far more common for /ʃ/ and /ʒ/. You can gauge the degree of similarity between the two sets of sibilants by producing a lip-rounded [s] and slowly retracting

your tongue until you hear [ʃ]. Because of the similarity in articulation, some speakers may substitute the postalveolar fricatives for the alveolar fricatives. The alveolar constriction for /s/ averages about 1 mm and the incisor constriction about 2 to 3 mm, according to radiographic studies. A wide range of constrictions larger than those for /s/ will result in /ʃ/-type sounds. It is therefore not surprising that the prevailing substitution is /ʃ/ and /ʒ/ in place of /s/ and /z/ and not the other way around.

Another fricative fits less neatly into the scheme of articulatory phonetics. The *aspirate* /h/ is a fricative with the constriction in the larynx at the glottis. It is usually voiceless, as in "hat," but can be voiced when embedded between phonated sounds, as in "ahead," particularly when the syllable following the voiced /h/ is more heavily stressed than the syllable preceding it. The only required movement is the approximation of the vocal folds, controlled by the laryngeal adductors and abductors. The vocal tract takes the shape of whatever vowel is to follow. During the production of the [h] in "heat" and "hot," the vocal tract takes the shape of [i] and [ɑ], respectively, which has caused some phoneticians to characterize /h/ as a voiceless vowel.

Fricatives are *continuants*. Unlike stops, they can be prolonged. In common with all speech sounds, fricatives are the product of a sound source (sometimes two sources) modified by a resonator and by the effect of the sound radiating at the mouth opening. The fricative noise originates at the articulatory constriction. Research has shown that the spectrum of the fricative sound at the lips is determined largely by the resonant characteristics of the constriction and portion of the vocal tract anterior to the noise source. Figure 6.9 shows sound spectrograms of the fricatives. The bands of noise in these spectrograms have been enhanced to make them easily visible. Typically, however, fricative energy is very low in intensity for /f/, /v/, /θ/, and /ð/, mainly because there is no appreciable resonating cavity anterior to the point

Frequency in kHz

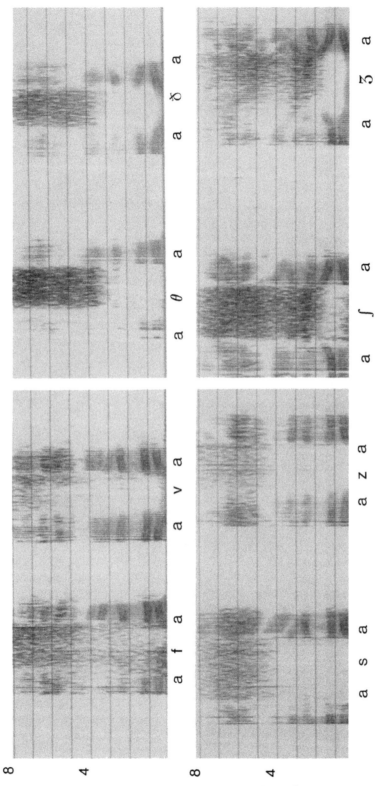

**FIGURE 6.9** Sound spectrograms of the fricatives. (Digital spectrograms courtesy of Kay Elemetrics.)

of constriction. Despite the low level of energy, the frequency band is broad. A narrower band of high-frequency, high-energy noise characterizes the alveolar fricatives /s/ and /z/. Most of the sound energy for /s/ is above 4 kHz, whereas for /ʃ/ it is around 2,000 Hz and above for a male speaker. Because the point of articulation for /ʃ/ is farther back in the mouth than for /s/, the resonating cavity anterior to it is longer than that for /s/, resulting in its lower frequencies. The lip rounding and protrusion that are more usually associated with /ʃ/ also lengthen the front cavity and contribute to its lower resonant frequency. This acoustic effect of lip posture is much the same as we have seen for the back vowels.

As an example of the source–filter account of consonant production, let us detail the acoustic production of /s/ much as we did with /i/, /ɑ/, and /u/ for the vowels. The resonances for /s/ are derived from the natural resonant frequency of the constriction and the natural resonant frequency of the cavity in front of the constriction. Figure 6.10 shows

a vocal tract configuration appropriate for /s/ production. The narrow constriction resonates like a tube open at both ends in which the lowest resonant frequency has a wavelength ($\lambda$) twice the length of the tube. Using the measurements given above for the alveolar constriction, we can calculate that the natural resonant frequency for such a tube would be about 6,800 Hz.

$$f = \text{velocity of sound}/\lambda \text{ (wavelength)}$$
$$= 34{,}400 \text{ cm/s}/5 = 6{,}880 \text{ Hz}$$

The source of the fricative noise is at the anterior edge of the constriction. The air-filled cavity in front of the noise source can be likened to a tube closed at one end, because the constriction is extremely narrow at the source. Because tubes closed at one end and open at the other are quarter-wave resonators rather than half-wave resonators, the resonance for the anterior cavity approximates 8,600 Hz.

$$f = \text{Velocity}/\lambda = 34{,}400 \text{ cm/s}/4 \text{ (1 cm)}$$
$$= 8{,}600 \text{ Hz}$$

Because of the narrowness of the constriction, the back cavity resonances are severely attenuated and therefore not perceptually salient. Thus, spectrograms generally show little energy below 4,000 Hz. The resonances that would have been produced below 4 kHz have been attenuated by the back cavity antiresonances. We have seen that most of the perceptually significant energy for /s/ lies above 4,000 Hz. For /ʃ/, the perceptually significant energy lies above 2,000 Hz.

Uldall (1964) reported that when /s/ precedes a voiceless stop (/p/, /t/, or /k/, as in "spill," "still," or "skill"), the lower border of the fricative noise changes, reflecting vocal tract adjustments being made during the fricative. The border lowers in frequency as the tract approaches labial closure (/sp/), increases in frequency during the approach to alveolar stops (/st/), and remains stable for the palatal–velar stop (/sk/).

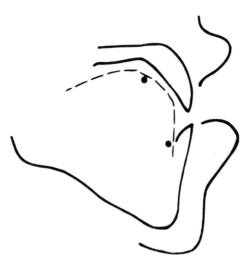

**FIGURE 6.10** Tracing made from a lateral radiograph of the vocal tract in position for [s] production. The *black dots* represent lead pellets. Movements of the tongue were analyzed by following the movements of the pellets from frame to frame.

## Nonresonant Consonants II: The Stops

We turn now to the class of sounds articulated with the greatest degree of obstruction to the breath stream: the stop consonants, /p/, /t/, and /k/ (voiceless) and /b/, /d/, and /g/ (voiced). The term "stop" is an apt designation because the essential distinguishing characteristic of these sounds is the momentary cessation of emitted airflow caused by the complete occlusion of the vocal tract.

The articulators form the occlusion at the end of what is usually called the "closing phase" of stop formation. In fact, two simultaneous occlusions are essential for each of the six stop-consonant phonemes. One is the velopharyngeal closure that seals off the nasal cavities from the rest of the vocal tract and the other is an occlusion formed by the lips or tongue within the oral cavity. The locations of the oral occlusions are identical to those made for the nasals: bilabial for /p/ and /b/, lingua-alveolar for /t/ and /d/, and linguapalatal/velar for /k/ and /g/ (Fig. 6.11).

The occlusions are maintained throughout the second phase of stop articulation, the "hold" or "closure" phase, during which they prevent air from flowing out of the vocal tract, resulting in the increase in intraoral pressure necessary to produce the stop consonants.

The final phase in most stop articulations is the "release." In this phase, one of the two occlusions, usually the oral occlusion, is broken, releasing the pent-up air pressure and allowing the resumption of airflow out of the vocal tract. It is also possible to release a stop by lowering the velum. This strategy, called nasal release, is normally used when a stop is followed by a *homorganic* nasal (one with the same place of articulation as the stop). The most obvious occurrence of nasal release is when the nasal is syllabic, as in a word such as "hidden" ([hɪdn̩]). If you say this word slowly, consciously maintaining the alveolar contact for the /d/ until you hear the /n/, you should be able to sense the movement of the velum that releases the stop.

When stops are orally released, there is an audible burst of noise caused by the outward rush of the air that was blocked by the occlusion. This burst of noise, which is part of the release phase, is another example of an aperiodic sound source produced in the supraglottal vocal tract. It is analogous to the frication generated in the production of fricatives, but it differs from frication in that it is transient rather than prolongable. Stops, then, differ from all other sounds we have discussed thus far in that they are not continuants.

Because stop articulation usually ends with the release of a transient burst of noise, the term *plosive* is sometimes used as a label for this class of sounds. We have avoided using the label "plosive" because the release phase of articulation is omitted in certain phonetic contexts. Release does not usually occur, for instance, when two homorganic stop sounds occur in sequence, as in "hot dog." In this context, the /t/ closure is maintained unbroken and serves for the /d/ closure as well. It is thus the /d/, not the /t/, that is released. Many phoneticians have noted that stops in absolute final position are often unreleased in English, although some recent research has suggested that release, even if not audible, is more likely to occur than not. It is certainly possible to maintain the closure for the final bilabial and alveolar stops in sentences such as "He worked in his lab" and "She wore a hat." It is much less likely,

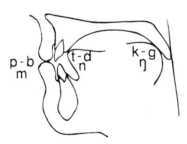

**FIGURE 6.11**  The place of articulation for bilabial, alveolar, and palatal–velar stops and nasals.

however, that the final velar stop in "They ate some cake" will be unreleased.

The muscular activity underlying the articulation of stops obviously varies considerably from one place of articulation to another, with the exception of that for the velopharyngeal closure that accompanies each of the sounds. Activity of the orbicularis oris and other facial muscles contributes to labial closure for /p/ and /b/. The alveolar stop /t/ and its voiced cognate /d/ are produced by moving the tip or blade of the tongue forward and up to contact the alveolar ridge. The superior longitudinal muscle, fibers of which course under the superior surface of the tongue from front to back, aids in producing this closure of the oral cavity. It, like the other tongue muscles, is innervated by the hypoglossal (twelfth cranial) nerve. Closure for /k/ and /g/ results from elevating the dorsum of the tongue so that it comes in contact with the back of the hard palate or with the velum. The place of articulation often depends on the context. For example, the place of articulation for the /k/ preceding the front vowel /i/ in "keep" is farther forward than for the /k/ preceding the back vowel /u/ in "coop." Thus, although /k/, /g/, and /ŋ/ are often classified as velar consonants, palatal–velar is sometimes a more accurate description. The styloglossus and palatoglossus muscles are instrumental in the tongue backing and elevation necessary for this closure. The mylohyoid muscle (Fig. 6.12), a flat trough-like muscle attached to the inner sides of the mandible, serves as the floor of the oral cavity. This muscle is innervated by the motor component of the mylohyoid branch of the trigeminal (fifth cranial) nerve, which is normally considered to be a sensory nerve serving the facial area. Contraction of the mylohyoid fibers elevates the floor of the oral cavity, assisting in raising the heavy back of the tongue for /k/, /g/, and /ŋ/.

There is a seventh stop, called the glottal stop ([ʔ]), that occurs with some frequency in English. Unlike the other stop sounds, the glottal stop is not classified as a phoneme of English. In American English, the glottal stop

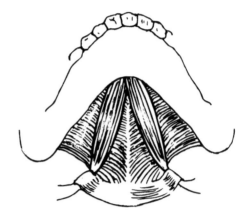

**FIGURE 6.12** The mylohyoid muscles form the floor of the mouth and contract to help elevate the tongue. The paired muscles lying below the mylohyoids are the anterior bellies of the digastric muscle, which act in lowering the jaw.

is sometimes used to initiate vowels, as we mentioned earlier in our discussion of glottal attack in the section on phonation. The sound also has currency as an allophone of /t/ or /d/ in certain dialects. For instance, it is the sound some New Yorkers substitute for the /t/ in "bottle," [baʔl̩], and for the /d/ in "wouldn't" [wʊʔn̩t]. Speakers of some British dialects, such as Cockney, commonly use the glottal stop as a substitute for all of the stop consonants.

The glottal stop, as its name indicates, is articulated at the glottis by tightly approximating the vocal folds. Although the folds are the articulators for this sound, they do not vibrate during its production, and so it is classified as voiceless. The folds behave analogously to the lips and tongue in the production of the oral stops, forming an occlusion, holding it, and then releasing the airstream when they are abducted. Because the occlusion is below the level of the velopharyngeal port, velopharyngeal closure is irrelevant to its production, although it normally occurs as it does in the articulation of the other stops.

We now turn our attention to the acoustic features that characterize stop production. Let us first consider those features that are a function of stop manner of articulation. There are four of these. The first and most pervasive is what is usually termed a "silent gap." This period of silence is a result of the "hold" period in articulation, during which there is no flow of air out of the vocal tract. In point of fact, the silent gap is not always literally silent. In the cases of the voiced stops, /b/, /d/, and /g/, a low-intensity harmonic, the fundamental frequency ($f_o$), may run through all or part of the duration of the stop closure. Nonetheless, the term "silent gap" is often used to describe the closure for all of the stop consonants. In any case, the gap is always devoid of appreciable formant structure or noise. Figure 6.13 shows examples of the silent gaps, both those that are truly silent and those in which an $f_o$ is evident (at the baselines of the spectrograms of /b/, /d/, and /g/).

The second acoustic feature associated with stop production is a noise burst at the moment of release. This burst, which appears in spectrograms (Fig. 6.13) as a vertical spike following the silent gap, is somewhat more intense and thus more conspicuous for the voiceless than for the voiced stops. Release bursts are very brief (10 to 35 ms) but often cover a broad range of frequencies with varying intensity. The frequencies at which the bursts are most intense are relevant to the place of articulation and will be considered below.

A third identifying acoustic feature is the speed with which the acoustic signal attains maximum intensity (for syllable-initial stops) or falls to minimum intensity (for syllable-final stops). These are called, respectively, *rise time* and *fall time*. Rise and fall times are both very rapid for stops, compared with other consonants. The reason for this is the relatively rapid opening and closing gestures associated with stop articulation. The increased air pressure behind the point of occlusion, when it is released, also contributes to the rapid rise time of stops in syllable-initial position.

The final identifying acoustic feature of stop manner is the change in the first for-mant frequency that occurs as the vocal tract changes shape after the release of syllable-initial stops and before the occlusion is completed for syllable-final stops. The first formant rises rapidly after the release of initial stops and falls rapidly before completion of the closure for the final stops. There is an articulatory basis for this acoustic feature, just as there is for all the acoustic features of speech sounds: You will recall that the frequency of the first formant is positively correlated with the size of mouth opening. This means that the $F_1$ frequency should be minimal during stop articulation, as the oral cavity is completely occluded. Opening the tract raises the frequency of $F_1$ in the case of initial stops, and closing the tract will force the frequency down in the case of final stops. The degree of rise or fall varies considerably, depending on the $F_1$ frequency of the neighboring sounds. For example, the increase or decrease in $F_1$ is much greater when a stop precedes or follows a vowel such as /ɑ/, which has a high first formant frequency, than when it precedes or follows a vowel with a low first formant frequency, such as /i/.

Two acoustic features are associated with the place of articulation of stop consonants. We have mentioned that the most intense frequency of the transient burst of noise associated with stop release is a function of the point in the oral cavity where the occlusion is made. The bursts of the labial stops, /p/ and /b/, generally exhibit peaks in their spectra at low frequencies, around 600 Hz and below. The high frequencies (around 3,000 Hz) are characteristically most intense in the spectra of the bursts of the alveolar stops, /t/ and /d/. The palatal–velar stops, /k/ and /g/, present a more variable picture: Spectral peaks for the bursts are linked to the $F_2$ frequency of the vowel after the stop. For the velars, the intense portion of the burst usually extends upward a few hundred hertz from the frequency of the second formant of the adjacent vowel.

A second acoustic feature associated with the place of articulation is the direction of

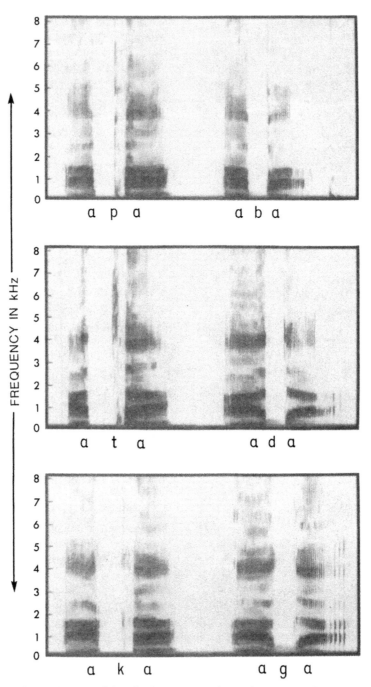

**FIGURE 6.13**   Wideband spectrograms of vowel–stop–vowel
disyllables. Note the truly silent gap in the closure for /ptk/ and the
voicing (phonation) during the closure for /bdg/. Each closure is
followed by a characteristic burst of transient noise as the tongue
releases the air trapped behind the closure at the alveolar ridge.

frequency change of the second formant of the vowel following or preceding a stop. During the formation (closing phase) of a stop occlusion and just after an occlusion is released, the rapid movements of the articulators cause sudden changes in the resonance peaks of the vocal tract. We have already discussed such changes in connection with the feature of $F_1$ change associated with stop manner. Because these changes in formant frequencies occur during the transition from one speech sound to another, they are referred to as *formant transitions*.

You will recall that in our discussion of vowels we indicated that the frequency of $F_2$ was correlated with the length of the front cavity. In general, this correlation holds for the stops, and so $F_2$ is a reflection of the movement of the tongue or lips from or to a place of stop occlusion. Unfortunately, because the destination (for prevocalic stops) or origin (for postvocalic stops) of $F_2$ varies with the neighboring vowel, there is no simple way of associating a particular direction or degree of transition change with a particular place of articulation. We consider these transitions more fully in the discussion of speech perception in Chapter 10.

There remains the topic of the acoustic features that are associated with the voicing classes of stop consonants. Recall that the stops of English can be grouped into cognate pairs by the place of articulation (/p-b/, /t-d/, /k-g/), with one member of each pair being classified as voiceless (/p/, /t/, or /k/) and the other as voiced (/b/, /d/, or /g/). In many contexts, such as the intervocalic context shown in Figure 6.13, this simply means that phonation continues throughout the period of articulatory closure for /b/, /d/, and /g/ and ceases during the closure for /p/, /t/, and /k/—a classic example of the voiced–voiceless difference. We should point out that, although no air is emitted *from* the vocal tract during the closure phase of stops, it is still possible for air to flow *within* the tract. Thus, in the case of intervocalic /b/, /d/, and /g/, when the vocal folds are adducted, a pressure difference can be created across the glottis and the vocal folds can be set into vibration for a brief period of time.

In other contexts, however, the difference between the members of the cognate pairs is less straightforward. For instance, in stops in syllable-initial position before a vowel or resonant consonant, speakers of English do not normally phonate during the closures of either /p/, /t/, and /k/ or /b/, /d/, and /g/. In this context, the opposition between the two sets of stops is maintained by a difference in the timing of the onset of phonation relative to the release burst of the stop: Phonation for /b/, /d/, and /g/ begins at or very shortly after stop release, whereas there is a delay of at least 50 ms before phonation begins after the release of /p/, /t/, and /k/. This relative timing of stop release and the initiation of phonation has been termed *voice onset time (VOT)* by Lisker and Abramson (1964). On wideband spectrograms VOT is measured in milliseconds as the duration between the vertical spike marking the transient burst of stop release and the first vocal pulse that can be observed at the baseline. If the onset of phonation follows stop release, VOT values are positive; if voicing onset precedes stop release, VOT values are negative. Thus, if phonation begins 75 ms after stop release, the VOT value is given as +75; if phonation onset occurs 85 ms before stop release, the VOT is −85.

VOT, then, can be understood as an acoustic measurement, but, as always, one that is the result of a coordinated articulatory strategy. Let us inspect that strategy. Figure 6.14 shows both labial and glottal adjustments used to produce initial prevocalic /p/ and /b/ in English. Notice that at the moment of labial occlusion, the vocal folds have begun to adduct for /b/. Adduction continues during the hold period, so that by the time the /b/ is released, the folds are in phonatory position, ready to vibrate. This accounts for the low, positive VOT values (between 0 and 10 ms) that characterize /b/.

In contrast, the folds do not begin to adduct for /p/ until sometime during the hold period, so that at the moment of stop release,

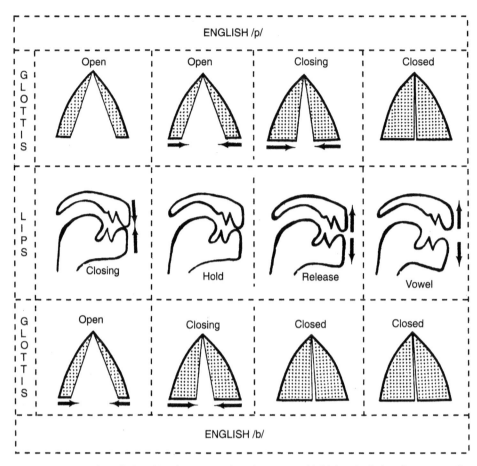

**FIGURE 6.14** The relationships between glottal states and labial articulation for prevocalic /p/ and /b/ in English.

the glottis is still partially open. Vocal fold adduction is not complete until sometime after the release of the stop, during the articulation of the following vowel. This accounts for the long positive VOT values (about +60 to +70 ms or more) that characterize /p/. It also accounts for the presence of another acoustic feature that differentiates the voiced from the voiceless stops: aspiration.

Aspiration, a period of voicelessness after stop release, is associated only with /p/, /t/, and /k/ in English. It is present after those stops because the open glottis at the moment of stop release allows the breath stream to flow freely into the upper vocal tract without generating phonation. The reverse is true for /b/, /d/, and /g/: the closed glottis at the moment of stop release forces the breath stream

to set the vocal folds into vibration and to carry the periodic phonated vibrations into the upper vocal tract. Phonation and aspiration are therefore complementary phenomena in English. The VOT differences between /p/, /t/, and /k/ and /b/, /d/, and /g/ and the presence versus absence of aspiration in those stops are clearly visible in Figure 6.13.

Other languages use different timing contrasts to distinguish between voicing classes of stop consonants. Spanish, Italian, and French /b/, /d/, and /g/, for example, display negative values of VOT. That is, phonation commences during the hold period for the stops because vocal fold adduction begins during the closing phase of stop articulation. This ensures that the folds will be in phonatory position during the hold period,

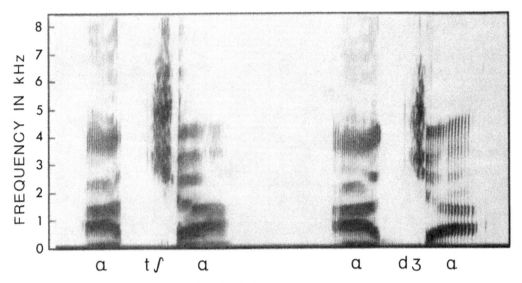

**FIGURE 6.15**  Spectrograms of [atʃa] and [adʒa].

so that phonation can commence. In contrast, the VOT values for /p/, /t/, and /k/ in these languages are much like the values for /b/, /d/, and /g/ in English. In fact, speakers of Spanish, Italian, and French often appear to English-speaking listeners to produce only voiced stops: none of the stops in these languages is significantly aspirated because the glottis is always closed at or very shortly after the moment of stop release and does not allow the free flow of a voiceless breath stream.

It should be clear from our discussion of VOT that differentiating voiced from voiceless stops requires complex and highly coordinated motor activity. The timing of the activity of the abductor and adductor muscles of the larynx must be precise, not only with respect to each other but also with respect to the muscles controlling the articulators of the supraglottal vocal tract.

## Nonresonant Consonants III: The Affricates

English has only two affricates, [tʃ] (voiceless) and [dʒ] (voiced), as in "chair" and "jar." An affricate is simply a stop with a fricative release. An alveolar closure is made for the [t] or [d], and when the speaker releases the clo-

sure, the tongue is retracted to the postalveolar region of the palate and shaped appropriately for the production of sounds that are essentially identical to the fricatives [ʃ] and [ʒ]. The lips are usually rounded slightly during the articulation of the fricative portions of the affricates and often during the stop portions as well. Acoustically, as you would expect, the affricates present a combination of stop and fricative features. Figure 6.15 shows the "silent" gaps of stop closures (both with and without phonation striations at the baseline of the spectrogram for /dʒ/ and /tʃ/, respectively). It also shows the bursts of noise marking stop release and the extended durations of aperiodicity (frication) that are characteristic of fricatives.

## Summary

Now that we have surveyed the consonant sounds of English, it may be helpful to show how they are related to each other as a function of the parameters of production. A traditional way of doing this is to chart the consonants according to the place and manner of articulation (Fig. 6.16). The various places of articulation are conventionally displayed across the top of the chart, with the most anterior articulations (labial) at the left and

| | Both Lips (bilabial) | Lip-Teeth (labio-dental) | Tongue-Teeth (lingua-dental) | Tongue-Ridge (alveolar) | Tongue-Hard Palate (post-alveolar) | Tongue-Blade Palate (palatal) | Tongue-Velum (velar) | Glottis (glottal) |
|---|---|---|---|---|---|---|---|---|
| Stops | p   b | | | t   d | | (k)   (g) | k   g | ? |
| Fricatives | | f   v | θ   ð | s   z | ʃ   ʒ | | | h |
| Affricates | | | | n | tʃ   dʒ | | | |
| Nasals | m | | | ɪ r | | | ŋ | |
| Semivowels | w | | | | r | | j | (w, r) |

**FIGURE 6.16** Classification of the American English consonants. Voiceless consonants appear to the left in each column, voiced consonants to the right. Secondary forms of the same sound are shown in parentheses.

the most posterior articulations (velar, glottal) at the right. The manners of articulation are listed vertically at the left, arranged in either increasing or decreasing order of degree of constriction. Figure 6.16 uses the latter arrangement, beginning at the top with the stops and proceeding to the semivowels.

Peterson and Shoup (1966) have adapted this type of consonant chart in an interesting way, making it a less abstract analog

of the vocal tract. Their adaption includes the places of constriction of the vowels, as well as the consonants, to show how the articulations of consonants and vowels, normally charted separately (Fig. 5.22), are related to each other. Figure 6.17 is an adaptation of their chart from which all non-English sounds have been deleted. The vertical axis represents complete vocal tract closure at the top and proceeds to an open tract at the

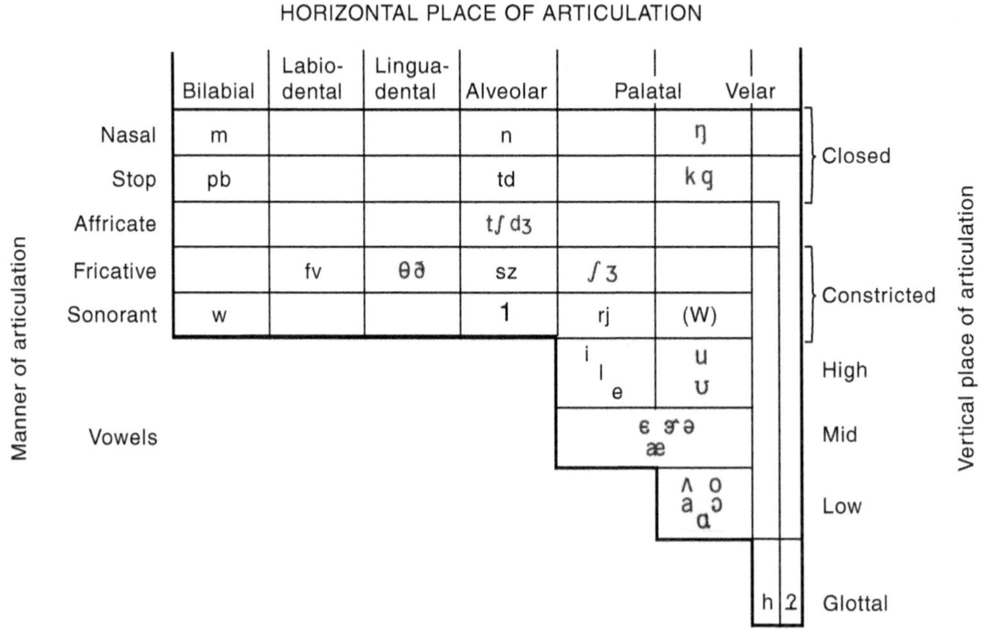

**FIGURE 6.17** Peterson and Shoup's chart for the sounds of American English. (Adapted with permission from Peterson, G. E., and Shoup, J. E., A Physiological Theory of Phonetics. *J. Speech Hear. Res. 9*, 1966, 5–67.)

bottom, with sounds having a common manner of articulation arranged in horizontal rows. For example, the row for stops begins with /p/ and /b/, continues with /t/ and /d/, descends as a column after /k/ and /g/, and ends at the glottal stop. The place of articulation is represented as it was in Figure 6.16. The parameter "vertical place of articulation" at the right of the chart unites the tongue height and manner of articulation description of vowels and consonants.

Charts of this sort serve several purposes. For instance, they remind us that all segmental speech sounds, both consonants and vowels, are produced by a single articulatory system and a single vocal tract. In addition, the systematic relationships among various sounds are easy to discern: the relationship of one sound's place of articulation to those of others as well as the similar pattern of distribution of the places of articulation of stops and nasals. Moreover, inclusion of the vowels reveals that the place of articulation of the "front" vowels is well posterior to the position of the front-articulated consonants and reminds us of the similarities between the high front vowels /i/ and /u/ and the initiation of the glides /j/ and /w/.

## THE EFFECTS OF CONTEXT ON THE PRODUCTION OF SPEECH SOUNDS

Up to this point, we have discussed most speech sounds as if they were produced one at a time, independently of each other. This is not, of course, the case. The sounds of speech occur in context and are affected and altered by neighboring sounds. An understanding of the nature of the alterations caused by context is critical to the understanding of speech because the effects of context influence every aspect of production—muscular activity, articulatory movement, and the acoustic signal. We shall identify two basic types of context effects in this section and will differentiate them from each other on the basis of (1) the number of articulators and (2) the number of speech sounds involved in each effect.

## Assimilation

The most basic type of sound change involves an alteration in the movement of a single articulator. In a sense, the articulator takes a shortcut. Let us consider an example. You intend to say, "Eat the cake." Normally, you articulate /t/ with your tongue tip on your alveolar ridge and /ð/ with your tongue tip against your upper incisors. Articulating this sequence of sounds in the usual way would require that you move the tip of your tongue from one place of articulation to the other. Obviously, it is more efficient for you to place your tongue tip directly on your incisors for the /t/ and to leave it there, in the position required for the following /ð/. In other words, you have created a shortcut, producing what is called a dentalized /t/.

Let us be clear about what has occurred. The fricative sound has influenced its neighbor, /t/, so that the /t/ becomes more like /ð/ in its articulation. We say that the /t/ has been *assimilated* to the place of articulation of the /ð/. Notice that in this example the change is phonetic: from one allophone of the phoneme /t/ (alveolar) to another allophone (dental) of the *same* phoneme. We call this type of assimilation *partial*, as there is no phonemic change.

Radiographic and palatographic studies (see Chapter 14) have provided specific evidence of the effect of articulatory position on articulator movement in partial assimilation: Tongue–palate contact for the [k] in preceding the front vowel in "key" is often farther forward than for the [k] preceding the back vowel in "caught," as the consonant is assimilated to the vowel. MacNeilage (1970) has given a different sort of example: speaking with a pipe clenched between the teeth. Tongue elevation for an alveolar stop would have to assimilate to this higher mandible position compared with the movement required were the mandible lower and the mouth more open for a preceding low vowel, such as /ɑ/. In either case, we would expect that the intended phoneme would be produced, and that the assimilation would then be partial.

Assimilation can, however, involve a change from an allophone of one phoneme to an allophone of a *different* phoneme. We call this type of change *complete* assimilation. Consider the utterance "ten cards." In this context, the alveolar /n/ in "ten" will be articulated with the dorsum of the tongue on the velum, in anticipation of the lingua-velar /k/. But this, of course, will produce the lingua-velar nasal /ŋ/, a different phoneme from the /n/ we normally expect to occur at the end of "ten." The complete assimilation of /n/ to the place of articulation of a following velar stop is one that has occurred many times in the history of English. Words such as "think," "bank," and "anger," although they are all spelled with the letter "n," have been pronounced with the nasal /ŋ/ for hundreds of years.

Assimilations, both complete and partial, can be subclassified in many ways. When a sound is influenced by a following sound, as in the examples we have just considered, *anticipatory* (also called right-to-left) assimilation is the result. When a sound is influenced by a preceding sound, *carryover* (left-to-right) assimilation will occur. Carryover assimilation is exemplified by the voicing class of the plural morpheme after nouns ending in voiced consonants: the voiceless /s/ following the voiceless [t] in "cats" remains an [s], but the plural marker following the [g] in "dogs" is voiced: The phonation for the /g/ is carried over to the plural marker, producing [z].

Assimilations can also be categorized according to the way articulation is affected. We have already seen examples of assimilations of place of articulation ("eat the cake," "ten cards") and voicing ("dogs"). Assimilations of manner of articulation, although less common than the other types, do occasionally occur. The word "educate," once pronounced with a sequence of stop plus glide—/dj/ ([ɛdjuket])—a pronunciation still favored by some educators, is now pronounced almost universally with an affricate ([ɛdʒuket]).

This manner change has occurred because of what was originally an assimilation of place of articulation: the assimilation of the /d/ to the palatal place of articulation of the /j/. The movement of the tongue back toward the palate as the stop was released generated a fricative release and thus resulted in the affricate that we usually hear in this word. This type of assimilation is called *palatalization*.

So far, we have described assimilation only in terms of articulatory movement. Let us turn to muscular activity and acoustics and see how they cause and reflect the effects of assimilation.

On the level of muscle activity, electromyographic recordings associated with a given speech sound vary with phonetic context. MacNeilage and De Clerk (1969) found pervasive influences of adjacent vowels or consonants on the EMG signal associated with a particular speech sound. An example of partial assimilation, drawn from the work of Bell-Berti and Harris (1982), is the activity of the genioglossus muscle, which, you will recall, fronts and elevates the mass of the tongue. Genioglossus muscle activity (Fig. 6.18) was found to be greater for the high vowel [u] following the low vowel [ɑ] than it was following the high vowel [i]: To

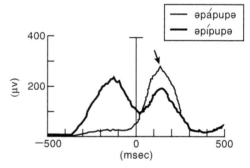

**FIGURE 6.18** Genioglossus muscle activity for [u] after [ɑ] and [i]. The amount of activity is greater after [ɐ] because the tongue must move farther. *Arrow* indicates peak activity for [u]. (Reprinted with permission from Bell-Berti, F., and Harris, K. S., *Some Aspects of Coarticulation.* Leeds, England: VIII International Congress of Phonetic Sciences, Aug. 1975.)

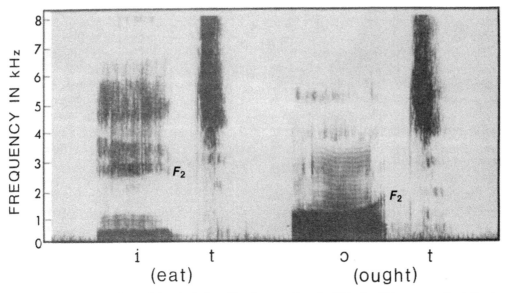

**FIGURE 6.19**  Acoustic partial assimilation. The $F_2$ transition for [t] in "eat" is very small relative to the $F_2$ transition for [t] in "ought".

attain the high back articulatory position for [u], the tongue had to move farther from the low back position for [ɑ] than from the high front position for [i]. We can see, then, that articulatory positions at a given time affect the muscle activity necessary to produce forthcoming movements.

Figure 6.19 shows an acoustic effect of partial assimilation. To produce the [t] closure for the [t] of "eat," a relatively small change in oral cavity shape is made, resulting in a small $F_2$ transition. That is, the tongue does not have to move far to get from its location for the high, front vowel [i] to the location of [t]. In contrast, the [t] closure following the low, back vowel [ɔ] requires a shortening of the vocal tract (which was lengthened for [ɔ]) and an extensive tongue elevation, resulting in a second formant transition that displays an extensive rise in frequency. Thus, the method of producing each [t] has been assimilated to its vowel environment.

Acoustic evidence also exists for the assimilation of vowels caused by a change in the rate of speaking. Faster speaking rates cause the tongue to fall short of its target positions. Lindblom (1963) has provided spectrographic analyses showing that increased

speaking rate neutralizes the formant patterns of vowels, making them more like those of adjacent sounds. Usually, the neutralization is rather subtle, but you can hear the difference between the nonneutralized and neutralized versions of a vowel if you compare the /æ/ in the protest "But you **have**!" with a quickly delivered, "You have **seen** it," with primary stress on "seen."

## Coarticulation

Another kind of phonetic influence is called coarticulation. A strict definition of coarticulation is that two articulators are moving at the same time for different phonemes. This differs from assimilation (one articulator modifying its movements because of context), although these two types of context effect are related. An example of coarticulation is when a speaker, saying "two" [tu], rounds the lips (first articulator) for [u] at the same time that the tongue (second articulator) is approaching or is already in contact with the alveolar ridge for [t].

Coarticulation results because of the temporal overlap between the articulatory gestures for the vowels and the consonants. It has been observed in studies of acoustics, articulatory movement, and muscular activity. Kozhevnikov and Chistovich (1965) found that lip rounding for [u] can start at the beginning of a consonant–consonant–vowel (CCV) syllable if none of the intervening sounds requires a movement that is antagonistic to it. So, for example, a speaker saying the word "stoop" (/stup/) may begin the lip-rounding gesture for /u/ during the production of the word-initial /s/.

Radiographic investigations also present evidence of coarticulation. Perkell (1969) cites an example in which the mandible lowers earlier for the sequence of sounds /n/ + /ɑ/ than for a sequence such as /t/ + /ɑ/. The reason for this is that lowering the mandible during stop production would increase oral cavity size, lowering intraoral air pressure; because stops require high intraoral pressure, mandible lowering is deferred until after the completion of the alveolar closure for /t/. In contrast, because high intraoral air pressure is not needed to produce /n/, the mandible is free to lower before the completion of the alveolar closure.

If an articulator is free to move, it often does. Daniloff and Moll (1968) found that the lips begin to round for /u/ several phones before the vowel. Bell-Berti and Harris found orbicularis oris muscle activity for the /u/ at a relatively fixed time before the vowel sound, during the activity for the consonant or consonant cluster preceding it, but unaffected by the number of consonants intervening.

Öhman's (1966) observations of spectrograms led him to theorize that the tongue may act as three somewhat independent articulators, with the tip, blade, and dorsum coarticulating with each other. Borden and Gay (1979), in a cinefluorographic study, verified this theory with movement data. Whatever part of the tongue was free to lower for /ɑ/ during stop production did lower. If the tip of the tongue was elevated for /t/, the back of the tongue lowered simultaneously for the /ɑ/. If the dorsum was involved with /k/ closure, the front of the tongue got a head start in lowering. Stone (1992) has presented ultrasound and x-ray data showing

that portions of the tongue move independently of each other. The available evidence thus indicates quite strongly that it is possible for parts of the tongue to coarticulate with each other. There are, however, individual differences in the patterns of coarticulation.

Coarticulation and assimilation of one articulatory movement to another are pervasive in running speech. It is what Liberman (1967) has called, in both perception and production of speech, *parallel processing*. The combination of assimilation and coarticulation is what makes speech transmission rapid and efficient. As we shall see in the chapter on speech perception, the extent to which speech sounds are encoded in the acoustic signal depends on such processes as assimilation and coarticulation.

The segmental modifications necessary for rapid transmission should not be confused with the different, but interesting, kinds of sound changes and differences associated with dialects and idiolects. These include deletions, such as the omission of the first [r] in "library," additions such as the intrusive or linking [r] before the "of" in "idea of," and *metathesis* (reversals in the sequencing of sounds), such as [æks] for "ask" or [lɑrnɪks] for "larynx." All sound influences, however, demonstrate that speech sounds are not produced in the same manner as beads are put on a string, one after another with no change in their form regardless of which beads are surrounding them.

It is important to remember this, because in a great deal of our introductory discussion it was necessary to treat phonemes as if they were isolated segments of speech. This mistaken notion is further reinforced when we write or read phonemic transcriptions. Such transcriptions record speech sounds as isolable and permutable segments. Yet we know that phonemes exist as independent units only in our minds and perhaps as symbolic representations on paper in transcriptions. It is our mental ability to segment the unbroken stream of speech that leads us to identify individual speech sounds, assign them to families (phoneme classes), and refer to them as *segmental* phonemes.

# *C*LINICAL NOTE

Two disorders may result from failure to make perceptually acceptable adjustments of the velopharyngeal mechanism: *hypernasality* and *hyponasality*, with too much nasal resonance in the first instance and too little nasal resonance for /m/, /n/, and /ŋ/ in the second instance. The problem of hypernasality is most apparent in speakers who are born with a *cleft palate*, a condition in which part or all of the palate has failed to fuse. Even after surgery to close the palate, the velum may be too small or lack the muscle force to close off the nasal cavities adequately. This condition not only results in too much nasal resonance for the vowels but also prevents the speaker from building up sufficient pressure in the oral cavity for stops and fricatives because of the unchecked escape of air through the nose. Persons with degenerative disorders of the nervous system may also produce inappropriate degrees of nasal resonance for a different reason: muscle weakness in the levator palatini.

Too little nasal resonance often accompanies nasal congestion caused by colds. In some cases, hypernasality and hyponasality occur in the same speaker at different times because both raising and lowering of the velum are variously mistimed in relation to other articulators. People with cerebral palsy sometimes evidence this disorder.

The mistiming of articulator movements is a symptom of many motor speech disorders and is likely to affect the production of any speech sounds, depending on the contexts in which they occur. Good control over interarticulator coordination is especially important for those articulatory maneuvers that are subject to tight timing constraints, such as those we have described with regard to voice onset time (VOT).

Without precise interarticulator timing, a speaker is likely to produce VOT values that deviate from the expected norms. Clinical researchers have, in fact, investigated VOT in a great number of speech disorders that involve poor motor control. Many studies of VOT in stuttering, apraxia, Parkinson's disease, and other disorders have appeared in recent years and continue to appear in the literature with great regularity.

When we know a language, we know which families of sounds contrast with each other. Speakers of English, for example, understand that the family of /p/ sounds contrasts with the family of /t/ sounds in utterances such as "pie" and "tie." In running speech, however, these segments rarely exist independently. Sometimes we use a speech sound alone, as when we exclaim "Oh!" or we quiet someone with "shhh." In utterances such as "pie," however, the production is never accomplished by saying [p] and then quickly saying [aɪ]. If the sounds are produced independently of each other, no matter how quickly the [aɪ] follows the [p], the utterance is not heard as a normal production of [paɪ], because the speaker has not coarticulated, that is, has not produced more than one phoneme at the same time. In a coarticulated production of "pie," the lips are closed for the [p] in [paɪ], while the tongue is lowering for the beginning of the [aɪ], and while the lips are opening to release the burst, the tongue is fronting and elevating for the second part of the diphthong. The sounds thus overlap and merge into one continuously changing acoustic stream, further bonded by the suprasegmental or prosodic features of speech.

## REFERENCES AND SUGGESTED READING

### General Acoustics of Speech

Denes, P. B., and Pinson, E. N., *The Speech Chain*, 2nd ed. New York: W. H. Freeman, 1993.

Fant, G., *Acoustic Theory of Speech Production*. The Hague, The Netherlands: Mouton, 1960.

Fry, D. B. (Ed.), *Acoustic Phonetics: A Course of Basic Readings*. New York: Cambridge University, 1976.

Fry, D. B., *The Physics of Speech*. Cambridge: Cambridge University Press, 1979.

Kent, R. D., and Read, C., *The Acoustic Analysis of Speech,* 2nd ed. Albany, NY: Singular, 2002.

Lehiste, I. (Ed.), *Readings in Acoustic Phonetics*. Cambridge, MA: MIT Press, 1967.

Olive, J. P., Greenwood, A., and Coleman, J., *Acoustics of American English Speech: A Dynamic Approach*. New York: Springer-Verlag, 1993.

Pickett, J. M., *The Acoustics of Speech Communication*. Boston: Allyn & Bacon, 1999.

Potter, R. K., Kopp, G. A., and Green, H. C., *Visible Speech*. New York: Van Nostrand Co., 1947.

Stevens, K. N., *Acoustic Phonetics*. Cambridge, MA: MIT Press, 1998.

## Articulation and Resonance: Consonants

Andrésen, B., *Pre-Glottalization in English Standard Pronunciation*. New York: Humanities Press, 1968.

Bell-Berti, F., *The Velopharyngeal Mechanism: An Electromyographic Study. Haskins Laboratories Status Report (Suppl.)*. New Haven, CT: Haskins Laboratories, 1973.

Bell-Berti, F., Control of Pharyngeal Cavity Size for English Voiced and Voiceless Stops. *J. Acoust. Soc. Am. 57,* 1975, 456–461.

Bell-Berti, F., and Hirose, N., Palatal Activity in Voicing Distinctions: A Simultaneous Fiberoptic and Electromyographic Study. *J. Phonet. 3,* 1975, 69–74.

Fritzell, B., The Velopharyngeal Muscles in Speech: An Electromyographic and Cinefluorographic Study. *Acta Otolaryngol. (Stockh.) Suppl. 250,* 1969.

Fujimura, O., Analysis of Nasal Consonants. *J. Acoust. Soc. Am. 34,* 1962, 1865–1875. Reprinted in Kent et al., 1991 (q.v.), 301–311.

Heinz, J. M., and Stevens, K. N., On the Properties of Voiceless Fricative Consonants. *J. Acoust. Soc. Am. 33,* 1961, 589–596.

Kuehn, D. P., and Dalston, R. M., Cleft Palate Studies Related to Velopharyngeal Function. In *Human Communication and Its Disorders*. H. Winitz (Ed.). Norwood, NJ: Ablex, 1988.

Ladefoged, P., *A Course in Phonetics,* 3rd ed. New York: Harcourt Brace Jovanovich, 1993.

Ladefoged, P., *Vowels and Consonants,* 2nd ed. Malden, MA: Blackwell Publishing, 2005.

Lisker, L., and Abramson, A. S., A Cross-Language Study of Voicing in Initial Stops: Acoustical Measurements. *Word 20,* 1964, 384–422.

Lubker, J. F., An Electromyographic-Cinefluorographic Investigation of Velar Function During Normal Speech Production. *Cleft Palate J. 5,* 1968, 1–18.

Moll, K., and Daniloff, R. G., Investigation of the Timing of Velar Movements During Speech. *J. Acoust. Soc. Am. 50,* 1971, 678–684.

Netsell, R., Subglottal and Intraoral Air Pressures During the Intervocalic Contrast of /t/ and /d/. *Phonetica 20,* 1969, 68–73.

Peterson, G. E., and Lehiste, I., Transitions, Glides, and Diphthongs. *J. Acoust. Soc. Am. 33,* 1961, 268–277.

Shadle, C. H., Articulatory-Acoustic Relations in Fricative Consonants. In *Speech Production and Speech Modelling*. W. H. Hardcastle and A. Marchal (Eds.). Dordrecht, The Netherlands: Kluwer Academic Publishers, 1990, pp. 187–209.

Stone, M., Faber, A., Raphael, L., and Shawker, T., Cross-Sectional Tongue Shape and Lingua-Palatal Contact Patterns in [s], [ʃ], and [l]. *J. Phonet. 20,* 1992, 253–270.

Subtelny, J. D., Oya, N., and Subtelny, J. D., Cineradiographic Study of Sibilants. *Folio Phoniatr. (Basel) 24,* 1972, 30–50.

Tuller, B., Harris, K. S., and Gross, B., Electromyographic Study of the Jaw Muscles During Speech. *J. Phonet. 9,* 1981, 175–188.

## English Speech Sounds

## Context Effects: Assimilation and Coarticulation

Bell-Berti, F., and Krakow, R., Anticipatory Velar Lowering: A Coproduction Account. *J. Acoust. Soc. Am. 90,* 1991, 112–123.

Bell-Berti, F., and Harris, K. S., Temporal Patterns of Coarticulation: Lip Rounding. *J. Acoust. Soc. Am. 71,* 1982, 449–454. Reprinted in Kent et al., 1991 (q.v.), 599–604.

Bell-Berti, F., Krakow, R. A., Gelfer, C. E., and Boyce, S. E., Anticipatory and Carryover Effects: Implications for Models of Speech Production. In *Producing Speech: Contemporary Issues for Katherine Safford Harris*. F. Bell-Berti and L. J. Raphael (Eds.). New York: American Institute of Physics, 1995, pp. 77–97.

Borden, G. J., and Gay, T., Temporal Aspects of Articulatory Movements for /s/-Stop Clusters. *Phonetica 36,* 1979, 21–31.

Daniloff, R. G., and Hammarberg, R. E., On Defining Coarticulation. *J. Phonet. 1,* 1973, 239–248.

Daniloff, R. G., and Moll, K., Coarticulation of Liprounding. *J. Speech Hear. Res. 11,* 1968, 707–721.

Fowler, C. A., and Saltzman, E., Coordination and Coarticulation in Speech Production. *Lang. Speech 36,* 1993, 171–195.

Kent, R. D., and Minifie, F. D., Coarticulation in Recent Speech Production Models. *J. Phonet. 5,* 1977, 115–135. Reprinted in Kent et al., 1991 (q.v.), 651–669.

Kozhevnikov, V. A., and Chistovich, L. A., *Rech artikulyatsiya i vospriyatie.* Moscow-Leningrad, 1965. Translated as *Speech: Articulation and Perception.* Springfield, VA: Joint Publications Research Service. U.S. Department of Commerce, 1966.

Lindblom, B. E. F., Spectrographic Study of Vowel Reduction. *J. Acoust. Soc. Am. 35,* 1963, 1773–1781. Reprinted in Kent et al., 1991 (q.v.), 517–525.

MacNeilage, P. F., Motor Control of Serial Ordering of Speech. *Psychol. Rev. 77,* 1970, 182–196. Reprinted in Kent et al., 1991 (q.v.), 701–715.

MacNeilage, P. F., and De Clerk, J. L., On the Motor Control of Coarticulation in CVC Monosyllables. *J. Acoust. Soc. Am. 45,* 1969, 1217–1233.

Marchal, A., Coproduction: Evidence from EPG Data. *Speech Commun. 7,* 1988, 287–295.

Öhman, S. E. G., Coarticulation in VCV Utterances: Spectrographic Measurements. *J. Acoust. Soc. Am. 39,* 1966, 151–168. Reprinted in Kent, R. D., et al., 1991 (q.v.), 567–584.

Perkell, J. S., *Physiology of Speech Production: Results and Implications of a Quantitative Cineradiographic Study.* Cambridge, MA: MIT Press, 1969.

Peterson, C. E., and Shoup, J. E., A Physiological Theory of Phonetics. *J. Speech Hear. Res. 9,* 1966, 5–67.

# The Acoustics of Prosody

**7**

*Language resembles music in making use of both the musical and unmusical qualities of sound.*

–Dwight Bolinger, Aspects of Language

So far we have been investigating the articulation and acoustic features of what are called the *segmental* features of speech. The study of prosody, in contrast, focuses on what are called the *supra*segmental sounds of speech. These suprasegmental features include, among other things, intonation (the variations in fundamental frequency during an utterance) and stress (the relative emphasis placed on syllables). In order to understand why such features are called suprasegmentals, we need to explain first why the consonants and vowels that were discussed in the preceding chapters are referred to as segmental sounds.

Suppose, for example, that you were asked to transcribe the phonemes you heard when someone spoke the word "role." The transcription would look like this: /rol/. That is, you would have identified three *segments*: /r/, /o/, and /l/, even though a wide-band spectrogram of the utterance (Fig. 7.1) reveals no clear division or separation of the acoustic signal into three discrete sections that correspond to the three phonemes of the transcription.

Next, consider the two possible ways in which stress or emphasis can be placed on the syllables of the word "record." A speaker might place more stress on the first than on the second syllable (REcord), in which case the word will be understood as a noun. Alternatively, the speaker might place more stress on the second syllable (reCORD) than on the first, in which case the word will be understood as a verb. The point is that both syllables consist of more than one segment. Thus, stress, which is assigned to whole syllables, is a *supra*segmental feature.

Perhaps the suprasegmental nature of intonation is even more obvious than that of stress. Speakers use intonation for several

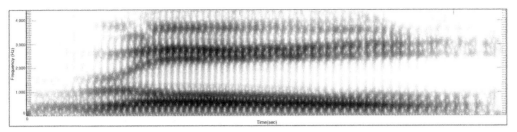

**FIGURE 7.1** Spectrogram of the word "role." Note that the continuous formant structure makes it impossible to recover three acoustic segments that correlate with the linguistic segments (/rol/) that listeners report hearing.

purposes, some of which we will discuss below. One of those purposes is to contrast statements with questions. By varying the way pitch changes over the duration of a sentence, especially near the end, a speaker can indicate that "I like taking tests" is either a statement (however unlikely) or an ironic question. Those variations in pitch, caused by changes in the fundamental frequency of vibration of the vocal folds, "cover" all of the phonetic segments of the sentence, thus making intonation, like stress, a suprasegmental feature of speech and language.

## SOME ELEMENTS OF PROSODY

As we have seen, the prosodic, or suprasegmental, features of speech usually occur simultaneously with two or more segmental phonemes. They are overlaid on syllables, words, phrases, and sentences. The suprasegmental features that we shall consider are stress, intonation, duration, and juncture.

### Stress

The coarticulation of consonants and vowels is what binds sounds together into syllables, and it is the *syllable* that is the unit of stress. Consideration of *lexical stress*, the pattern of stress within words, reveals that utterances may be monosyllables, such as "bat," "eat," and "tea," disyllables, such as "beyond," "hidden," and "table," and polysyllables, such as "unicorn" (three syllables),

"immediate" (four syllables), and "unsophisticated" (six syllables). Listeners can usually count the number of highly resonant centers (the *syllabic nuclei*) in an utterance, to determine the number of syllables in a word, even though they are not aware of the basis of this determination. Each syllabic nucleus can be counted, regardless of the degree of stress it has received.

We can also analyze stress as it occurs in phrases and sentences: The following passage contains 13 syllables, but only four of them receive the highest level of stress, called primary stress. Read the passage aloud and see if you can count the number of syllables in the sentence and identify the four syllables that receive primary stress.

> *What wisdom can you find that is greater than kindness?*
>
> –Emile, On Education,
> Jean Jacques Rousseau, 1762

If you responded as do most listeners, you counted 13 syllables, and perceived four syllables with primary stress: (1) the first syllable in "wisdom," (2) the monosyllabic word "find," (3) the first syllable of "greater," and (4) the first syllable of "kindness."

In English, as in other languages, stress functions as a "pointer" by indicating which information in an utterance is most important. Let's see how this pointing function works in sentences, clauses, and phrases. Here is a series of questions and statements:

1. WHICH one of those green books is yours?
2. That's NOT your green book!
3. WHOSE green book is this?
4. Is that your RED book?
5. WHAT is that?

Respond to each of the questions and statements by repeating the following sentence, *in its entirety:*

THIS IS MY GREEN BOOK.

In each succeeding repetition, you will find that the heaviest stress moves from one word to the next, starting with "THIS" and ending with "BOOK," in response to the information that is requested or provided by each of the five sentences above. For example, question number 3 is likely to be answered with: "This is MY green book," with the monosyllabic word "my" receiving the greatest level of stress in the sentence. Native speakers usually can place stress accurately on syllables within sentences without any conscious effort. Moreover, they are quite sensitive to stress that is misplaced. For instance,

"This is my green BOOK" as a response to the question (number 3 again) "WHOSE green book is this?" will sound peculiar to them because the information being called for in question number 3 concerns the ownership of the book and not what is owned.

Lexical stress points to the most important syllable or syllables in words and thus performs several important functions. One is to differentiate nouns and verbs. For example, the word "PERmit," with the first syllable stressed, is a noun meaning "a document of authorization," but "perMIT," with the second syllable stressed, is a verb meaning "to allow." "Permit" is unusual in this regard because the vowel in its lesser stressed syllable is often produced without being noticeably neutralized. More typical examples, which do evidence vowel neutralization (i.e., the vowels in the more weakly stressed syllable become more schwa-like), are pairs such as "OBject" (noun) versus

"obJECT" (verb); "DIgest" (noun) versus "diGEST" (verb); and "REcord" (noun) versus "reCORD" (verb). In words of more than two syllables, there is a tendency to retain a second stress for verbs ['ɛstə'meɪt] as "to 'EStiMATE" but to lose the secondary stress for the noun, ['ɛstəmət] as "an EStimate."

There are instances, in English, of syllables that are normally only weakly stressed becoming important because of the contrasts they provide. Thus, the meaning of the sentence "I told you to REceive the guests, not to DEceive them" requires that the first syllables of "receive" and "deceive" be heavily stressed, because these are the syllables that differentiate the two words. Normally, of course, the second syllable of each word is the one that receives primary stress. This use of stress is called *contrastive* because the contrastive elements of the words are made explicit by speakers.

But all uses of stress rely on contrasts, even if they are only implied. In some instances, the implied contrast is with something that was not said. When you stressed "green" in "This is my GREEN book," you implied the contrast with the name of any other color that might have been said (but was not), as well as the contrast with any other syllable in the sentence that might have been stressed (but, again, was not). The contrast between strongly and weakly stressed syllables in English is what makes the pointing function of stress possible. In a sense, the more weakly stressed syllables are as important as the strongly stressed syllables, because without them, there would be no contrast between the more important and the less important information.

The alternation between heavily and weakly stressed syllables in English gives the subjective impression that the stressed syllables occur at fairly regular intervals, a phenomenon called *isochrony* (iso = equal; chron = time) or *stress-timing*. Recent research, however, has cast doubt on the physical reality of isochrony, particularly on the acoustic level of analysis.

How does a speaker use his vocal mechanism to generate the different degrees of stress required? The general answer is that the more stress a speaker wishes to place on a syllable, the more effort he or she will expend in producing the syllable, and the less stress, the less effort. This answer, however, must be made more specific in terms of the use of respiratory, phonatory, and articulatory behaviors. Interestingly, these behaviors were first inferred from acoustic analyses.

The three acoustic characteristics that are most often associated with heavily stressed syllables are (1) higher $f_0$, (2) greater duration, and (3) greater intensity than weakly stressed syllables. Let us see how each of these characteristics arises from the use of the vocal mechanism.

The higher $f_0$ associated with stressed syllables is, as we have seen in Chapter 4, a function of increased tension on the vocal folds. This extra effort within the larynx on the part of the cricothyroid muscle may be supplemented by increased expiratory effort, which raises subglottal pressure and so also assists in raising $f_0$. It also drives the folds farther from their rest position, causing the higher intensity associated with stressed syllables.

The greater duration of stressed syllables indicates that more muscular effort must be used in their production, most particularly within the articulatory system. The increased amount of time used to articulate highly stressed syllables allows the articula-

tors to approximate the target positions for the vowels in those syllables. This is reflected in the formant frequencies of stressed vowels as compared with the neutralized formants of lesser-stressed syllables that display the effects of articulatory undershoot—the failure of the articulators to attain their target positions.

Studies of the contributing factors to the production of stress have shown that the fundamental frequency has the greatest effect. That is, small changes in $f_0$ will override changes in duration or intensity. Most often, when speakers produce greater degrees of stress, they raise $f_0$ on a syllable, but increased stress can be signaled simply by producing a syllable in which $f_0$ is simply out of line, higher or lower, with surrounding syllables. If you say "This is MY green book" first with a high $f_0$ and then with a low $f_0$, on "MY," you can observe how both strategies can cause the syllable to receive heavy stress.

Duration is second to $f_0$ as a contributing factor to the production of stress. Relatively small increases in syllable duration can override decreases in the intensity of a syllable. Syllable intensity is least effective in the production of heavily stressed syllables. It should be noted, however, that in most instances, a speaker will employ all of these factors, producing greater stress on a syllable by raising $f_0$ and by increasing syllable duration and intensity. Figure 7.2 illustrates how the three factors co-occur in stressed syllables.

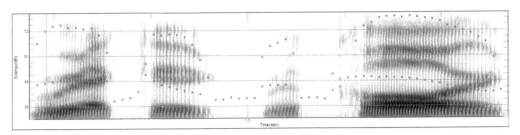

**FIGURE 7.2**   $f_0$ contours, wideband spectrograms, and amplitude displays of the noun "REcord" and the verb "reCORD." Note the higher $f_0$ peak, greater duration, and greater intensity for the first syllable in "REcord" than for the first syllable in "reCORD." Similarly, there is a higher $f_0$ peak, greater duration, and greater intensity for the second syllable in ".reCORD" than for the second syllable in "REcord".

## *C*LINICAL NOTE

In recent years, the prosodic or suprasegmental features of language have become increasingly relevant as accent reduction has fallen within the scope of practice of speech-language pathologists. This is because of the fact that faulty production of stress, intonation, and juncture can seriously affect a speaker's intelligibility, and such faulty production is a hallmark of much foreign-accented speech. The negative effects of non-native <u>supra</u>segmental features can, in fact, render speak less intelligible than the production of non-native segmental features. Listen, for instance, to the production of a sentence that contains few segments that are typical of American English pronunciation. Most native speakers of English have little difficulty understanding this sentence as "Arthur failed the mathematics exam." In contrast, listen to the production of a sentence that is very difficult for native speakers of English to understand, even though the segmental sounds are fairly typical of those produced by native speakers. The reduced intelligibility is caused by the fact that the stress patterns, both lexical and phrasal, are very different from those that might be produced by a native English speaker. Even after repeated hearings, listeners may still not understand the sentence as "Patrick followed orders." The effect of using atypical levels of stress in the case of foreign accent is more profound than simply causing confusion between, for example, a noun (REcord) and a verb (reCORD), for several reasons. The most important of these reasons is the fact that changing the degree of stress on a syllable affects the quality of the vowel and resonant consonants that it contains. Thus, for instance, the vowels in the word "money," which normally has a heavily stressed first syllable and a weakly stressed second syllable, will change significantly if the second syllable is heavily stressed and the first syllable is weakly stressed. The result is a production that is not recognizable as an English word ([məni]) in contrast with the two pronunciations of "record," mentioned above.

## Intonation

The suprasegmental features can reveal the attitudes and feelings of the speaker in ways the segmental information alone can never do. Stress, for example, when used for emphasis, can express disdain for children in general—"not that CHILD!"—or dislike of a particular child—"not THAT child!" The use of changing $f_0$, perceived as the pitch pattern or *intonation* contour of a phrase or sentence, is particularly effective in expressing differences in attitude. For instance, in this example, the stressed words (either "child" or "that") would most likely be marked by a sharp rise in $f_0$.

In addition to conveying information about attitudes, intonation can also signal differences in meaning. "Today is Tuesday," said with a rising intonation contour (the pitch increasing during "Tuesday"), turns a statement into a question (Fig. 7.3). We see

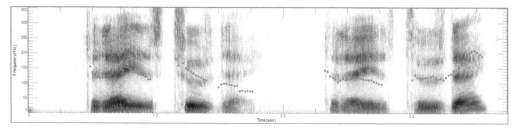

**FIGURE 7.3** Intonation contours for the sentence "Today is Tuesday," spoken as a statement (terminal fall in $f_0$) and as a question (terminal rise in $f_0$).

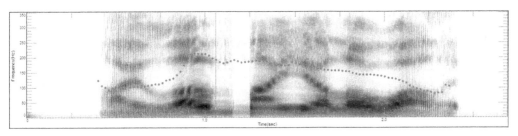

**FIGURE 7.4**  A basic rise–fall intonation pattern, used for statements, questions that cannot be answered with a "yes" or "no," and for certain kinds of special emphasis.

that it is possible for the prosodic information that is transmitted along with the segmental information to override the literal meaning of the words being spoken. The sentence "That's a pretty picture!" can be said in such a way that it conveys genuine admiration of the picture or a sarcastic and negative evaluation of its artistic worth. It is even possible to use intonation to convert a grammatically constructed question to a statement (the opposite of what we saw for the sentence "Today is Tuesday"). Try saying "Am I a good tennis player" in such a way as to let your listeners know that you could make them forget Venus Williams in a minute.

Intonation patterns (perceived changes in $f_o$) can be imposed on a sentence, a phrase, or even a word. American English sentences are often characterized by a rise–fall intonation curve (Fig. 7.4). The pitch rises during the first part of an utterance and falls at the end. This is generally true of declarative sentences and of questions that are impossible to answer with yes or no.

Declarative sentence:

He left an hour ago.

[hilɛftən ˀaʊɚ əgoʊ]

Question impossible to answer with yes/no:

How do you like it here?

[haʊdəju laɪk ɪth ɪɚ]

Special emphasis:

Wow!

[waʊ]

Another intonation contour common in English is the end-of-utterance pitch rise. Pitch rise indicates a question to be answered with a "yes" or "no." It may also indicate that a sentence is incomplete or that a response is expected. For instance, if a speaker wants to prompt a listener to supply information, he might say "And the name of the movie you are recommending is . . .," with a rise in pitch at the end of the utterance.

Yes/no question:

Is it ready?

[ɪzɪt redɪ]

Incomplete sentence:

As I think about it...

[æzaɪθ ɪŋk əbaʊt ɪt]

Because it signals incompletion, a pitch rise can be used by speakers to "hold the floor" during a discussion. If a speaker pauses to think in the midst of a phrase, with the pitch rising, he will most likely be understood as signaling that he is not yet done speaking, and so a polite discussant would be less likely to interrupt than if the pause occurred at a fall in intonation.

The rise–fall intonation pattern, especially the terminal fall in $f_0$, is found in virtually all languages. It may well be that this universal feature is physiologically conditioned. Phoneticians and linguists have noted that infant cries follow this intonation pattern and explain it in terms of the falling subglottal pressure that occurs as the child readies himself for an inhalation. The relatively rapid pressure fall drives the vocal folds more slowly, decreasing $f_0$. In other words, superimposing phonation on the exhalation portion of the normal respiratory cycle naturally causes $f_0$ to fall and listeners to perceive a lowering of pitch. The rise–fall pattern persists in adults and children who speak and is used for utterances such as simple declarative sentences. It is often referred to as an *unmarked breath group*, signifying its status as a default pattern for neutral utterances which have no special meanings that would have to be signaled by deviations from the unmarked pattern.

There are, however, as we have seen, utterances which require modification of the rise–fall pattern. The "yes–no" questions and incomplete sentences that we discussed above are examples of such utterances because they require a terminal rise in $f_0$ and perceived pitch. These modifications result in what is called a *marked breath group* because they call attention to some special meaning that the speaker intends to convey. Terminal rises (as well as those that occur at other places in an utterance) result chiefly from increased cricothyroid muscle activity intonation that tenses the vocal folds, causing them to vibrate faster, and that overrides the effect of falling subglottal pressure. Speakers may, of course, also lower $f_0$ at various places before the end of an utterance in order to mark it as special. This can be accomplished by relaxing the cricothyroid muscle which causes the vocal folds to vibrate more slowly. Relaxation of the cricothyroid muscle can also occur at the end of an utterance along with a decrease in subglottal pressure, and it should be noted that both of these features contribute not only to a fall in $f_0$ but also to a decrease in intensity.

The portion of the unmarked breath group during which $f_0$ falls, called the declination, can vary in many ways. The decline of $f_0$ may be relatively unbroken, or, quite often, can display momentary $f_0$ peaks that mark stressed syllables. The location of declination onset can also vary considerably from one utterance to another. If the heavi-

est stress in a sentence occurs early, the declination may occupy many syllables; a later-occurring sentence stress will cause a more rapid declination, even, in some instances, on a single syllable. Despite this variation in the location of the onset of declination, if one measures the natural declination of $f_0$ for each of many unmarked breath groups, one finds that although $f_0$ may vary considerably in its higher starting points, it falls to about the same frequency at the end of each breath group. Cooper and Sorensen (1981) regard this as evidence of some degree of planning. We saw a similar phenomenon in our discussion of respiration in Chapter 3: There is a tendency for each breath group to end at about 35% to 40% vital capacity despite large variations in starting volumes.

It seems, therefore, that the decrease in subglottal pressure at the end of a phrase is the most important factor in the overall declination of $f_0$ but that the elevation of $f_0$ for each stressed syllable is the combined result of cricothyroid muscle and internal intercostal muscle activity, elevating both $f_0$ and the intensity of the voice.

You can demonstrate the natural declination of $f_0$ by producing an audible sigh. Notice that the pitch falls as the lung volume decreases. Now add the alternating stressed and unstressed syllables typical of English:

**Jack** and **Jill** went **up** the **hill**
To **fetch** a **pail** of **wa**ter.
**Jack** fell **down** and **broke** his **crown**,
And **Jill** came **tum**bling **af**ter.

You will observe that each stressed syllable is higher in $f_0$ and intensity than its neighboring unstressed syllables, but that each succeeding stressed syllable in a phrase is a bit lower in $f_0$ than its predecessor (Fig. 7.5). Although a case may be made that a pattern of falling intonation is natural to the speech system, we can override the system for linguistic reasons. We could choose to emphasize that Jack broke his crown instead

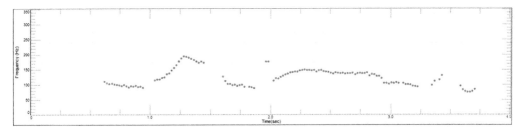

**FIGURE 7.5** A typical example of $f_0$ declination in a spoken English sentence.

of his leg or to turn "Jill came tumbling after" into a question. Intonation thus functions to mark syntactic contrasts (phrase endings, interrogation vs. declaration), to change meaning and to signal attitudes and feelings. Excitement, including some kinds of anger and states of enthusiasm, is often accompanied by large shifts in intonation, whereas calm, subdued states, including some forms of grief, anger, peacefulness, and boredom, are characterized by a narrow range of variation in intonation. We know how people feel as much by the way they say their messages as by the messages themselves.

## Duration

Segmental duration has been mentioned in the discussion of vowels. Speech sounds vary in intrinsic duration. In general, the diphthongs and tense vowels (that are most often diphthongal) are described as intrinsically "long" sounds. The lax vowels, in contrast (that are most often monophthongs), are described as intrinsically "short" sounds. The continuant consonants (fricatives, nasals, and semivowels) frequently exceed the durations of the stop consonants even if the closure is included in the overall stop duration.

In addition to possessing intrinsic durations, sounds may vary in duration because of context. For example, vowels in English are of greater duration when they occur before voiced consonants, as in "leave," than when they occur before voiceless consonants, as in "leaf." They are also longer before continuants, as in "leave," than be-

fore stops, as in "leap." This pattern of differences is found across languages, suggesting that it is conditioned by physiology. English, however, shows unusually large differences between the durations of vowels preceding voiced and voiceless consonants, suggesting a learned overlay that may supplement an underlying physiologic difference. In English, vowels preceding voiced consonants in isolated words can be more than half again as long as those preceding voiceless consonants. This is in marked contrast with the voicing-conditioned differences found in some other languages. In Spanish, for instance, research has shown a small average difference (18 ms) between vowels preceding voiced and voiceless consonants.

We have seen that falls in intonation are used by speakers to signal the completion of a thought or sentence and that rising intonation is used to signal incompletion and an implied request for a listener to respond. These rises and falls in intonation will occur most frequently before the pauses that occur at the end of phrases and sentences. Durational information is also used to supplement these changes in intonation: Speakers will lengthen syllables that occur at the ends of phrases and sentences, to provide additional information about the syntax of their utterances. Such *phrase-final* or *pre-pausal lengthening* is thus another example of redundancy in the production of speech. For instance, the monosyllabic word "hot" in the sentence "Yesterday it was really hot" will have a greater duration than in the sentence "It was really hot yesterday," because of its position at the end of the sentence. The speaker thus provides intonational and durational cues for the listener.

## Juncture

The suprasegmental feature of juncture takes several forms, but we will focus here only on the type of juncture that is relevant to the syllable affiliations of speech sounds—that is, the signaling of which sounds belong to which syllables. We should begin with an example of what is meant by syllable affiliation. Consider the following pair of two-word sequences: "peace talks" and "pea stalks." A transcription of the phonemes (in the authors' dialect) in these sequences would be identical: /pistɔks/. Despite the identical phonemes, most speakers have no difficulty indicating that /s/ is the last sound of the word "peace" in "peace talks," or that /s/ is the first sound of the word "stalks" in "pea stalks." In other words, the meaning intended by the speaker is dependent on the syllable with which the /s/ is affiliated.

How, then, does the speaker indicate the intended meaning? In this particular example, the speaker will distinguish the utterances by controlling the degree of aspiration following the release of the /t/. In "peace talks," where the /t/ is in syllable-initial position before a stressed vowel, there is, as is normally the case in English, a relatively long period of aspiration; in "pea stalks," the syllable-initial /s/ preceding the /t/ causes the stop to be virtually unaspirated. To put this in terms of the previous chapter, the speaker has produced a much longer VOT for the initial /t/ in "talks" than for the /t/ preceded by the /s/ in "stalks."

Using aspiration in this way is only one strategy than can be used to specify the syllable affiliation of sounds, and we should make it clear that speakers use this and other strategies automatically and that listeners are normally unaware of the particular strategy being used by a speaker. We should also emphasize that the rather unlikely pair of utterances we have used as an example are not likely to be confused with each other even

when spoken in isolation. Spoken in the context of a sentence, confusion would be virtually impossible. After all, even if the /t/ did receive aspiration, a listener would not be likely to misunderstand the anomalous sentence to be "The farmer watered the peace talks."

Let's look at another example, one which relies on a slightly different strategy to signal the syllable affiliation of a sound. Consider that in normal conversational speaking style, there will be only one /s/ articulation in sentences such was "We miss Sally" and "We miss Tom." The /s/ in the first sentence must represent two phonemes: the syllable-final /s/ in "miss" and the syllable-initial /s/ in "Sally." That is, the /s/ must be affiliated with two syllables. In the second sentence, the /s/ represents only the final /s/ in "miss." Acoustic analysis reveals that in the first sentence, speakers maintain the frication for the articulated [s] for a longer period of time than in the second sentence. The speaker is thus able to use a single articulation either to represent two phonemes by making a longer /s/-closure, or to represent a single phoneme with a briefer closure. A similar lengthening or shortening can occur for stop closures: The /g/ closure will be longer in "big gun" than in "begun."

Not all articulatory strategies deal exclusively with duration. For instance, consider the following sequence of sounds: /əneɪm/. If the /n/ is affiliated with the preceding schwa, the speaker will have signaled that "an aim" was intended; if the /n/ is affiliated with the second syllable, than the speaker's intention will have been to say "a name." Although durational differences can play a role in differentiating the utterances, many speakers insert a glottal stop before the vowel of the second syllable of "an aim" in order to convey that the /n/ is affiliated with the first syllable.

In this section, we have been able only to provide a sample of the phonetic features that speakers produce in order to establish the syllable affiliation of speech sounds. There are many others. We should conclude, however, by restating that many of these features of juncture co-occur with the other prosodic features we have mentioned, including stress, duration, and intonation. Indeed, although we can neatly categorize and separately discuss each of the prosodic features, they are often inter-related and co-occur. Thus, for example, durational features (phrase-final lengthening) and intonational features (terminal falls of $f_0$) can both convey information about the syntax. Similarly, raising $f_0$ and increasing the intensity and duration of a syllable provide information about stress and about utterance types (statement vs. question). The co-occurrence of features, as we have seen, results in the redundancy that makes speech resistant to the misperceptions and misinterpretations that can occur when listening conditions are less than optimal.

## BIBLIOGRAPHY

### General Works on Speech Production

Bell-Berti, F., and Raphael, L. J. (Eds.), *Producing Speech: Contemporary Issues: For Katherine Safford Harris*. New York: American Institute of Physics, 1995.

Kent, R. D., Atal, B. S., and Miller, J. L. (Eds.), *Papers in Speech Communication: Speech Production*. Woodbury, NY: Acoustical Society of America, 1991.

Lieberman, P., and Blumstein, S. E., *Speech Physiology, Speech Perception and Acoustic Phonetics*. New York: Cambridge University Press, 1988.

Hardcastle, W. J., and Laver, J. (Eds.), *The Handbook of the Phonetic Sciences*. Oxford: Blackwell Publishers, 1997.

### General Acoustics of Speech

Denes, P. B., and Pinson, E. N., *The Speech Chain*, 2nd ed. New York: W. H. Freeman, 1993.

Kent, R. D., and Read, C., *The Acoustic Analysis of Speech,* 2nd ed. Albany, NY: Singular, 2002.

Pickett, J. M., *The Acoustics of Speech Communication*. Boston: Allyn & Bacon, 1999.

Stevens, K. N., *Acoustic Phonetics*. Cambridge, MA: MIT Press, 1998.

### Suprasegmentals

Atkinson, J. E., Correlation Analysis of the Physiologic Features Controlling Fundamental Voice Frequency. *J. Acoust. Soc. Am. 63*, 1978, 211–222.

Bolinger, D. L., *Intonation and Its Parts: Melody in Spoken English*. Stanford: Stanford University Press, 1986.

Collier, R., Physiological Correlates of Intonation Patterns. *J. Acoust. Soc. Am. 58*, 1975, 249–255.

Cooper, W. E., and Sorensen, J. M., *Fundamental Frequency in Sentence Production*. New York: Springer-Verlag, 1981.

Crary, M. A., and Tallman, V. I., Production of Linguistic Prosody by Normal and Speech-Disordered Children. *J. Commun. Disord. 26*, 1993, 245–262.

Cruttenden, A., *Intonation*. Cambridge: Cambridge University Press, 1986.

Crystal, T. H., and House, A. S., The Duration of American English Vowels. *J. Phonet. 16*, 1988, 263–284.

Crystal, T. H., and House, A. S., Segmental Duration in Connected Speech Signals: Syllabic Stress. *J. Acoust. Soc. Am. 84*, 1988, 1574–1585.

Cutler, A., Lexical Stress. In *The Handbook of Speech Perception*. D. B. Pisoni and R. E. Remez (Eds.). Malden, MA: Blackwell Publishing, 2005, pp. 264–289.

Erickson, D., Articulation of Extreme Formant Patterns for Emphasized Vowels. *Phonetica 59*, 2002, 134–149.

Fear, B. D., Cutler, A., and Butterfield, D., The Strong/Weak Syllable Distinction in English. *J. Acoust. Soc. Am. 97*, 1995, 1893–1904.

Fry, D. B., Duration and Intensity as Physical Correlates of Linguistic Stress. *J. Acoust. Soc. Am. 27*, 1955, 765–768.

Fry, D. B., Experiments in the Perception of Stress. *Lang. Speech 1*, 1958, 126–152.

Gay, T., Physiological and Acoustic Correlates of Perceived Stress. *Lang. Speech 21*, 1978, 347–353.

Gelfer, C. E., Harris, K. S., Collier, R., and Baer, T., Is Declination Actively Controlled? In *Vocal Fold Physiology, Biomechanics, Acoustic, and Phonatory Control*. I. Titze and R. Scherer (Eds.). Denver, CO: Denver Center for the Performing Arts, 1983, pp. 113–126.

Klatt, D., Linguistic Uses of Segmental Duration in English. *J. Acoust. Soc. Am. 59,* 1976, 1208–1221.

Lehiste, I., *Suprasegmentals.* Cambridge, MA: MIT Press, 1970.

Lehiste, I., Suprasegmental Features of Speech. In *Principles of Experimental Phonetics.* N. Lass (Ed.). St. Louis, MO: Mosby, 1996, pp. 226–244.

Sanderman, A., and Collier, R., Prosodic Phrasing at the Sentence Level. In *Principles of Experimental Phonetics.* N. Lass (Ed.). St. Louis, MO: Mosby, 1996, pp. 321–332.

# Feedback Mechanisms and Models of Speech Production

# 8

*So sings man, and every fateful
Echo bears his amorous speech*

—Heinrich Heine, O Die Liebe Macht Uns Selig

## FEEDBACK MECHANISMS IN SPEECH

Speech scientists are interested in how a speaker controls the production of speech. To what degree does the speaker monitor his actions, and to what degree and under what situations might he produce speech with little or no information on how he is proceeding?

To answer this question, we must consider the science of self-regulating machines, called *cybernetics*. The term, coined by Norbert Wiener, from the Greek word meaning "steersman," refers to the study of systems that control themselves on the basis of their actual performance rather than being controlled by an external operator who compares the system's performance with the performance expected of it. A thermostat that turns off the furnace when the temperature reaches a specified value is an example of a *servomechanism*, the engineering term for a self-regulating machine. If a device controlling the temperature in your home were not a servomechanism, you would have to consult a thermometer periodically and make the required adjustments according to your preference.

In a servomechanism, the output of a device is fed back to a point in the system where the feedback information may be used to adjust the continuing performance. The feedback may indicate that the performance of the device is within prescribed limits and should *not* be changed, or that the performance is outside the prescribed limits and, thus, *should* be changed. In a biological system such as the speech mechanism, the feedback that does *not* call for a change is called *negative feedback*; whereas the feedback that indicates there *is* need for a change in performance is called *positive feedback*. Systems operating under feedback control are described

**155**

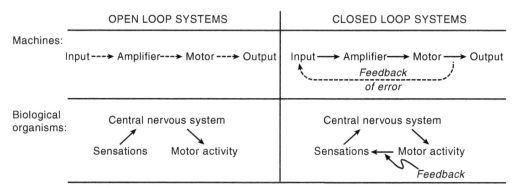

**FIGURE 8.1**   Open and closed loop control for machines and biologic systems.

as *closed loop* systems. Figure 8.1 contrasts *open loop* and closed loop systems in machines and in biological organisms. The difference between them is that in open loop systems, the output is preprogrammed and does not require feedback, whereas in closed loop systems, the performance of the system is fed back to be matched with the program. If there is a discrepancy between the program and the performance, adjustments are made to bring the performance in line with the program.

The production of speech requires the simultaneous and coordinated use of respiratory, phonatory, and articulatory mechanisms, an activity so complex that some method of feedback control seems likely. At least four kinds of information are available to a speaker that could be used in feedback control: auditory, tactile, proprioceptive, and central neural feedback.

## Auditory Feedback

Simply put, auditory feedback is hearing our own speech. Unlike the solely air-conducted acoustic signal that our listeners hear, auditory feedback is both air- and bone-conducted. Because a great deal of our own speech is conducted to our hearing mechanism by way of the bones in the skull that emphasize low frequencies, we do not sound to ourselves the way we sound to others. This is why speakers are often surprised at what they hear when a recording of their speech

is played back to them and often protest that "I don't sound like that!"

Interest in the role of feedback mechanisms in the control of speech was aroused by an accidental discovery made by a New Jersey engineer, Bernard Lee, in 1950. While he was recording himself on a tape recorder, he noticed that under some circumstances, the auditory feedback from his own speech could make him disfluent. That happened because in a tape recorder, the record head ordinarily precedes the playback head, as shown in Figure 8.2. If a speaker listens to his own previously recorded speech through a headset plugged into the playback head, which provides a slight time delay, fluent speech sometimes becomes disfluent, syllables are repeated, or inappropriately prolonged. It is also true that disfluent speakers, such as stutterers, may become more fluent under such conditions of *delayed auditory feedback* (DAF). The DAF effect can now be produced by digitally recorded and computer-processed speech in which both the recording and the amount of delay are electronically controlled.

This DAF effect provoked much excitement and a flurry of studies in the 1950s. The DAF effect was interpreted by many as proof that speech acts as a servomechanism, with auditory feedback as the chief control channel. This theory has been challenged by some, who note that some speakers can continue to speak fluently under DAF by attending to the printed page and ignoring the

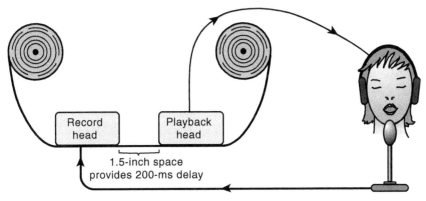

**FIGURE 8.2**    The delayed auditory feedback effect. A speaker records his or her own voice while listening to the recording at a time delay by monitoring the playback head of the tape recorder. A 1.5-inch space provides a 200-ms delay at a tape speed of 7.5 inches per second. This delay leads to maximum speech interference in adults.

acoustic signal, that the duration of the error corrections, when they occur in the form of stalls, are not linearly related to the amount of delay time, and that DAF is disruptive only at high intensity. An alternative interpretation of the DAF effect is that it is a result of forcing a speaker to attend to auditory feedback information that conflicts with information received from articulatory movements. It is a case of your muscles telling you "Yes," you have said something, but your ears telling you "No." In any case, it is important to remember that DAF is a very abnormal feedback condition, and that forcing a speaker to function under abnormal conditions of feedback is not the same as depriving him or her of the sort of feedback he or she normally receives. In other words, DAF does not reveal how a speaker might perform if he or she simply could not hear himself or herself.

There are ways of interfering with auditory feedback other than delaying it. In general, the speakers attempt to normalize any distortion. For example, if the air-conducted sound is amplified, speakers decrease vocal intensity; if it is attenuated, they increase vocal intensity. If they cannot hear themselves at all, they increase intensity (the *Lombard effect*) and prolong phonation, as you know if you have ever tried to talk to someone

sitting under a hair dryer. Even filtering out frequency regions of the speech that is fed back causes speakers to make articulatory adjustments to modify some of the resonance characteristics of the speech they produce. Garber (1976) found that speakers who hear their own speech through a low-pass filter respond by decreasing the low-frequency nasal resonance and raising $f_o$, presumably in an attempt to restore the missing high-frequency information.

These effects demonstrate that audition does operate as a feedback system for speech control, but they fail to settle the question of whether auditory feedback is essential for a skilled speaker. If so, is it used continuously or only in difficult speaking conditions? Adventitiously, deafened speakers suffer little immediate effect on the intelligibility of their speech; however, after an extended period of deafness, certain sounds deteriorate, notably /s/, and the suprasegmental structure of speech suffers. Despite evidence that speakers attempt to compensate for distortions in auditory feedback, audition may not serve effectively as a feedback mechanism to monitor ongoing, skilled articulation because the information it provides to the speaker arrives too late; he or she has already spoken and can only make corrections after the fact. Speakers do use audition, however, to sharpen their speech sound targets and, if they are attending to themselves, to notice errors they have already made and to revise what they have previously said.

## Tactile Feedback

Tactile feedback is the information you receive from your sense of touch. The act of speaking can generate perceptions of touch in many ways. The articulators, for instance, are continually coming into contact with one another, the lower lip touching the upper lip, the tip or blade of the tongue touching the alveolar ridge, the dorsum of the tongue touching the roof of the mouth, and the velum touching the pharyngeal walls. Even air pressure differences caused by valving the breath stream at the glottis or in the supraglottal cavities will impinge on the walls of the vocal tract and induce sensations of touch.

Tactile sensations include the perception of light touch, mediated by free nerve endings of sensory fibers lying near the surface of articulators, and the perception of deeper pressure, mediated by more complex nerve bodies farther from the surface. When touch receptors are stimulated, the responsiveness of surrounding cells is inhibited, which aids in localizing and sharpening sensations. The lips, alveolar ridge, and anterior tongue are highly endowed with surface receptors responsive to light touch. The tongue dorsum contains more sensory fibers than any other part of the human body. In addition to touch, some of these receptors are responsive to taste, temperature, and pain.

A method of measuring tactile sensation is to explore *two-point discrimination* with an instrument called an esthesiometer. A subject can feel two separate points on the tip of the tongue when the points are only 1 to 2 mm apart, but farther back on the tongue or on its lateral margins, the points must be nearly 1 cm apart to be differentiated. There are more touch receptors on the superior surface of the tongue than on the inferior surface and more in the alveolar ridge area of the hard palate than on the posterior part of the palate. Tactile sensation from the anterior two thirds of the tongue is transmitted by sensory fibers in the lingual branch of the trigeminal (fifth cranial) nerve. The trigeminal nerve also transmits impulses from touch receptors of the lips and palate. The glossopharyngeal (ninth cranial) nerve carries sensory information from the posterior third of the tongue. It is thought that some of the sensory fibers of the lingual nerve may course with the motor nerve to the tongue, the hypoglossal (twelfth cranial) nerve.

A second method of evaluating tactile sensation in the mouth is to test *oral stereognosis* by putting objects of various shapes into the mouth of a subject for either identification or discrimination. The ability to identify (name) the shapes (e.g., triangles, circles) by feeling them with the tongue and palate and then pointing at the appropriate pictures was found to have little or no relation to speech proficiency. On the other hand, the ability to discriminate two shapes (i.e., to tell whether they are the same or different) was found by Ringel (1970) to bear some relation to the ability to articulate speech sounds with normal proficiency.

There have been attempts to determine the importance of tactile information by interfering with normal tactile feedback and determining whether and how the interference has affected speech. Using the same techniques that dentists use to block the conduction of nerve impulses from the oral area, speech scientists have anesthetized various branches of the trigeminal nerve, thus depriving the speaker of tactile feedback. Such nerve blocks often result in distorted articulation of speech, especially the consonant /s/, but, in general, speech remains highly intelligible. Even when the ability to perform oral stereognosis and two-point discrimination tasks is markedly impaired or absent, subjects can move the tongue in all directions and feel its points of contact with other articulators. When auditory masking is added to the nerve block, no significant increase in articulation errors occurs.

Several theories have been advanced to account for the speech distortions that result from the application of sensory anesthesia, but, as yet, none has been adequately tested because of the difficulty in controlling variables inherent in the nerve block technique.

Audition and taction are called *external feedback* systems because the information they provide is delivered to external receptors. These receptors are classified as external because they are located on the surfaces of the organs of the vocal tract and of the hearing mechanism: The flow and pressure exerted by the airstream and the points of contact between articulators stimulate the tactile receptors in the vocal tract. Analogously, the sound waves produced by the speech mechanism are first delivered to and processed by the peripheral organs of hearing.

Although auditory and tactile information are both generated by muscle activity, they do not contain feedback about the muscle activity itself. Such feedback, which is available to the speech production mechanism, is our next topic of discussion.

## Proprioceptive Feedback

Direct feedback from muscles, a type of *response* feedback, is delivered more quickly than either type of external feedback, auditory or tactile. In general, proprioception allows us to sense the velocity, the direction of movement, and the position of body structures such as arms or legs. Specifically with regard to speech, proprioception provides information about the velocity, the direction of movement, and the location of the organs of speech, including articulators such as the tongue, lips, and mandible.

Among the primary sources of proprioceptive information are (1) sensors in joints that transmit information about bone angles and (2) receptors along tendons that respond to muscle contractions and transmit data about both muscle stretching and shortening. These data translate, on a functional level, to the ability to perform a task such as touching your forefinger to the tip of your nose while your eyes are closed.

The receptors embedded in striated (voluntary) muscles are of special interest to speech physiologists. These receptors are called *muscle spindles* because they are often shaped like the slender fiber holders from which thread is twisted in spinning. Muscle spindles are more complex in their innervation than tendon and joint receptors. They have efferent (motor) as well as afferent (sensory) neurons. The spindles (Fig. 8.3) are

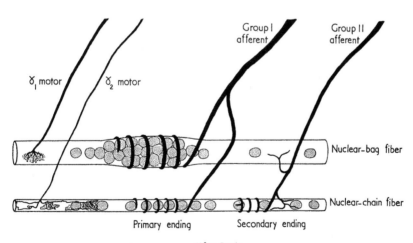

(After Boyd)

**FIGURE 8.3**  The central region of two types of muscle spindles. (Reprinted with permission from Matthews, P. B. C., Muscle Spindles and Their Motor Control. *Physiol. Rev. 44*, 1964, 219–288.)

## *C*LINICAL NOTE

As you've discovered from reading about external feedback, both auditory and tactile feedback provide information needed for the normal acquisition and development of speech and language. The amplification devices for children (and adults) with impaired hearing are designed primarily to increase the amplitude and quality of the speech of others, rather than of their own speech. Feedback can, to some extent, be augmented through the use of such devices as cochlear implants, hearing aids, and FM frequency-modulated systems (if a transmitter is located near the speaker's mouth—a technique not widely used), but there are few data on how such augmented auditory feedback affects the speech of hearing-impaired speakers. Clearly, this is an area that is ripe for a team research effort by speech-language pathologists and audiologists.

Tactile feedback of the acoustic signal that is recoded into vibrations applied to different parts of the skin surface (left and right sides of the abdomen; locations along the arm) has been used to help hearing-impaired speakers differentiate self-produced speech sounds on the basis of their most salient component frequencies. Such vibrotactile devices enable speakers to distinguish sounds with high-frequency components, such as /s/, from sounds such as nasals or vowels that are characterized by lower component frequencies. Finer sound distinctions can be made with vibrotactile devices with multiple channels keyed to smaller ranges of frequency.

Auditory feedback can also be recoded visually using real-time frequency tracking devices. Fundamental frequency, for instance, can be tracked on computer monitors by speakers and related to tactile and proprioceptive feedback from the muscles and organs that are active during phonation. Analogously, the generation of real-time wideband sound spectrograms can provide information that may allow speakers to relate articulatory behavior to the resonances that mark vowels and consonants.

---

encapsulated muscle fibers (intrafusal fibers) lying parallel to the main muscle fibers (extrafusal fibers). When the efferent neurons that stimulate the main muscle fire, the smaller efferent neurons that supply the muscle spindles are activated simultaneously. In effect, the intrafusal fibers of the muscle spindle mimic the activity of the main muscle fibers. The motor neurons to the main muscle are larger (8 to 20 μm in diameter) and are therefore called *alpha* (α) motoneurons, in contrast to the smaller motoneurons (2 to 8 μm in diameter), called *gamma* (γ) motoneurons, which innervate the spindle fibers at each end. Primary (Ia) and secondary (IIa) afferents are stimulated by and provide information about the lengthening of the intrafusal fibers and by the rate at which the length of the fibers changes. This information is fed back to the central nervous system.

The primary afferents from spindles are among the largest of human neurons, ranging from 12 to 20 μm in diameter, conducting impulses at rates as fast as 120 m/s. The velocity with which the spindles convey the feedback information makes them attractive as possible mechanisms for ongoing control of rapid motor activities, including speech. Muscle spindles are found in the intercostal muscles, all of the laryngeal muscles, the genioglossus muscle, the intrinsic muscles of the tongue, and, sparsely, in the facial muscles. Thus, muscles involved in speech production seem well supplied with spindles, which can be tuned to feed back information on muscle length changes.

Although the neural pathways for spindle information from some muscle systems are known, the route for the tongue is not clear. Spindle afferents from the tongue are believed to course along the otherwise motor hypoglossal (twelfth cranial) nerve and to enter the brainstem by way of the dorsal cervical nerves C1 through C3.

The proprioceptive feedback system may operate on both reflex and voluntary levels. Some pathways go to the spinal cord, but others go to the cerebral cortex and the cerebellum. Although the sensation of muscle activity is usually unconscious, it can be made conscious, but only under carefully designed and controlled experimental conditions. Goodwin, McCloskey, and Matthews (1972) mechanically stimulated the arm of a man who was blindfolded. The man was instructed to flex his other arm to match the position of the arm under stimulation. The subject misjudged the position, thinking the muscles in the stimulated arm were more extended than they were. The investigators then paralyzed the joint and cutaneous afferents in the index finger of a subject to see whether spindles alone were consciously perceived without information from joint receptors. As one of the investigators manipulated the finger, the subject could sense the movement and the direction of the movement; hence, the spindle output could be consciously perceived.

Proprioception for speech is difficult to investigate directly. Indirectly, proprioceptive feedback has been investigated by mechanically interfering with normal positional relationships and articulator movements to study compensatory adaptations. Subjects try to speak with bite blocks interfering with normal jaw raising; with metal plates unexpectedly pressing against the lips, interfering with labial closure; or with palatal prostheses in the mouth, altering the width of the alveolar ridge. There is still much to be learned about the nature of speakers' reactions to compensate for such mechanical interference. One thing that is known, however, is that speakers compensate immediately in response to such experimental perturbations of the speech production mechanism. They continue to speak intelligibly and at a normal rate, with no need to pause or rehearse new or alternative

strategies of articulation. It is not clear what feedback information—auditory, tactile, proprioceptive, or some combination of these—is instrumental in directing the compensations observed.

Two interesting attempts have been made to block $\gamma$ motoneurons from speech muscles directly. Critchlow and von Euler (1963) paralyzed the $\gamma$ fibers to the external intercostal muscles. The Ia fibers stopped firing during inspiration, firing during expiration only because of passive stretch of the inspiratory muscles. Although this had no effect on speech, it did indicate that the $\gamma$ and $\alpha$ motoneurons are activated together, because the spindle afferents are normally active from the inspiratory muscles during inspiration. Had the experiment involved paralysis of the less accessible expiratory intercostals, any effect on speech would have become apparent.

In another study, Abbs (1973) attempted to selectively block the $\gamma$ motoneurons to the mandibular muscles by anesthetizing the mandibular branch of the trigeminal nerve bilaterally, blocking both the large fibers ($\alpha$ motoneurons to main muscle fibers and afferents from tactile and proprioceptive receptors) and small fibers ($\gamma$ motoneurons and afferents for pain and temperature). Because large fibers recover before smaller fibers, it was assumed that when muscle force and touch returned to normal while pain and temperature senses were still blocked, the motor supply to the spindles would be blocked. In this condition, subjects lowered the mandible with less velocity and acceleration. There were, however, no perceptually obvious effects on speech.

Experimenters have carried out direct studies of proprioception in animals. Investigations of monkeys that underwent bilateral deafferentation from muscles of the limbs or from jaw muscles suggest that purposeful movements can be performed without either vision or somatic sensation from the involved muscles. Further study is needed to establish whether control of fine motor adjustments is perfect despite the deafferentation. Well-learned motor patterns are maintained, at least grossly, but the ability to adjust to unexpected change should be explored further, as should the ability to learn new motor patterns.

Thus, normal human adult speakers compensate immediately (with no trial and error) for any perturbation such as an unexpected load on an articulator or the insertion of a bite block; monkeys can perform learned movements without proprioceptive (stretch reflex) information. Apparently, learned motor performance can proceed without proprioceptive feedback. Polit and Bizzi (1978) suggest, furthermore, that when a monkey is blocked from pointing to a target as it has been taught to do, the limb can store the energy needed, in the form of some equilibrium point previously set, so that when the limb is released, it simply springs forward to the target without a reprogramming of the gesture.

The idea that speech, too, may be controlled automatically at the level of the coordinating muscle groups is inherent in a mass-spring model of motor behavior known as action theory, developed by Fowler, Turvey, Kelso, and others (1980, 1983). According to this theory, the system acts like a series of functionally coupled oscillators, so that if one of the vibrators is constrained, one or more of the others automatically compensates. We have already seen a possible example of this type of compensation in our discussion of front cavity length for the back vowels. Let us assume that you are the subject in an experiment and have been asked to produce the vowel [u]. Your intention is to lengthen the front cavity to produce an appropriately low $F_2$ by using the muscle group that rounds and protrudes the lips. The experimenters, however, foil your plan by placing a metal plate in front of your lips just as you begin to protrude them. Your response will be to resort to the use of another muscle group, either the lingual muscles that can retract the tongue and thus lengthen the front resonating cavity, or the strap muscles of the neck that can lower the larynx, thus increasing

the length of the vocal tract which will lower all the formant frequencies, including $F_2$. Whichever plan you adopt to enlarge the resonating cavities and lower $F_2$, the compensation is virtually immediate and below the level of consciousness.

## Internal Feedback

Internal feedback is the conveyance of information within the brain about motor commands before the motor response itself. Feedback of this type is possible because in addition to information fed back from the periphery, the nervous system can convey information in loops that are central, that is, entirely within the brain.

In light of the many neural connections among the motor areas of the cerebral cortex, the cerebellum, and the thalamus, neurophysiologists have suggested that the control of the type of skilled patterns of movement found in piano playing or speech may operate under a feedback system housed in the central nervous system. Learned patterns under cerebellar control may be activated by the midbrain in association with the motor strip of the cerebrum. Accordingly, information could then be returned to the cerebellum from the motor cortex about whether the neural messages were dispatched as intended. This information would be received and processed well before the muscle response.

There is as yet no direct evidence for internal feedback. Although it is known that the cerebellum and the thalamus are active about 100 ms before movement, current techniques do not allow experimenters to relate this activity to a specific feedback loop.

In summary, several kinds of feedback are available to the speaker (Fig. 8.4). These include the theoretically rapid central internal feedback systems in the central nervous system, capable of feed-forward (prediction) and high-level feedback of initiated motor commands; the relatively fast proprioceptive response feedback systems of the peripheral nervous system, capable of movement

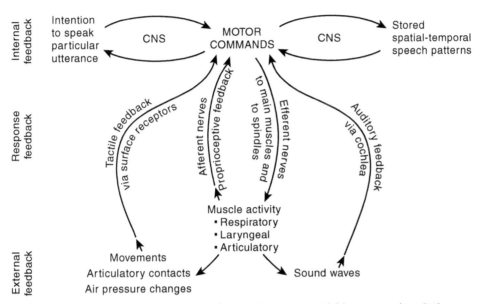

**FIGURE 8.4**  A conceptualization of the feedback systems available to a speaker. CNS, central nervous system.

and positional feedback for the fine control needed in skilled motor acts; and the slower external feedback of the results of motor acts, including, for speech, the acoustic signal, the air pressure variations within the vocal tract, and the physical contact between articulators. The more central the system, the earlier it can feed back information and the more effective it can be for ongoing control of rapid and complex motor patterns. The more peripheral systems, operating after the motor response, can be effective for comparing result with intention and may therefore be important for learning a new motor pattern.

## Developmental Research on Feedback Mechanisms

As we have seen, most of the experimental evidence provided by normally skilled speakers seems to indicate that feedback is not essential for the maintenance of speech production. But we ought to consider the possibility that infants and young children who are learning to speak may be more dependent on feedback than adolescents and adults are.

No one who is aware of the difficulty encountered by children with profound hearing loss in learning speech can doubt the importance to the developing speaker of comparing his own auditory output to the speech of the community in which he lives. People deafened later in life may suffer relatively minor losses to the intelligibility of their speech. Moreover, among the hearing population, children are more adept than adults in acquiring the stress and intonation patterns of a new language. This suggests a more adaptable auditory–motor linkage in young speakers than among older people. Siegel and his colleagues (1976, 1980) found that normal 5-year-olds are more affected by DAF than 8-year-old children. Adults were found to be least affected. Under DAF, the 5-year-olds displayed the greatest reduction in the number of syllables produced per second and the greatest increase in the number of nonfluencies per sentence. This indicates that children may monitor their speech more closely than adults and so are less able to ignore the delay in feedback. An investigation by MacKay (1968) showed that the speech of younger children was most affected by a different delay than adults—500 ms for the 4- to

6-year-olds and 375 ms for the 7- to 9-year-olds, compared with the 200-ms delay that maximally affects adults. It seems that children are more affected than adults when there is a mismatch between auditory and proprioceptive information. When feedback information is simply diminished, there is no marked difference between children and adults. When speaking in the presence of noise, children increase their vocal intensity as adults do, and interference with the sense of taction by nerve block produces the same minor effect on the speech of 4-year-olds as it does on the speech of adults.

The essential combination for learning coordinated speech gestures is perhaps proprioception and audition. Proprioceptive information is available during muscle length changes, and the child need not wait for the result of the movement to get the feel of the gestural pattern. The sense of movement can then be associated with its acoustic and tactile results, and the whole sensation can be compared with the intended sound pattern. Thus, a child trying to perfect production of the word "ball" makes a stab at it based on previous trials, senses the movements and positions of the articulators, which he quickly associates with their tactile and acoustic results, and compares this output with the adult sound of "ball," a stored sound pattern. It is difficult to test the importance of proprioception. Auditory or tactile masking alone is insufficient to disrupt speech when testing linguistic items that the child already knows. Future studies should focus on the effects of interference with feedback channels while subjects, both children and adults, are learning new speech patterns.

## MODELS OF SPEECH PRODUCTION

When we partially understand a system, such as the speech production mechanism, we sometimes make a model of it. A model is a simplification of a system or some part of it. By testing the model under various conditions, we can discover whether or not it behaves like the system and thus learn something about how the system may function.

Many types of models can be fashioned. Perhaps the most obvious type is the mechanical model, a physical version of the system to be tested. von Békésy (1949), for example, constructed a mechanical model of the cochlea in which the basilar membrane was represented by a sheet of rubber of varying thickness. The model looked like a tank of water with a flexible shelf in it. No attempt was made to have it look like the cochlea. Yet it served as the model of von Békésy's traveling wave theory of hearing. At high frequencies of vibration, the waves set up in the tank produced maximum vibrations in the thinnest part of the flexible shelf, and at low frequencies of vibration, the displacement of the membrane was greatest for the thickest portion.

If von Békésy were constructing his model today, he most likely would use a computer to create a representation of his mechanical "cochlea." This type of model can be generated by feeding a physical description of the system into a computer along with the rules by which the system is presumed to operate. The rapid calculating and graphics capabilities of the computer can then be used to determine the changes in the system under various conditions and to display them visually for inspection. An example of this type of computer modeling is Flanagan's (1972) work on a cover-body (two-mass) model of the vocal folds in which the outer (cover) and inner (body) parts vibrate more or less differently from each other (see Chapter 4). Computers are also used today for purely mathematical modeling. This type of computer modeling is, of course, a much faster and more complex extension of the sort of work that was once done with pencil and paper, slide rules, and mechanical calculating machines.

We should note that the validity of all modeling depends to a great extent on the accurate description of the system. If von Békésy's model of the structure of the basilar membrane had been faulty, the vibratory pattern of his rubber sheet might have been very different from that found within the human cochlea. The same would be true for the vibratory patterns that Ishizaka and Flanagan (1972) found for the vocal folds if either his description of the folds or the rules he projected for their response had been incorrect.

Although mechanical and computer modeling have been used in connection with speech, most speech production models are expressed in natural language. They consist of verbal descriptions, charts, definitions, and rules. We shall discuss several models of this type, including those with a strong linguistic basis and emphasis, those that view the goal of speech production as the attainment of targets of one sort or another, those that focus on the role of timing, and those that take a stand on the role of feedback in speech production.

## Linguistically Oriented Models

Linguistic and phonetic analysis has long been concerned with the structure of the sound systems of languages. Indeed, one of the outcomes of such an analysis, the International Phonetic Alphabet (IPA), can be understood as an implied model of speech production because the symbols it uses are tacit representations of the parameters of articulation (e.g., manner of articulation, place of articulation, and voicing for consonants, and, for vowels, tongue, lip, and jaw position).

In 1966, Gordon Peterson and June Shoup, taking the IPA as a starting point, attempted to describe all of the sounds of spoken language, using physiologic and acoustic data from experimental phonetics as their basis. The physiologic component of their model is built from 19 preliminary definitions, 22 axioms, and 77 definitions, followed by two phonetic charts, the first (see Fig. 6.17) representing eight manners of articulation in 13 horizontal and 13 vertical places of articulation and the second chart representing 12 secondary phonetic parame-

ters. In addition, they described three parameters of prosody. The acoustic component of their model comprises verbal and mathematical descriptions of six types of speech waves, six types of acoustic phonetic parameters, and three acoustic parameters of prosody. Finally, the authors relate acoustic phonetics to physiologic phonetics by discussing the transformations possible between the physiologic and acoustic characteristics of speech.

Another linguistically based model is based on a distinctive feature analysis of speech sounds. Early work on this type of model was done by Roman Jakobson, Gunnar Fant, and Morris Halle (1963). Their model attempted to account for the phonetic features of all known languages. An account of the model, *Preliminaries to Speech Analysis*, posited a set of 12 pairs of feature oppositions (e.g., voiced versus voiceless) that were largely derived from the inspection of sound spectrograms and then related to articulation. Each speech sound was specified by assigning to it a single feature from each of 12 pairs.

In 1968, with the publication of *The Sound Pattern of English*, Noam Chomsky and Morris Halle redesigned the binary distinctive feature system in articulatory rather than acoustic terms. For example, instead of the Jakobson, Fant, and Halle opposition of grave versus acute, in which the grave feature refers to sounds that occupy the lower frequency regions of the spectrum and the acute feature refers to the high-frequency regions of the spectrum, Chomsky and Halle reformulated the distinctive features in terms of such binary articulatory features as ± "rounded," ± "high tongue body," and ± "back tongue body." They posited a total of 27 features, divided among the categories of major class features, cavity features, manner of articulation features, and source features.

Because each sound in a sequence is described by a (unique) set of distinctive features, this model is essentially static. It cannot account for the dynamic nature of speech without a supplementary set of rules to generate the acoustic results of the sequencing of articulatory features, including the assimilative and coarticulatory effects of context (see Chapter 6). To be fair, the authors are more interested in the phonologic competence of speakers than in the realization of their phonetic output, and even though they do not specify the role of timing and the effects of context, the Chomsky and Halle features are more useful to a speech production model than is a purely acoustic set of features.

Students should be aware that there is no one set of distinctive features that is universally accepted for use in speech analysis or in modeling speech production. Individual linguists and phoneticians have proposed different feature inventories, often to meet different requirements. Clearly, someone interested in phonology will make different decisions about the number and types of features that are important as opposed to someone interested in specifying the physiologic, articulatory, or acoustic output of the speech mechanism. There is even a disparity of opinion concerning the binary nature of the features. Ladefoged (1972), for instance, proposes a system in which each occurrence of a feature is specified by a percentage, indicating the extent to which it is used. This strategy permits both a phonological characterization of each sound and a phonetic characterization of each sound as it varies in context.

The final group of linguistically oriented models of speech production that we consider stems from work on speech perception. It was first presented in a paper by Liberman, Cooper, Shankweiler, and Studdert-Kennedy in 1967. As we shall see in our discussion of speech perception, this paper linked speech perception to speech production. The authors maintained that speech sounds are encoded in the acoustic signal because of the way they are produced by the speech mechanism. They therefore found it necessary to project a model of speech production that explained the process by which the speech sounds become encoded. The model (Fig. 8.5) depicts the encoding process as a series of transformations, from

the phonemes (or the sets of features they comprise) to the acoustic signal that transmits them in their encoded forms to the listener. This model rejects the notion that there is a simple and direct conversion from phoneme to sound. It holds, rather, that there is acoustic "smearing" of the phonemes resulting from the coarticulation of two or more phonemes simultaneously.

According to this model, the appropriate neuromotor rules govern the simultaneous transmission of neural signals to many muscles. The articulatory gestures produced when these muscles contract cause variations in the vocal tract shape that conform to a set of articulatory rules. The time-varying changes in cavity shape are converted into what we hear as speech by a set of acoustic rules. The point is that, in these multiple conversions, the phoneme as a static entity is modified by its context because more than one phoneme is being transmitted by the motor system of the speaker at one time. The acoustic signal must therefore reflect the overlap in muscle activity and articulatory movements. We will describe this model more fully in the chapter on speech perception.

The models discussed above are strongly influenced by linguistic considerations. Other models of speech production emphasize neurophysiologic considerations more strongly.

## Target Models

It is not difficult to think of speech production as a process in which speakers attempt to attain a sequence of targets corresponding to the speech sounds they are attempting to produce. Theorists have used this concept to construct models of speech production, although there is some disagreement over whether the targets are spatial, auditory–acoustic, or somewhat more abstract.

Let us first consider models that propose spatial targets as the basis of speech production. Peter MacNeilage, in a 1970 paper "Motor Control of Serial Ordering of Speech,"

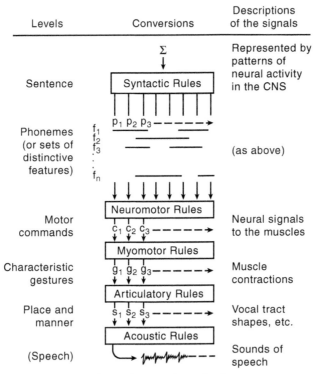

| Levels | Conversions | Descriptions of the signals |
|---|---|---|

**FIGURE 8.5** A schema for speech production as conceptualized by Liberman. Perception is conceived as the reverse of the process shown here. CNS, central nervous system. (Modified with permission from Liberman, A. M., Cooper, F. S., Shankweiler, D. P., and Studdert-Kennedy, M., Perception of the Speech Code. *Psychol. Rev. 74*, 1967, 431–461.)

presented a speech production model compatible with Hebb's (1949) idea of motor equivalence and the then-current work on γ loop control in motor systems. An example of motor equivalence is the fact that if you can write the letter B with your right hand, you can write it with your left hand or even with your toes. Although the muscles used are different and you may be clumsier some ways than others, your production will retain some aspects of your individual style. A specific example of motor equivalence in speech, given by MacNeilage, is the ability of any speaker to produce speech while holding an object, such as a pipe stem, between his teeth, even though the jaw, tongue, and lip movements and underlying muscle activity must be altered. You can sense the changes in muscular and articulatory behavior by saying "hot" first in a natural manner while your jaw is lowered and your mouth open, and then again with your jaw immobilized as you hold a pencil or pipe between your teeth. MacNeilage argues that this sort of motor equivalence demonstrates that speakers do not issue an invariant set of motor commands for each speech segment, because speakers must approach the vocal tract shapes for a particular segment from many different starting positions. Rather, the goal of the speaker is a spatial target. The brain has an internalized spatial representation of the areas of the vocal tract within which the articulators move. To reach a desired spatial target, the speaker must adapt articulatory movements to the target position in relation to the particular starting position of the articulators at a given time. The theory posits speech production as an essentially open loop system with a series of targets specified in advance, although it is likely that the γ loop feedback mechanism facilitates the articulatory adjustments required in varying contexts by monitoring muscle behavior.

Acoustic–auditory targets (as opposed to spatial targets) have also been used as a basis for modeling speech production. These targets are presumably specified in terms of invariant vowel formant frequencies for which the speaker aims with varying degrees of success: as we have seen, weakly stressed vowels are reduced, becoming more schwa-like as the result of articulatory undershoot. Nonetheless, listeners are able to compensate perceptually for the reduction and so recover the identity of the vowel as if the targets had, in fact, been attained. Hence, the target is idealized psychologically by the listener and is not a function of motor equivalence in the articulation of the speaker.

It is also possible to construct models that use both spatial and acoustic–auditory targets. Sibout Nooteboom (1992) concurs with MacNeilage's target theory, finding an internalized spatial coordinate system more efficient than stored motor patterns for each possible action, but he proposes that Mac-Neilage did not go far enough in his model. MacNeilage proposes spatial targets as the goals with γ loop control of muscle activity to facilitate the articulatory adjustments that are conditioned by context and required to achieve motor equivalence. Nooteboom, however, cautions that the goal of the speaker is to be understood, and is therefore primarily perceptual. Spatial targets sometimes vary, and so motor equivalence is not always required for the speaker to produce a given sound in a variety of phonetic contexts. Nooteboom offers the example of speakers producing [u] with and without lip rounding. If lip protrusion is not used to lengthen the tract for the lowering of formants, tongue retraction or depression of the larynx may be substituted to achieve the de-

sired acoustic result. The spatial targets thus differ from one production strategy to the other, but both generate the same phoneme, /u/. Nooteboom's speech production model would include an internal representation of an auditory perceptual space. Accessing both the auditory and spatial representations, the brain of the speaker uses rules relating these representations to calculate the motor commands necessary to attain a target starting from any current articulatory state.

Ladefoged has also suggested an acoustic–auditory theory of speech production, at least for vowels. He implies that control of production may differ between consonants and vowels.

Targets of a more abstract nature than articulatory–spatial configurations or formant frequencies have been proposed by action theorists. They posit a model of speech production that directly transforms phonologic targets into sound without multiple conversions. A target in this view is a minimally specified vocal tract adjustment. Self-regulated functional units of muscle groups and articulators control both the active and passive forces required to attain the target. This theory has an ecologic emphasis that takes into account both the inherent mechanical properties of the speech production system (the momentary tension, elasticity, and inertia acting on the muscle groups involved) and the potential external mechanical influences on the system (as when a child places a hand on a speaker's chin).

Browman and Goldstein's (1992) articulatory (or gestural) phonology provides a model that is related to the linguistic and target models described earlier and, in certain respects, to the timing models described later in the chapter. The basic units of the model are articulatory gestures, such as lip opening and pharyngeal width, that can cause differences in the phonological classification of speech sounds. To some extent, then, these gestures are reminiscent of distinctive features. They differ from distinctive features, however, in at least two important ways. First, the gestures are physiological entities and not specific features of vowels or consonants. Second, they are specified with regard to their relative timing. This enables the model to account for coarticulatory effects in a way that most distinctive feature systems cannot do.

## Timing Models

The search for the invariant correlate of the phoneme, whether physiological–articulatory or acoustic, is not the only concern of the experimental phonetician. The fact that speech is ordered in time has led to several speech production models that emphasize timing. Lashley's classic 1951 paper succeeded in discrediting associate chain theories of speech production in the minds of most theorists who have followed him. An associate chain theory holds that each movement serves as the stimulus for the movement that follows it. In contrast, Lashley theorized that speech production incorporates several interacting but independent systems corresponding to the speaker's intention, the store of images and words, the motor organization, and a temporal ordering mechanism. The important point is that although the temporal ordering is not inherent in the idea, the word, or the motor organization, it can control their ordering. The temporal ordering device is a syntax, an integrating schema, that orders the words and the motor activity of speech production. Lashley's is an open loop model, comprising continually interactive systems.

Sven Öhman (1966) has constructed a mathematical model of the articulation of vowel–consonant–vowel (VCV) utterances in which the vocal tract is sectioned by 50 radial planes. Using the highest point of the palate and the beginning of the curved oral cavity as coordinates, the model mathematically summarizes the coarticulation that Öhman described from spectrograms. The model includes static properties of phonemes and dynamic rules that blend the phonemes into running speech. Öhman views the temporal ordering of motor activity as the result

of the speaker superimposing consonant articulations on what is essentially a string of vowel-to-vowel articulations. This assumption accounts for the coarticulatory effects he observed in the VCV syllables and also implies separate control mechanisms for vowels and consonants.

William Henke (1966) has developed a computer model based on articulatory data. The timing component of the model is a scan-ahead mechanism for motor control. Motor commands may be initiated simultaneously for a sequence of segments, as long as no intervening segment in the sequence requires a contradictory command. For example, according to this sort of model, the scan-ahead mechanism, operating on the intended production of the word "strew" (/stru/), would permit lip rounding for the [u] to begin with the articulation of the [s], because none of the sounds before the /u/ requires some other lip posture. The model thus generates a string of phonemes with coarticulation resulting from the spread of features from one sound to other, adjacent sounds. Research by Bell-Berti and Harris (1981) suggests that the features for a target phone simply begin at a fixed time before that phone and so do not simply migrate without constraints. This finding explains why a feature does not occur in an unlimited number of neighboring segments.

Rhythm is another temporal aspect of speech that has provided the basis for a model. James Martin (1972) has proposed a model of speech rhythm in which the timing of the more highly stressed syllables in a phrase is planned first and given primary articulatory emphasis by the speaker, whereas the timing and articulation of the lesser-stressed syllables receive secondary consideration in planning and articulation. The production mechanism is under central nervous system control. Although some languages, including English, appear to be more obviously stress-timed than others, Martin considers such relative timing patterns, or rhythms, to be universal. Stress timing (isochrony) is the tendency for primary

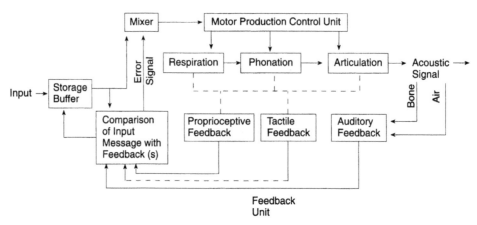

**FIGURE 8.6** Fairbanks's model of speech production. (Adapted with permission from Fairbanks, G., A Theory of the Speech Mechanism as a Servosystem. *J. Speech Hear. Disord. 19*, 1954, 133–139.)

stresses to occur at equal intervals in an utterance. Listeners seem to sense the rhythm of speech and use it to help predict the rest of a message.

However, when one sets out to measure the rhythm of speech in the laboratory, isochrony turns out to be as elusive as the phoneme. It may be that it exists in the mind of the speaker but is temporally blurred as it is transformed to the acoustic stream of speech, much as the features of segmental phonemes are smeared by coarticulation. The listener, however, according to Martin, is capable of perceptually reconstructing the intended isochronous timing (perhaps in a process analogous to the one in which the identities of reduced vowels are recovered), despite the irregularities in the speaker's rate or in other factors that contribute to the perception of rhythm.

## Closed Loop and Open Loop Models

The status of feedback in the production of speech has motivated a number of models. As shown in our discussion of feedback, that status has recently been questioned. A number of years ago, however, it was more or less generally assumed that feedback is an essential component of speech production, and the models of that period reflected that assumption. A classic (and the first) example

of a closed loop model was developed by Grant Fairbanks and published in 1954. Fairbanks depicted the speech mechanism as a servomechanism in which auditory, tactile, and proprioceptive feedback played prominent roles.

The model is depicted graphically in Figure 8.6. The storage buffer holds in memory the utterance that is to be produced. The comparison unit performs two tasks: it relates the intended signal to the feedback of the actual output for correction and it uses a predicting device so that speech production need not be delayed until the error signal disappears. When a discrepancy between the intended and the obtained signal appears in the comparison unit, it is sent to the mixer, so that the motor production control unit can be adjusted.

Among the first models to depict speech production as an open loop process was the one published by Kozhevnikov and Chistovich (1965) of the Pavlov Institute in Leningrad. It stimulated thought on speech organization by presenting a model of speech timing and syllable control. By measuring the durations of phrases separated by pauses, the investigators showed the pauses to be much more variable in duration than the intervals of speech between the pauses. They concluded that time can be measured meaningfully only within a phrase. When the rate

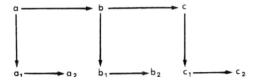

**FIGURE 8.7** Commands for syllables a, b, and c. The syllable commands include consonant commands ($a_1$, $b_1$, and $c_1$) and vowel commands ($a_2$, $b_2$, and $c_2$). Commands for consonants and vowels may be issued simultaneously, though they are realized sequentially. (Adapted from Kozhevnikov, V. A., and Chistovich, L. A., *Speech: Articulation and Perception*. Springfield, VA: U.S. Department of Commerce, 1966.)

of speech is changed within a phrase, they found that the relative durations of the syllables and words remained constant; only by measuring the changes in consonants and vowels within each syllable did they find a significant difference in relative durations. The durations of the consonants change little at faster or slower rates, but the durations of the vowels change considerably. Kozhevnikov and Chistovich concluded that the organization of articulatory timing was contained in motor commands specifying complete syllables. Thus, for example, the commands for a CV syllable (e.g., "a" in Fig. 8.7) include instructions for both the consonant ("$a_1$") and the vowel ("$a_2$") of that syllable. Furthermore, as Henke's model predicted, movements required by different segments within the syllable may be initiated simultaneously, unless they are contradictory.

The control of the syllable commands was hypothesized to be open loop on the basis of a comparison of predictions from an open loop and a closed loop model. Figures 8.8 and 8.9 contrast the alternative

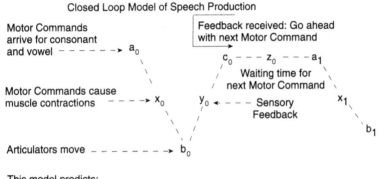

Closed Loop Model of Speech Production

This model predicts:

Basic rate:      | ----Syl. 1 ----| ---- Syl. 2----| ----Syl. 3--|

Slower Syl. 2:  | ---- Syl. 1 ----| ----- Syl. 2----|----- Syl. 3---|

Faster Syl. 2:  | ---- Syl. 1 ----| --- Syl. 2 --|----- Syl. 3 | ----

**FIGURE 8.8** Hypothesis of closed loop control. The command to begin the next syllable is issued in response to an afferent impulse indicating the beginning of the preceding syllable. $a_0$ and $a_1$ are the moments of arrival of the syllable commands; $b_0$ and $b_1$ are the moments of the beginning of the corresponding movements; and $c_0$ is the moment of entry into the nervous system of the afferent impulse indicating the beginning of the movement. (x and y indicate time for motor and sensory transfer, z, the interval between movement and the next command.) (Adapted from Kozhevnikov, V. A., and Chistovich, L. A., *Speech: Articulation and Perception*. Springfield, VA: U.S. Department of Commerce, 1966.)

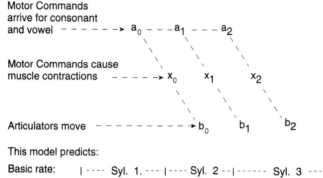

Open Loop Model of Speech Production

Motor Commands
arrive for consonant
and vowel   – – – – – –→  $a_0$  – – –$a_1$  – – – $a_2$

Motor Commands cause
muscle contractions   – – – – –→ $x_0$     $x_1$        $x_2$

Articulators move   – – – – – – – – –→$b_0$     $b_1$      $b_2$

This model predicts:

Basic rate:   | – – – – Syl. 1. – – – | – – – – Syl. 2 – –| – – – – – – Syl. 3 – – –

Slower Syl. 2:   | – – – – Syl. 1 – – – | – – – – – Syl. 2 – – – –| – – – – – Syl. 3 – – –

Faster Syl. 2:   | – – – – – – Syl. 1 – – – –| – – Syl. 2 – –| – – – – – Syl. 3 – – – –

**FIGURE 8.9** Hypothesis of open loop control. Commands for successive syllables are centrally issued. Afferent impulses do not affect the onset of successive syllables. (Adapted from Kozhevnikov, V. A., and Chistovich, L. A., *Speech: Articulation and Perception*. Springfield, VA: U.S. Department of Commerce, 1966.)

hypotheses. In the closed loop hypothesis, the command to begin each syllable awaits sensory feedback indicating that the preceding syllable command was issued (Fig. 8.8). This is a form of closed loop control. The open loop hypothesis holds that syllable commands are issued without sensory feedback from the muscle response (Fig. 8.9). Testing these two hypotheses by measuring the inevitable durational variability obtained when a phrase is repeated about 150 to 200 times, Kozhevnikov and Chistovich tentatively concluded the first hypothesis of closed loop control to be less probable. The phrase was "Tonya topila banyu," which means "Tonya heated the bath." The investigators found that the variation in syllable duration was greater than the variation for the whole phrase and that the durations of the adjacent syllables were negatively correlated. They concluded that the data support an open loop model in which syllables are articulatory events independent of adjacent syllables, in the sense that each syllable command is automatically initiated under the guidance of an unspecified rhythm generator in the nervous system.

At this point, it seems likely that speech operates as a system (Figs. 8.4 and 8.10) in which the more general speech goal (the kind of sound stream the speaker intends to produce) is roughly planned by a feed-forward predictive flow of information within the brain. This internal feedback is based on the speaker's knowledge of the acoustics of speech and of his or her own speech production system. The details of muscle activity and coarticulation are the natural result of muscle groups cooperating to perform a unified function. The flow of proprioceptive information among these groups of muscles is normally available and is important to the establishment of speech patterns in children but may be largely redundant for those who have learned to speak. Much of the tactile and auditory feedback (external feedback) available to the speaker is not thought to be used for ongoing control but rather is reserved for identifying and correcting errors after they have been made and for maintaining an internal schema. This model does not support the notion that the speech production mechanism of the established speaker acts like a servomechanism.

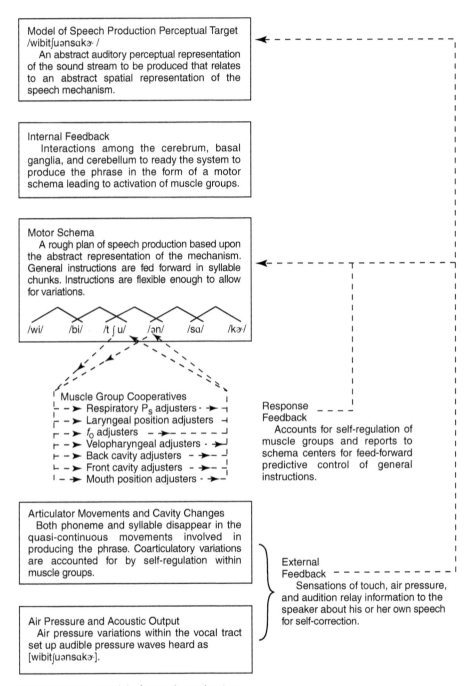

**FIGURE 8.10**   Model of speech production.

Questions of the role of closed and open loop control systems for speech remain unresolved today. So, too, do the principles governing motor programming, as they are revealed in speech rhythm and coarticulation. As our knowledge increases, the models, the feature systems, and even the definitions will continue to be modified. There is no better way to realize both how much and how little we know and how complex speech

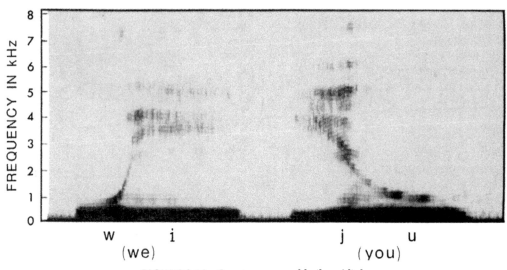

**FIGURE 8.11**    Spectrograms of [wi] and [ju].

production is than to describe just the peripheral events that occur in the production of a short utterance. The last section of this chapter is such a description.

## PRODUCTION OF A SENTENCE

We beat you in soccer:

['wi' bi'tjuən'sakɚ] or ['wi'bi'tʃuən'sakɚ]

Having been soundly defeated by a rival college football team, a member of the defeated team retorted to a comment by one of the victors with "We may have lost in football, but we beat you in soccer." If we were inside the brain of that speaker pushing buttons to produce "we beat you in soccer," what might be the order and integration of the commands to the speech production mechanism? The phrase is appealing because it contains stops, fricatives, a nasal, semivowels, and our favorite vowels [i], [a], and [u]. Also, when said with the [ju] unassimilated to the [t] as in one of the alternative pronunciations, there is a pleasing symmetry in having [wi] and [ju], which are not only opposites in that they refer to the rival teams but also spectrographic mirror images of one

another, [wi] starting at an acoustic [u] and gliding to [i], while [ju] starts at an acoustic [i] and glides to [u] (Fig. 8.11).

Whatever intentions the speaker may have had—retribution, a desire to inform, or merely offering a friendly but slightly barbed joke—we shall not attempt to determine. Nor shall we trace the interactions of syntactic and semantic recall and decision. Presuming that "we beat you in soccer" was put momentarily in a buffer for output and that the timing and prosodic control were imposed on it as it was fed out into motor commands, we shall indicate some of the motor events peripheral to the more general motor goals, whatever they may have been. The logical way to indicate the motor events is in terms of neural activity, muscle contraction, articulator movements, changes in resonating cavities, air pressure changes, and acoustic results. Omissions outnumber inclusions. Not included are all the constantly effective passive forces of elasticity, gravity, mass, and inertia. Only some of the obvious active muscle forces are included. Auxiliary muscle activity and agonist–antagonist relationships are not described. Also omitted are the many possible transmissions of sensory information from changes in muscle length, from contact between articulators, and from

**TABLE 8.1** Production of a Sentence (*An explanation of the abbreviations can be found in a footnote at the end of the table*)

| Innervation | Muscles | Movements | Pressure Changes | Result |
|---|---|---|---|---|
| Phrenic n. | → Diaphragm | → Lowering thoracic floor | → Thoracic vertical volume increase, pressure decrease | → Inhalation |
| Thoracic n. (T₁–T₁₁) | → EIm and interchondral IIm | → Ribs elevated and expanded | → Lateral and antero-posterior thoracic volume increase, pressure decrease | → Inhalation (~65% VC) |
| C. N. XII | → GGm | → Tongue elevated to "ready" position | | |
| C. N. VII | → OOm | → Lip protrusion for [w] | | |
| C. N. XI | → LPm | → Velum raised and backed to block nasal resonance during [wibiʤu] | | |
| C. N. XII | → SGm | → Tongue dorsum elevated to [u] position for [w] | → Lower the resonance characteristics by elongated vocal tract | |
| C. N. X | → IAm | → Adduction of vocal folds for [wibi] | | |
| C. N. X | → LCAm | → Aids in adduction of vocal folds | | |

(*Continued*)

175

**TABLE 8.1** Production of a Sentence (*Continued*)

| Innervation | Muscles | Movements | Pressure Changes | Result |
|---|---|---|---|---|
| | Diaphragm relaxes gradually | Thorax and lungs slowly restored by elasticity, gravity, and torque | Decrease in vertical thoracic volume; pressure increase | Exhalation of about 7 cm $H_2O$ $P_s$ during utterance |
| | | Folds part as high-velocity air flows between them | $P_s$ opens glottis | |
| | | Adducts folds | Bernoulli effect (negative pressure between vocal folds) | |
| | | | $P_s$ builds and opens glottis again | Repetition of this cycle releases a rapid train of air pulses that excite air (voicing) in broad band of freq. ($f_0$ and harmonics) during [wibi] |
| | | | Source sound amplified and filtered by resonance of vocal tract set for [u] | Onset of [w]; low-freq. periodic sound |
| C. N. XII | GGm contracts as SGm relaxes | Tongue moves from high back to high front for [wi] and remains for [bit] | Phonated sound pressure resonated in changing tract [u] → [i] | $F_2$ glides up from low resonances of [u] tract to high resonances of [i] tract, producing [wi] |
| C. N. VII | Rm contracts as OOm relaxes | Lips move from rounded to spread for [wi] | | |

176

C. N. X ⟶ IAm continues to contract but LCAm relaxes ⟶ Glottis more open, continues to vibrate ⟶ More $P_s$ air released into tract for stop

C. N. VII ⟶ OOm ⟶ Lips close ⟶ Pressure builds behind closure ⟶ Vocal tract resonances damped

OOm relaxes ⟶ Lips part for [b] ⟶ Sharp air pulse released without aspiration ⟶ Transient aperiodic burst added to phonation for [b]

$T_1$–$T_{11}$ ⟶ IIm ⟶ Depresses ribs ⟶ Adds pressure to $P_s$ ⟶ Increases intensity for stressed [i]

C. N. XII ⟶ GGm remains contracted ⟶ Tongue blade high in oral cavity; pharyngeal cavity larger, oral smaller than neutral ⟶ Pressure wave from glottis amplified by resonances of vocal tract ⟶ Low $F_1$; high $F_2$ and $F_3$ owing to small oral cavity [i]

C. N. X ⟶ PCAm ⟶ Abduct vocal folds; vibration stops ⟶ Increased airflow into oral cavity for stop/affricate

C. N. XII ⟶ SLm added to GGm ⟶ Tongue tip and blade up for alveolar contact ⟶ Intraoral pressure builds behind occlusion ⟶ Silence during closure

(*Continued*)

**TABLE 8.1** Production of a Sentence (*Continued*)

| Innervation | Muscles | Movements | Pressure Changes | Result |
|---|---|---|---|---|
| C. N. XII | SLm relaxes | Contract released | Sharp air pulse released with aspiration | Transient aperiodic high-freq. burst [t] |
| C. N. X | IAm and LCAm | Adduct vocal folds to resume phonation | Sudden reduction in intraoral pressure | $f_0$ and [i] resonance |
| C. N. XII | GGm still active, giving way to SGm contraction | Tongue remains high for [i] shape at onset of [i] and shifts to high back [u] shape | Resonances change from [i] to [u] | $F_1$ stays low; $F_2$ goes from high to low freq. [ju] |
| C. N. VII | OOm | Lips protrude | | |

Or alternative pronunciation: [tʃuən]

| Innervation | Muscles | Movements | Pressure Changes | Result |
|---|---|---|---|---|
| C. N. XII | GGm still active, giving way to SGm contraction | Slow release of blade into palatal constriction | Higher velocity airflow through constriction | [ʃ] turbulence at release of stop: [tʃ] affricate |
| C. N. XII | GGm still active, giving way to SGm contraction | Tongue backing and elevating to [u] position | Lower resonances | Lower formants |
| C. N. X | IAm and LCAm | Adducts vocal folds; resumes phonation for [uən] | Reduced intraoral pressure | $f_0$ and [u] resonances |
| C. N. VII | OOm | Lip protrusion | Lengthen tract, lowering resonances | Lower formants |

C. N. XII inactive ——→ Tongue returns to neutral ——→ Evenly spaced formants

C. N. XII active ——→ SLm ——→ Blade raised to alveolar ridge ——→ Small pressure increase within oral cavity ——→ $F_2$ rising

C. N. XI decreases activity ——→ LPm relaxes ——→ Velum lowers; opening to nasal cavities ——→ Pressure drop as tract volume increases ——→ Low-freq. nasal resonance added; also antiresonances [n]

Or alternative: /ŋ/

(Same as above but timing is different, with first alternative [ən] having oral to nasal resonance transition and second alternative [ŋ] having faster velar lowering.)

C. N. XII ——→ SLm ——→ Blade up to alveolar ridge ——→ Intraoral pressure increase ——→ $F_2$ rising

C. N. XI ——→ PGm ——→ Lowers velum ——→ Sudden pressure drop; nasal resonance ——→ Low-freq. nasal resonance; upper formant anti-resonances

(Continued)

179

**TABLE 8.1**. Production of a Sentence (Continued)

| Innervation | Muscles | Movements | Pressure Changes | Result |
|---|---|---|---|---|
| C. N. XI | LPm | Abrupt high elevation and backing of velum, especially for [s], but maintained for rest of utterance | | |
| C. N. X | PCAm | Abduction of vocal folds to stop phonation | Airflow increased for high-pressure fricative | |
| C. N. XII | GGm with SLm (or ILm if tip down) | Blade to palate constriction | High-pressure flow through constriction; turbulence | Aperiodic noise 4 kHz and higher [s] |
| C. N. XII | SLm (or ILm) remains active / HGm contracts | Blade remains high for [s] as / Dorsum starts to lower for [a] | Pressure reduced as oral cavity enlarges | |
| C. N. V | ABDm | Opens jaw | | |
| C. N. X | IAm and LCAm | Adducts vocal folds resume phonation | Sound pressure from glottis | |
| $T_1$–$T_{11}$ | IIm | Ribs depressed | $P_s$ increased; vocal fold opening increases amplitude | Increased intensity for stressed [a] |
| C. N. X | CTm | Lengthens vocal folds | Increased tension of folds; faster vibration | Raise $f_0$ for [sa] prominence |
| C. N. XII | Maintains HGm activity as GGm and tip muscles relax | Anterior tongue lowers, occupying space in pharyngeal cavity | Increased volume in oral cavity; open tract increases SPL at output | High $F_1$; low $F_2$ for [a] resonance |

180

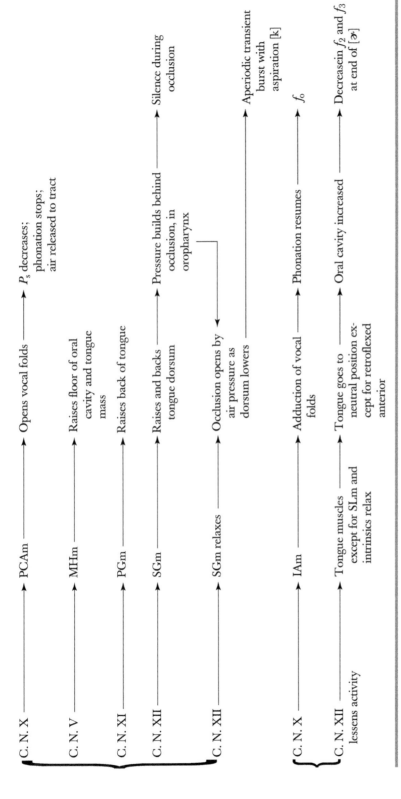

EIm, external intercostal; IIm, internal intercostal; GGm, genioglossus; OOm, orbicularis oris; LPm, levator palatini; SGm, styloglossus; IAm, interarytenoid; LCAm, lateral cricoarytenoid; Rm, risorius; PCAm, posterior cricoarytenoid; SLm, superior longitudinal; PGm, palatoglossus; ILm, inferior longitudinal; HGm, hyoglossus; ABDm, anterior belly of digastric; CTm, cricothyroid; and MHm, mylohyoid muscle. Other abbreviations include C. N., cranial nerve; SPL, sound pressure level; VC, vital capacity; $P_s$, subglottal pressure; $f_o$, fundamental frequency; $F_1$, $F_2$, $F_3$, first, second, and third formants; freq., frequency.

acoustic–auditory signals, which provide the speaker with information about his or her performance. We have made some specific assumptions, however, about the particular way (of many possibilities) in which the speaker has articulated the sentence to make the description concrete. Despite the omissions, the description is worth careful inspection, if only to demonstrate the interrelationships among the processes of respiration, laryngeal activity, and articulation (activities usually described separately) and to remind ourselves of the complexity of speech.

The speaker, let us say, needs a quick inhalation for the phrase to begin (Table 8.1). To avoid the mistaken notion that this attempt to interweave the respiratory, phonatory, and articulatory events of speech is the result of parallel but separate nerve-to-air pressure transformations or that there are direct phoneme-to-sound conversions, we shall frame the process another way with a model that may better represent the coordination among muscle groups involved in speech. Figure 8.10 shows the initial speech goal to be an auditory perceptual representation of "we beat you in soccer." We know the general sound of the phrase we plan to say. At this prespeech stage, there may be an internal loop of neural activity among the basal ganglia, the cerebrum, and the cerebellum of the brain, readying the system for speech output. The motor schema for producing the phrase may be in a rather abstract and flexible state, allowing for variations in the actual production. Rough specifications for changes in the speech mechanisms may form the schema. The general changes of the vocal tract for the utterance may be elicited from storage through cerebellar control of the motor areas of the cerebrum, and this representation may be fed forward in chunks of at least syllable size. The organization of particular muscle groups, such as the muscles that cooperate to regulate $f_o$, may be self-regulating via the response feedback of muscle spindles. We indicate how two chunks may overlap as the schema for [tʃuən] activates the muscle groups.

The muscle groups organized for a particular function not only are coordinated among themselves but also are coordinated with other muscle groups organized for a different function. This larger coordination may be made possible largely by feeding forward well-practiced interactions of specifications. The movements of articulators and the changes in cavity shapes are continuous, blurring phoneme and syllable boundaries as we perceive them. Variations in movement caused by context or by differences in initial position are the rule and are automatically produced as a result of the intimate coordination within each muscle group. Air pressure variations and the resultant acoustic stream are likewise dynamic in the ways they change across time. External feedback of the tactile and auditory feedback sensations may be too late to influence the peripheral motor patterns of muscle group activity, but they do influence the more general schema so that any mistake may be corrected on the next attempt.

The goal of the speaker, then, is to produce sounds that fit an auditory–perceptual target, to be understood by the perceptual system of a listener. In the following chapters, we will consider that perceptual system and the processes that may be involved in listening.

# BIBLIOGRAPHY

## Feedback

### General Readings

Borden, G. J., An Interpretation of Research on Feedback Interruption. *Brain Lang. 7,* 1979, 307–319.

Ringel, R. L., Oral Sensation and Perception: A Selective Review. *ASHA Rep. 5,* 1970, 188–206.

Wiener, N., Cybernetics. *Sci. Am. 179,* 1948, 14–19.

Wiener, N., *The Human Use of Human Beings,* 2nd ed. Rev. Garden City, NY: Doubleday, 1954.

## Auditory Feedback

Black, J. W., The Effect of Delayed Side-Tone Upon Vocal Rate and Intensity. *J. Speech Hear. Disord. 16,* 1951, 56–60.

Borden, G. J., Dorman, M. F., Freeman, F. J., and Raphael, L. J., Electromyographic Changes With Delayed Auditory Feedback of Speech. *J. Phonet. 5,* 1977, 1–8.

Fairbanks, G., and Guttman, N., Effects of Delayed Auditory Feedback Upon Articulation. *J. Speech Hear. Res. 1,* 1958, 12–22.

Fairbanks, G., Selective Vocal Effects of Delayed Auditory Feedback. *J. Speech Hear. Disord. 20,* 1955, 333–346.

Garber, S. F., *The Effects of Feedback Filtering on Nasality.* Paper presented at ASHA convention, Houston, Nov. 1976.

Lane, H. L., Catania, A. C., and Stevens, S. S., Voice Level: Autophonic Scale, Perceived Loudness, and Effects of Side Tone. *J. Acoust. Soc. Am. 33,* 1961, 160–167.

Lane, H. L., and Tranel, B., The Lombard Sign and the Role of Hearing in Speech. *J. Speech Hear. Res. 14,* 1971, 677–709.

Lee, B. S., Effects of Delayed Speech Feedback. *J. Acoust. Soc. Am. 22,* 1950, 824–826.

Siegel, G. M., and Pick, H. L., Jr., Auditory Feedback in the Regulation of Voice. *J. Acoust. Soc. Am. 56,* 1974, 1618–1624.

Stromstra, C., Delays Associated With Certain Sidetone Pathways. *J. Acoust. Soc. Am. 34,* 1962, 392–396.

Von Békésy, G., The Structure of the Middle Ear and the Hearing of One's Own Voice by Bone Conduction. *J. Acoust. Soc. Am. 21,* 1949, 217–232.

Webster, R. L., and Dorman, M. F., Changes in Reliance on Auditory Feedback Cues as a Function of Oral Practice. *J. Speech Hear. Res. 14,* 1971, 307–311.

Yates, A. J., Delayed Auditory Feedback. *Psychol. Bull. 60,* 1963, 213–232.

## Tactile Feedback

Borden, G. J., Harris, K. S., and Catena, L., Oral Feedback II. An Electromyographic Study of Speech Under Nerve-Block Anesthesia. *J. Phonet. 1,* 1973, 297–308.

Borden, G. J., Harris, K. S., and Oliver, W., Oral Feedback I. Variability of the Effect of Nerve-Block Anesthesia Upon Speech. *J. Phonet. 1,* 1973, 289–295.

Gammon, S. A., Smith, P. J., Daniloff, R. G., and Kim, C. W., Articulation and Stress/Juncture Production Under Oral Anesthetization and Masking. *J. Speech Hear. Res. 14,* 1971, 271–282.

Hardcastle, W. J., Some Aspects of Speech Production Under Controlled Conditions of Oral Anesthesia and Auditory Masking. *J. Phonet. 3,* 1975, 197–214.

Horii, Y., House, A. S., Li, K. P., and Ringel, R. L., Acoustic Characteristics of Speech Produced Without Oral Sensation. *J. Speech Hear. Res. 16,* 1973, 67–77.

Hutchinson, J. M., and Putnam, A. H. B., Aerodynamic Aspects of Sensory Deprived Speech. *J. Acoust. Soc. Am. 56,* 1974, 1612–1617.

Leanderson, R., and Persson, A., The Effect of Trigeminal Nerve Block on the Articulatory EMG Activity of Facial Muscles. *Acta Otolaryngol. (Stockh.) 74,* 1972, 271–278.

Prosek, R. A., and House, A. S., Intraoral Air Pressure as a Feedback Cue in Consonant Production. *J. Speech Hear. Res. 18,* 1975, 133–147.

Putnam, A. H. B., and Ringel, R., A Cineradiographic Study of Articulation in Two Talkers With Temporarily Induced Oral Sensory Deprivation. *J. Speech Hear. Res. 19,* 1976, 247–266.

Putnam, A. H. B., and Ringel, R., Some Observations of Articulation During Labial Sensory Deprivation. *J. Speech Hear. Res. 15,* 1972, 529–542.

Scott, C. M., and Ringel, R. L., Articulation Without Oral Sensory Control. *J. Speech Hear. Res. 14,* 1971, 804–818.

## Proprioceptive Feedback

Abbs, J., The Influence of the Gamma Motor System on Jaw Movements During Speech: A Theoretical Framework and Some Preliminary Observations. *J. Speech Hear. Res. 16,* 1973, 175–200.

Bowman, J. P., *Muscle Spindles and Neural Control of the Tongue: Implications for Speech.* Springfield, IL: Charles C Thomas, 1971.

Cooper, S., Muscle Spindles and Other Muscle Receptors. In *The Structure and Function of Muscle,* Vol. 1. G. H. Bourne (Ed.). New York: Academic Press, 1960, pp. 381–420.

Critchlow, V., and von Euler, C., Intercostal Muscle Spindle Activity and Its Motor Control. *J. Physiol. 168*, 1963, 820–847.

Fitzgerald, M. J. T., and Law, M. E., The Peripheral Connexions Between the Lingual and Hypoglossal Nerves. *J. Anat. 92*, 1958, 178–188.

Folkins, J. W., and Abbs, J. H., Lip and Jaw Motor Control During Speech: Responses to Resistive Loading of the Jaw. *J. Speech Hear. Res. 18*, 1975, 207–220. Reprinted in Kent et al. 1991, 605–618.

Fowler, C. A., and Turvey, M. T., Immediate Compensation for Bite Block Speech. *Phonetica 37*, 1980, 307–326.

Goodwin, G. M., and Luschei, E. S., Effects of Destroying the Spindle Afferents From the Jaw Muscles Upon Mastication in Monkeys. *J. Neurophysiol. 37*, 1974, 967–981.

Goodwin, G. M., McCloskey, D. I., and Matthews, P. B. C., The Contribution of Muscle Afferents to Kinaesthesia Shown by Vibration Induced Illusions of Movement and by the Effects of Paralyzing Joint Afferents. *Brain 95*, 1972, 705–748.

Hamlet, S. L., Speech Adaptation to Dental Appliances: Theoretical Considerations. *J. Baltimore Coll. Dent. Surg. 28*, 1973, 52–63.

Higgins, J. R., and Angel, R. W., Correction of Tracking Errors Without Sensory Feedback. *J. Exp. Psychol. 84*, 1970, 412–416.

Kelso, J. A. S., Tuller, B., and Harris K. S., A 'Dynamic Pattern' Perspective on the Control and Coordination of Movement. In *The Production of Speech*. P. MacNeilage (Ed.). New York: Springer-Verlag, 1983.

Ladefoged, P., and Fromkin, V. A., Experiments on Competence, and Performance. *IEEE Trans. Audio Electroacoust. 16*, 1968, 130–136.

Locke, J. L., A Methodological Consideration in Kinesthetic Feedback Research. *J. Speech Hear. Res. 11*, 1968, 668–669.

Matthews, P. B. C., Muscle Spindles and Their Motor Control. *Physiol. Rev. 44*, 1964, 219–288.

Mott, F. M., and Sherrington, C. S., Experiments Upon the Influence of Sensory Nerves Upon Movement and Nutrition of the Limbs. *Proc. Roy. Soc. Lond. Biol. 57*, 1875, 481–488.

Polit, A., and Bizzi, E., Processes Controlling Arm Movement in Monkeys. *Science 201*, 1978, 1235–1237.

Smith, T. S., and Lee, C. Y., Peripheral Feedback Mechanisms in Speech Production Models. In *Proceedings of 7th International Congress of Phonetic Sciences*. A. Rigault and R. Charbonneau (Eds.). The Hague, The Netherlands: Mouton, 1972, pp. 1199–1202.

Taub, E., Ellman, S. J., and Berman, A. J., Deafferentation in Monkeys: Effect on Conditioned Grasp Response. *Science 151*, 1966, 593–594.

Vallbo, Å. B., Muscle Spindle Response at the Onset of Isometric Voluntary Contractions in Man: Time Difference Between Fusimotor and Skeletomotor Effects. *J. Physiol. (Lond.) 318*, 1971, 405–431.

### Internal Feedback

Eccles, J. C., *The Understanding of the Brain*. New York: McGraw-Hill, 1973.

Evarts, E. V., Central Control of Movement. *Neurosci. Res. Program Bull. 9*, 1971.

Stelmach, G. E. (Ed.), *Motor Control*. The Hague, The Netherlands: Mouton, 1976.

### Developmental Feedback

Borden, G. J., Use of Feedback in Established and Developing Speech. In *Speech and Language: Advances in Basic Research and Practice*, Vol. 3. N. Lass (Ed.). New York: Academic Press, 1980.

MacKay, D. G., Metamorphosis of a Critical Interval: Age-Linked Changes in the Delay in Auditory Feedback That Produces Maximal Disruption of Speech. *J. Acoust. Soc. Am. 43*, 1968, 811–821.

Siegel, G. M., Fehst, C. A., Garber, S. R., and Pick, H. L., Jr., Delayed Auditory Feedback With Children. *J. Speech Hear. Res. 23*, 1980, 802–813.

Siegel, G. M., Pick, H. L., Jr., Olsen, M. G., and Sawin, L., Auditory Feedback in the Regulation of Vocal Intensity of Pre-School Children. *Dev. Psychol. 12*, 1976, 255–261.

### Models of Speech Production

Bell-Berti, F., and Harris, K. S., A Temporal Model of Speech Production. *Phonetica 38*, 1981, 9–20.

Browman, C., and Goldstein, L., Articulatory Phonology: An Overview. *Phonetica 49*, 1992, 222–234.

Chomsky, N., and Halle, M., *The Sound Pattern of English*. New York: Harper & Row, 1968.

Fairbanks, C., A Theory of the Speech Mechanism as a Servosystem. *J. Speech Hear. Disord. 19,* 1954, 133–139.

Fant, G., Auditory Patterns of Speech. In *Models for the Perception of Speech and Visual Form.* W. Wathen-Dunn (Ed.). Cambridge, MA: MIT Press, 1967.

Fowler, C. A., Speech Production. In *Speech, Language and Communication.* J. L. Miller and P. D. Eimas (Eds.). San Diego: Academic Press, 1996, pp. 30–61.

Fowler, C. A., Rubin, P., Remez, R. E., and Turvey, M. T., Implications for Speech Production of a General Theory of Action. In *Language Production,* Vol. 1, Speech and Talk. B. Butterworth (Ed.). New York: Academic Press, 1980.

Hebb, D. O., *The Organization of Behavior.* New York: Wiley, 1949.

Henke, W., *Dynamic Articulatory Model of Speech Production Using Computer Simulation* [Ph.D. Thesis]. Cambridge, MA: Massachusetts Institute of Technology, 1966.

Jakobson, R., Fant, C. G. M., and Halle, M., *Preliminaries to Speech Analysis.* Cambridge, MA: MIT Press, 1963. (Originally published in 1952 as Technical Report No. 13, Acoustics Laboratory, Massachusetts Institute of Technology.)

Kozhevnikov, V. A., and Chistovich, L. A., *Rech: Artikulyatisiya i Vospriyatiye,* Moscow-Leningrad, 1965. Translated as *Speech: Articulation and Perception,* Vol. 30. Springfield, VA: U.S. Department of Commerce, Joint Publications Research Service, 1966.

Ladefoged, P., De Clerk, J., Lindau, M., and Papçun, G., An Auditory-Motor Theory of Speech Production. In *UCLA Work Papers in Phonetics 22.* Los Angeles: UCLA, 1972, pp. 48–75.

Lashley, K. S., The Problem of Serial Order in Behavior. In *Cerebral Mechanisms in Behavior.* L. A. Jeffress (Ed.). New York: Wiley, 1951.

Liberman, A. M., Cooper, F. S., Shankweiler, D. P., and Studdert-Kennedy, M., Perception of the Speech Code. *Psychol. Rev. 74,* 1967, 431–461.

MacNeilage, P., Motor Control of Serial Ordering of Speech. *Psychol. Rev. 77,* 1970, 182–196. Reprinted in Kent et al. 1991, 701–715.

Martin, J. G., Rhythmic (Hierarchal) Versus Serial Structure in Speech and Other Behavior. *Psychol. Rev. 79,* 1972, 487–509.

Nooteboom, S. G. and Eefting, W. To What Extent Is Speech Production Controlled by Speech Perception? Some Questions and Experimental Evidence. In Y. Tohkura, E. Vatikiotis-Bateson, and Y. Sagisaka (Eds.). *Speech Perception, Production and Linguistic Structure.* Amsterdam: IOS Press, 1992, pp. 439–450.

Ohman, S.E.G. Numerical Model of Coarticulation. *J. Acoust. Soc. Am., 41,* 1967, 310–320.

Weismer, G., Tjaden, K., and Kent, R. D., Speech Production Theory and Articulatory Behavior in Motor Speech Disorders. In *Producing Speech: Contemporary Issues for Katherine Safford Harris.* F. Bell-Berti and L. J. Raphael (Eds.). New York: American Institute of Physics, 1995, pp. 35–50.

# SECTION IV    Speech Perception

# Hearing: The Gateway to Speech Perception

# 9

*Warble, child; make passionate my sense of hearing.*

–William Shakespeare, *Love's Labour's Lost*

The only reason we understand one another at all–and there are those who argue that we do a poor job of it–is that the human mind has developed into a remarkable seeker of patterns. It receives the seemingly chaotic variety of sights, sounds, and textures, searches for common properties among them, makes associations, and sorts them into groups. In this sense, then, we all perceive in the same way. In speaking to one another, we seem to extract the essences of sound and meaning from utterances diverse in dialect, vocabulary, and voice quality.

There is a duality, however, in our perception of other speakers; although we seek common denominators, we also impose ourselves on what we perceive. Like the legend of the blind men describing an elephant, each having touched a different part of the animal, each person perceives the world a bit differently, depending on individual experiences and expectations. In perceiving the speech communications of others, we tend to impose our own points of view on the messages. Our perceptions often match our expectations rather than what was actually said and heard. If part of a word is missing, our mind supplies it, and we fail to notice its absence. Even the sounds of speech are heard within the framework of our particular language, so that if we hear a less familiar language being spoken, we try to fit the less familiar sounds into the categories of speech sounds we have in our own language. Adults trying to imitate a new language, for this reason, speak with an obvious "accent," retaining the sound categories of their first language. In trying to say "tu" in French, an English speaker might say /tu/ instead of /ty/ and not even perceive the difference between the vowels a French speaker would use in the words "tu" /ty/ and "vous" /vu/.

Yet we normally do perceive an elephant with enough common ground to agree that it is an elephant. In speech communication, although we retain our individual and language-based perspectives, we receive the same acoustic signal, and our ears act on this signal in similar ways. Thus, we have learned the acoustic patterns that correspond to the distinctive speech sounds in our language. We seem to learn these despite the fact that the acoustic cues for individual speech sounds overlap in time. Whatever problems we encounter in recognizing and interpreting speech, we must first hear the acoustic signal that is generated by those speaking to us before we can solve them. This chapter thus describes the outlines of the hearing mechanism and the way in which it works. In the two chapters that follow this one, we will discuss the acoustic cues to the perception of speech sounds and processes that listeners use to decode the complicated acoustic signal.

## THE LISTENER

Communication by speech is the transmission of thoughts or feelings from the mind of a speaker to the mind of a listener. The concepts and attitudes that the speaker intends to express are embodied within a linguistic frame and rendered audible by the physiologic processes that we considered in earlier chapters. We will begin our description of the final links in what Denes and Pinson (1963) have called the "speech chain" by exploring what happens when a listener hears the speech signal. That is, we will describe audition, the process of registering the sounds in the brain of the hearer.

Listeners use more than acoustic information when they receive a spoken message. They use their knowledge of the speaking situation and their knowledge of the speaker, as well as visual cues obtained by watching the face and gestures of the speaker. These nonacoustic cues used in speech perception are important, but they fall outside the range of most studies of speech science as we have defined it. In this chapter, we shall limit

ourselves to a discussion of what is known and conjectured about the perception of speech as it involves extracting the sounds of speech from acoustic information. This limitation means that we shall largely ignore other important areas of investigation: the processes by which listeners arrive at meaning through semantic and syntactic analyses of the message.

Usually, listeners are aware only of the meaning of speech and remain quite unconscious of the components of the message. Just as a person who sees a dog run by is conscious of perceiving a dog, not a changing pattern of light, so a person perceiving speech is aware of the meaning of the message, not the individual sounds or sound patterns that form it. Linguistic information seems to be stored by meaning or by imagery. For example, Bartlett (1932) found that people tested repeatedly on folk stories that they had read often used entirely different words to relate the tale than the words used in the original, but the story outline and prominent images were remembered.

As strongly as listeners seem to seek meanings, they must be extracting these meanings from the sound patterns of speech. We shall focus on the acoustic, phonetic, and phonological analyses that presumably form the basis for further linguistic decisions. It does seem unlikely, however, that a listener would take the auditory information and proceed up the ladder to make phonetic, then phonological, then morphemic, and finally syntactic decisions to arrive at the meaning of the message. More likely, operating on certain expectations of what the speaker may be saying, the listener hears some of the message, makes a rough analysis, and leaps to synthesize it into something meaningful, simultaneously verifying it at all the levels mentioned.

No matter how a listener analyzes a message, the data on which he or she operates are the acoustic patterns of speech. The essential step, then, is that the listener hears the speech. Because the hearing mechanism per se is somewhat removed from the main concerns of this book, we say only a few words about the peripheral reception of speech, as the auditory system itself imposes certain changes on speech sounds.

## HEARING

The human auditory mechanism analyzes sound according to changes in frequency and intensity as a function of time. As a receptor, the ear falls short of the eye in sensitivity, but it seems to be remarkably responsive to the sounds that humans produce, the sounds of speech. These sounds change not only in amplitude but also in their mode of transmission as they travel through the outer ear, middle ear, cochlea, and auditory nerve to the brain. Figure 9.1 differentiates these parts of the mechanism. As we know from Chapter 2, the pressure waves of speech are usually disturbances in air and thus they continue in the outer ear. In the middle ear, however, they are converted from pressure waves to mechanical vibrations by a series of small bones leading to the cochlea of the inner ear. In the cochlea, a snail-shaped cavity within the temporal bone of the skull, the vibrations are again transformed. This time the transformation is from mechanical vibrations to vibrations in the fluid with which the cochlea is filled. Finally, the nerve endings in the cochlea act to transform the hydraulic vibrations into electrochemical information that is sent to the brain in the form of nerve impulses.

### The Outer Ear

The outer ear is composed of two parts: the external part you can readily see–the auricle or pinna–and the ear canal, or external auditory meatus, that runs from the pinna to the eardrum. Meatus means "channel," and the channel of the outer ear is specified as "external," to distinguish it from the internal auditory meatus that runs from the inner ear out of the temporal bone to the brain. The

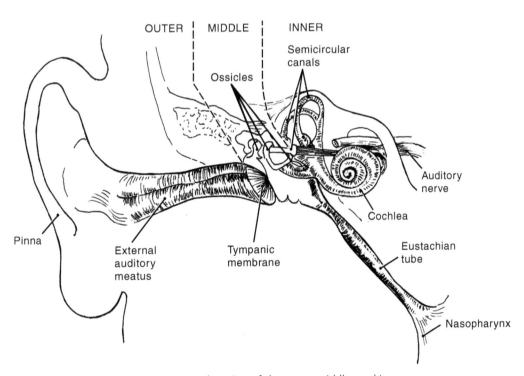

**FIGURE 9.1**  Frontal section of the outer, middle, and inner ear.

pinna funnels the sound somewhat, being a little more receptive to sounds in front of the head than behind it. The pinna also serves to protect the entrance to the canal, especially the small projection of the pinna, situated over the opening to the canal, called the tragus. One way to reduce the intensity of a loud sound is to press the tragus into the entrance to the auditory meatus with your finger.

The external auditory meatus protects the more delicate parts of the ear from trauma and from the intrusion of foreign objects. A waxy substance, cerumen, is secreted into the canal, and aided by the hairs (cilia) lining the canal, it filters out dust and any flying insects that intrude into the canal.

In addition to offering protection to the more critical parts of the ear, the external auditory meatus functions to boost the high frequencies of the sounds it receives. The meatus is an air-filled cavity about 2.5 cm long and open at one end. It therefore acts as a quarter-wave resonator, with a lowest resonant frequency of about 3,440 Hz.

$$f = \text{velocity of sound}/4 \text{ (length)}$$
$$= 34,400/10 = 3,440 \,\text{Hz}$$

A woman's or child's ear canal would probably be shorter than 2.5 cm and would resonate at higher frequencies. The high-frequency emphasis provided by the outer ear is useful for the perception of fricatives because much of the sound energy that distinguishes fricatives from each other is above 2,000 Hz.

To conclude our discussion of the outer ear, let us consider the advantage of having binaural hearing and ears on both sides of our heads. That advantage lies in our ability to localize a source of sound. A person who becomes deaf in one ear can hear perfectly well in a quiet environment but has difficulty monitoring a large group conversation because localization of sound is impaired. In a meeting room with voices coming from all directions, the unilaterally deaf person seeking

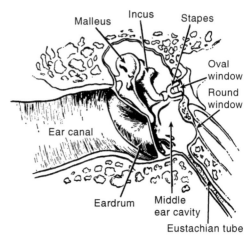

**FIGURE 9.2** Cross section of the middle ear and ossicles. (Modified with permission from Denes, P. B., and Pinson, E. N., *The Speech Chain.* New York: Doubleday, 1963.)

to locate the speaker may look in the wrong direction.

## The Middle Ear

The outer ear is separated from the air-filled middle ear cavity by the eardrum, more properly called the tympanic membrane (Figs. 9.1 and 9.2). The tympanic membrane is slightly concave as seen from the outer ear and is responsive to small pressure variations across a wide range of frequencies. The tension of the eardrum can be altered by a muscle, the tensor tympani, which pulls on the manubrium, or handle, of a small bone, the malleus, attached to the inside of the drum. At low frequencies, the tympanic membrane vibrates as a whole, but at high frequencies, different areas of the membrane are responsive to different frequency ranges.

On the internal side of the tympanic membrane is the ossicular chain, three tiny connected bones called the ossicles. The malleus (hammer), as we have mentioned, is attached to the tympanic membrane; the incus (anvil) acts as a fulcrum between the other two bones; and the stapes (stirrup) inserts into the membranous oval window

## CLINICAL NOTE

It is important for the clinician to understand and maintain the distinction between hearing and perception, especially with regard to speech. We can appreciate the difference between speech audition and speech perception when we compare the effects of deafness with those of developmental aphasia. When a child is born deaf or hard of hearing, the difficulty in learning language is based on dysfunction of the peripheral hearing mechanism. Without the auditory input of a normal-hearing child, the hearing-impaired child lacks the normal pool of information on which to base his or her own vocalizations and to match them, eventually, to a reasonable facsimile of the speech of others.

In contrast, when a child is born with brain damage that specifically interferes with speech perception, the child has normal hearing but is unable to interpret the sounds in any linguistically useful way. Although several syndromes are called by such terms as developmental aphasia or auditory agnosia, a common difficulty seems to lie in the processes leading to the discrimination and identification of speech sounds rather than in the auditory processes themselves. We can all, of course, experience the difference between hearing speech and perceiving the linguistic message it carries if we find ourselves in a place where the language being spoken is one we do not know. We hear exactly the same acoustic signal as the native speaker of the unknown language, but we are not sure how the sounds differ from those of our language, nor can we tell where phrases and words begin or end or, of course, what those words mean.

Given the differences between hearing sounds and perceiving speech and language, it is obvious that the clinical strategies used to ameliorate dysfunctions of the peripheral hearing mechanism must be largely different from those used to treat dysfunctions in the central nervous system. The clinician must always be aware of which type of disorder is presented by a patient so that an appropriate clinical regimen can be planned and administered.

---

leading to the inner ear. Thus, the ossicular chain bridges the space between the tympanic membrane and the cochlea. The chain is suspended in the air-filled cavity of the middle ear by ligaments and is held in such a delicate balance that no matter what position the body takes, the tiny bones are held in suspension, free to vibrate in response to sound. The vibrations in the outer ear take the form of disturbances of air molecules, but in the middle ear, they take the form of mechanical vibrations of the bony ossicles. The tympanic membrane and the ossicular chain taken together are especially responsive to the frequencies of acoustic signals that are important for speech.

Why have a middle ear at all? Why not have the fluid-filled cochlea on the other side of the tympanic membrane? The problem is a mismatch in impedance. Impedance is a force determined by the characteristics of a medium itself (gas, liquid, or solid) and is a measure of the resistance to transmission of signals. Liquid offers a higher impedance, or resistance, to sound pressure than does a gas such as air. When sound pressure waves traveling through air suddenly come to a fluid, most of the sound energy is reflected back, with very little admitted into the liquid. The cochlea is filled with fluid, and to overcome the difference in impedance between the air and the fluid, a transformer is needed to increase the sound pressure so that more of it will be admitted into the liquid. The middle ear is that transformer.

The middle ear increases sound pressure by approximately 30 dB. The ossicles by themselves cannot effect such a large amplification of the signal, although they do act as a lever to increase the sound pressure

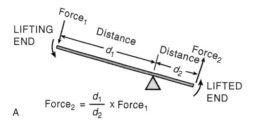

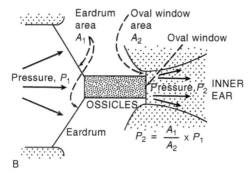

**FIGURE 9.3** *A*. The lever principle of the ossicles. *B*. The effect of the area difference between the tympanic membrane and the oval window. (Modified with permission from Denes, P. B., and Pinson, E. N., *The Speech Chain.* New York: Doubleday, 1963.)

by about 5 dB (Fig. 9.3). Leverage is the force long used by farmers to remove a heavy rock from a field. If the rock is too heavy for the farmer to lift, leverage can be used by placing a pole over a fulcrum, with the shorter part of the pole under the heavy object. A given pressure applied by the farmer results in a much larger pressure under the rock. In somewhat the same way, the pressures applied to the relatively long malleus are transmitted by the incus, which acts something like a fulcrum to the much smaller stapes. The result is an increase of a few decibels in transmission because of the increase in the pressure exerted on the oval window.

The leverage applied along the ossicles helps to overcome some of the impedance mismatch, but the larger part of the increase in pressure comes from the design of the tympanic membrane relative to the oval window.

The area of the tympanic membrane is about 0.85 cm$^2$ (although only about 0.55 cm$^2$ of that area is active in vibration), whereas the area of the oval window is 0.03 cm$^2$. When a given force $(F)$ is applied to a small area $(A)$, the pressure $(p)$ is greater than if it is applied to a larger area. This is expressed by the formula $p = F/A$. Thus, as area $(A)$ increases, the absolute value of the fraction $F/A$, which is the pressure, decreases.

Consider the following example: If your friend were to fall through the ice, you would be well advised to spread your weight over a large area in attempting to reach the victim. By lying flat or, better, by distributing your weight over an even larger area, by crawling along on a ladder, you are in much less danger of falling through the ice yourself. The pressure on any point is much less than if you were to attempt to walk to your friend on the ice, focusing all the pressure at the points on the ice beneath your feet. In an analogous manner, the sound vibrations occurring over the larger vibrating area of the tympanic membrane are focused by the stapes to the smaller area of the oval window, resulting in an increase in pressure of approximately 25 dB. Thus, the impedance-matching function of the middle ear is accomplished by the area difference between the tympanic membrane and the oval window and by the leverage afforded by the ossicular design, which adds a few more decibels.

Besides the important function of impedance matching between the air and the cochlear fluid, the middle ear serves two other functions. First, it attenuates loud sounds by action of the acoustic reflex. Second, by the action of the eustachian tube, it works to maintain relatively equal air pressure on either side of the eardrum despite any changes in atmospheric pressure.

The acoustic reflex is elicited when a sound having a pressure level of 85 or 90 dB reaches the middle ear. This causes a contraction of the smallest muscle in the body, the stapedius muscle, which is attached to the neck of the smallest bone in the body, the stapes. There are two theories to account for the function of this acoustic reflex. The first, that it protects the inner ear from loud sounds, posits that the contraction of the stapedius muscle pulls the stapes to one side, changing the angle of its coupling to the oval window and reducing the pressure it applies. The second theory is that the stapedius muscle, along with the tensor tympani muscle, stiffens the ossicular chain, thereby regulating intensity changes much as the eye adjusts to changes in light. In either case, the stapedius muscle takes a few milliseconds to act, allowing sounds with sudden onset to penetrate the inner ear before the reflex occurs. Also, like any muscle, it eventually fatigues, so that in a noisy environment, the reflexive attenuation of the sound will gradually lessen, allowing the full impact of the sound pressure to impinge again on the inner ear. The stapedius muscle is innervated by the facial (seventh cranial) nerve but is somehow associated with the innervation of the larynx (vagus; tenth cranial nerve), because phonation activates the acoustic reflex. The acoustic reflex attenuates frequencies below 1 kHz by about 10 dB; the spectral energy of the human voice is also largely below 1 kHz. Thus, the acoustic reflex may keep us from hearing ourselves too loudly, for we hear our own voice not only by the air-conducted sound coming through our outer ears but also by bone-conducted sound because our facial and skull bones vibrate in response to our own voices.

The middle ear also equalizes differences between internal and external air pressures. This is accomplished by the eustachian tube, which leads from the middle ear to the nasopharynx. The eardrum does not vibrate properly if the air pressure in the middle ear is different from the air pressure in the external auditory meatus. Relatively high pressure within the middle ear pushes out on the tympanic membrane, causes discomfort, and attenuates outside sounds. A sudden change in pressure, as when one drives up into the mountains or descends in an air-

plane, can create this pressure difference if the eustachian tube, normally closed, fails to open. The outside air pressure is suddenly lower whereas the air pressure in the middle ear cavity (containing the same air as when one was at sea level) is relatively higher. Swallowing, yawning, and chewing facilitate the opening of the tube, which is why airline passengers sometimes bring chewing gum on flights.

## The Inner Ear

Within the temporal bone of the skull are several coil-shaped tunnels filled with fluid called perilymph. The fluid is like seawater in many of its properties. Floating in the fluid are coiled tubes made of membrane and filled with a more viscous fluid called endolymph. Figure 9.4 depicts the membranous labyrinth. The snail-shaped coil is the cochlear duct, containing the sensory receptor for hearing, and the system of three coils is the vestibular system, consisting of the semicircular canals, which, along with the vestibule (utricle and saccule) connecting them, contain organs that sense changes in body position and movement.

We will limit our description to the cochlea, for audition is the first step in speech perception. As the footplate of the stapes vibrates in the oval window, the vibrations set up disturbances in the perilymph of the cochlea. These pressure waves in the perilymph surrounding the cochlear duct set up vibrations in the duct itself. Especially important are the resulting vibrations of the "floor" of the duct, which is called the basilar membrane.

The cochlea in humans is a cavity within the bone that coils around a bony core almost three times. The membranous duct (or cochlear duct) within is attached to the bony core on the inside and by a ligament to the bony wall on the outside. It is perhaps easier to visualize if we imagine the cochlear chambers uncoiled as in Figure 9.5. Pressure variations applied by the stapes

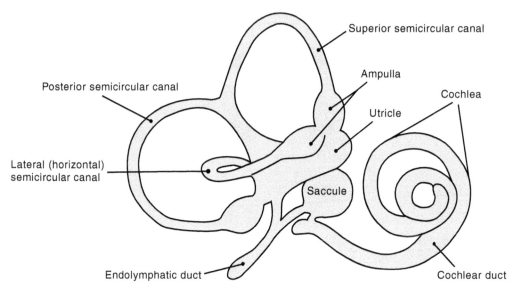

**FIGURE 9.4** The parts of the membranous labyrinth. The three semicircular canals, the ampulla, utricle, and saccule make up the vestibular organs, which sense body position and movement. The cochlea contains the organ of hearing. (Modified with permission from Durrant, J. D., and Lovrinic, J. H., *Bases of Hearing Science.* Baltimore: Williams & Wilkins, 1977.)

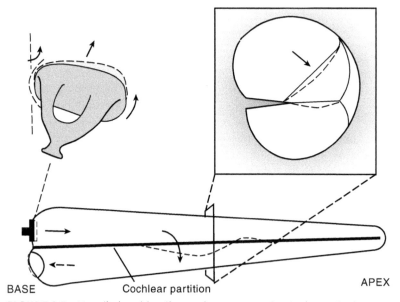

**FIGURE 9.5** Uncoiled cochlea (*bottom*); a cross section is shown in the upper right. The stapes, upper left, rocks in the oval window, leading to displacement of the cochlear partition, the basilar membrane in particular. (Modified with permission from Durrant, J. D., and Lovrinic, J. H., *Bases of Hearing Science.* Baltimore: Williams & Wilkins, 1977.)

rocking in the oval window are translated into pressure variations within the fluids of the cochlea, which, in turn, lead to displacements of the basilar membrane. The beauty of the system is that different parts of the basilar membrane respond to different frequencies. The membrane is narrow and stiff at the base, gradually getting wider and less stiff at the apex (the opposite of what one might expect). As a result, low-frequency sounds produce traveling waves in the fluid that stimulate the basilar membrane to vibrate with the largest amplitude of displacement at the wider, more flaccid tip. On the other hand, high-frequency sounds create pressure waves with the largest displacement of the basilar membrane at the thinner, stiffer base (Fig. 9.6).

The basilar membrane is not the sense organ of hearing, however. The organ of Corti, lying on the basilar membrane for the length of the cochlear duct, is the auditory receptor. It consists of rows of hair cells, along with other cells for support. Above the rows of thousands of hair cells is a gelatinous mass called the tectorial membrane. The basilar

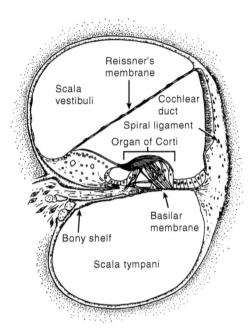

**FIGURE 9.7**  Cross section through the cochlea showing the scala vestibuli, the scala tympani, and the cochlear duct. The organ of Corti lies within the cochlear duct. (Modified with permission from Denes, P. B., and Pinson, E. N., *The Speech Chain.* New York: Doubleday, 1963.)

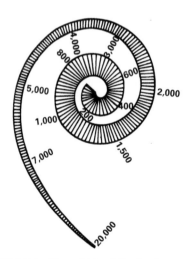

**FIGURE 9.6**  The width of the basilar membrane (somewhat exaggerated) as it approaches the apex. The approximate positions of maximum amplitude of vibration in response to tones of different frequency are also indicated.

membrane and the tectorial membrane are attached to the cochlear duct at different points and therefore move somewhat independently. Figure 9.7 shows a cross section of the cochlea. The scala vestibuli and scala tympani containing perilymph lie on either side of the cochlear duct. Pressure waves in the perilymph set up traveling waves within the cochlear duct. In some imperfectly understood way, the undulating motions of the basilar membrane cause the hair cells to be stimulated. The tectorial membrane above the hairs shears across the hairy endings of the cells, and the result is electrochemical excitation of the nerve fibers serving the critical hair cells.

The cochlea performs a Fourier analysis of complex sounds into their component frequencies. The sound of [i] as in "see" results in many traveling waves moving along the basilar membrane with at least two maxima of displacement: one near the apex for the lower resonance and one near the base of the cochlea for the higher resonance. If the speaker were to say [si] "see," the membrane displacement would initially be maximum even closer to the base of the cochlea for the high-frequency [s]. Also, the traveling waves would be aperiodic during [s] and become periodic during the phonated part of the word. Both the traveling wave theory and the description of the stiffness gradient of the basilar membrane are the result of the work of the late Georg von Békésy (1960).

Frequency information is extracted from the signal by the combined factors of the place of stimulation (which activates the sensory nerve fibers at a particular location along the basilar membrane—the place theory) and also by timing of impulses along the nerve fibers. Ernest Glen Wever (1954) theorized that at low frequencies, the displacement is not sharp enough to distinguish the frequencies by place; rather, they may be signaled by the number of cycles per second translated into a corresponding number of clusters of nerve impulses per second (Fig. 9.8). At high frequencies, place is probably important for indicating frequency, because neurons cannot fire at high frequencies. Another possibility is Wever's volley theory, by which several neurons would cooperate in the neural transmission of high frequencies (Fig. 9.9). The coding of intensity may well be as complicated as frequency coding. It is thought, though, that it is primarily transmitted by relative rate of nerve impulse spikes, as it is throughout the body.

## The Auditory Nerve

There are 30,000 nerve fibers serving the cochlea, each fiber coming from a few hair cells and each hair cell exciting several nerve fibers. They form a bundle known as the auditory nerve, or eighth cranial nerve. Another branch of the eighth cranial nerve relays information from the semicircular

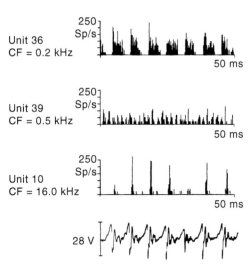

**FIGURE 9.8** Responses of single neurons of the auditory nerve of a cat to a presentation of a segment of the vowel [æ]. Bottom display shows the acoustic signal. The three upper displays show the number of spikes per second (Sp/s) for three neural units. Although different units have different firing frequencies, they maintain a fixed temporal relationship to the signal. (Modified with permission from Kiang, N. Y. S., and Moxon, E. C., Tails of Tuning Curves of Auditory-Nerve Fibers. *J. Acoust. Soc. Am. 55,* 1974, 620–630.)

canals. When the nerve fibers are excited by the stimulation of the hair cells, the frequency analysis performed by the organ of Corti is further refined because of lateral inhibition: when a certain place along the basilar membrane is maximally stimulated, to sharpen the effect, surrounding cells and nerve fibers are inhibited in their response.

The eighth cranial nerve does not have far to go between the cochlea and the temporal lobe of the brain. It exits the temporal bone by the internal auditory meatus and enters the brainstem where the medulla meets the pons. In the brainstem, most nerve fibers from each ear decussate (cross) to the contralateral pathway. At that point, comparisons can be made between signals from each ear to localize a sound source. It is thought that eighth cranial nerve fibers in the

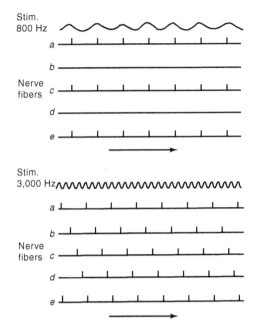

**FIGURE 9.9**  Wever's volley principle. At low frequencies (800 Hz), individual neurons can fire for each cycle of the stimulus, but at high frequencies (3,000 Hz), the organized firing of groups of neurons indicates frequency. (Modified with permission from Osgood, C. E., *Method and Theory in Experimental Psychology.* Oxford, England: Oxford University Press, 1953.)

brainstem may be specialized to detect certain auditory features. Such a specialization would be useful in detecting distinctions important to speech processing. From the brainstem, the eighth cranial nerve courses to the midbrain and then to the temporal lobe. Along the way, fibers go off to the cerebellum and to a network of the brainstem that acts to focus attention. Motor fibers of the auditory nerve also descend to control the sensitivity of the cochlea.

When signals arrive at the auditory cortex of the temporal lobe, the impulses have preserved the place–frequency arrangement of the basilar membrane. In a three-dimensional display along the superior part of the temporal lobe, low-frequency stimulation near the apex of the cochlea excites the layers of cortical cells along the lateral part of the primary auditory area, whereas high-frequency stimulation of the base of the cochlea is registered in columns of cells within the lateral fissure. This topographic representation is present in both temporal lobes. Most of the contribution to each lobe comes from the contralateral ear. Thus, hearing is accomplished, but the signals must be processed further if the hearer is to understand what is heard. Cortical processing of speech sounds will be discussed further in Chapter 11 when we consider the neurophysiology of speech perception.

## BIBLIOGRAPHY

### General Readings

Bartlett, F. C. Remembering. Cambridge, Great Britain: Cambridge University Press, 1932.

Denes, P., and Pinson, E. N., *The Speech Chain*, 2nd ed. New York: W. H. Freeman & Co., 1963.

Fant, G., Descriptive Analysis of the Acoustic Aspects of Speech. *Logos 5*, 1962, 3–17.

Kent, R. D., Atal, B. S., and Miller, J. L. (Eds.), *Papers in Speech Communication: Speech Production.* Woodbury, NY: Acoustical Society of America, 1991.

Pickett, J. M., *The Acoustics of Speech Communication.* Boston: Allyn and Bacon, 1999.

Plomp, R., *The Intelligent Ear.* Mahwah, NJ: Lawrence Erlbaum Associates, 2002.

### Hearing

Durrant, J. D., and Lovrinic, J. H., *Bases of Hearing Science,* 2nd ed. Baltimore: Williams & Wilkins, 1984.

Fletcher, H., *Speech and Hearing in Communication.* Princeton, NJ: van Nostrand, 1953. First published as *Speech and Hearing* in 1929.

Geldard, F. A., *The Human Senses.* New York: Wiley & Sons, 1953.

Helmholtz, H. L. F., *On the Sensations of Tone.* New York: Dover, 1961. Reprint of translation by A. J. Ellis, London: Longmans, Green, 1875.

Kiang, N. Y. S., and Moxon, E. C., Tails of Tuning Curves of Auditory-Nerve Fibers. *J. Acoust. Soc. Am. 55,* 1974, 620–630.

Stevens, S. S. (Ed.), *Handbook of Experimental Psychology*. New York: Wiley & Sons, 1951.

Stevens, S. S., and Davis, H., *Hearing: Its Psychology and Physiology*. New York: Acoustical Society of America, 1983. (Originally published by Wiley & Sons, 1938.)

Van Bergeijk, W. A., Pierce, J. R., and David, E. E., Jr., *Waves and the Ear*. London: Heinemann, 1961.

von Békésy, G., *Experiments in Hearing*. New York: McGraw-Hill, 1960.

Wever, E. G., and Lawrence, M., *Physiological Acoustics*. Princeton, NJ: University Press, 1954.

# The Acoustic Cues

**10**

*Clash forth life's common chord, whence, list how there ascend*
*Harmonics far and faint, till our perception end.*

—Robert Browning, "Fifine at the Fair"

---

## PERCEPTION OF SPEECH

There is evidence that the auditory system is especially tuned for speech, or, to look at it in evolutionary terms, that our speaking mechanisms and auditory mechanisms have developed together, so that we are best at hearing speech sounds. Looking at it from the perspective of historical linguistics, we can consider that human languages may have developed as they have by taking advantage of—and being constrained by—the mechanisms of speech production and perception. As we shall discover in the next chapter, infants categorize sounds of speech into groups similar to the distinctive groups (phonemes) that are used in many languages.

Many speech scientists believe that we are naturally equipped to perceive exactly those speech sounds that we are able to produce, although exactly how the perception process works is not yet entirely clear. The available evidence indicates that speech perception is a specialized aspect of a general human ability to seek and recognize patterns. In this case, the patterns are acoustic, and much of this chapter will describe acoustic patterns that listeners use as cues to the perception of speech.

The cues are often redundant. That is, there may be several cues to the identity of the same sound. Redundancy permits speech perception to take place under difficult conditions. Speech sounds are rarely produced in isolation, as we have indicated in earlier chapters. They overlap and influence one another as a result of their production. For perception, this means that speech sounds often are not discrete and separable, as the letters in a written word are. The listener, therefore, must use context to decode the acoustic message. Listeners often perceive speech sounds by using the acoustic information in neighboring segments. In addition, there is evidence that speech perception is a somewhat specialized and lateralized function in the brain, a subject we shall consider further.

## ACOUSTIC CUES IN SPEECH PERCEPTION

We know from the study of spectrograms that the acoustic patterns of speech are complex and constantly changing. Does the listener use all of the acoustic information available, or are some features of the acoustic patterns of speech more important than others? By synthesizing and editing speech, speech scientists have altered various features of the acoustic signal and then tested listeners to discover the effects of the alterations on perception.

In Chapters 5 and 6, we detailed the production of the general classes of speech sounds according to manner of articulation, starting with vowels, which are produced with the most open vocal tract, and concluding with the stops and fricatives, which are articulated with a more constricted vocal tract. We explained the production of each class of speech sound in terms of its articulatory features as well as its acoustic features. Following the same order, we shall consider the perception of the sounds of speech.

### Vowels

Vowels are among the most perceptually salient sounds in language. They are usually phonated (i.e., voiced) and thus relatively high in intensity; the vocal tract is usually more open for them than it is for consonants, producing prominent resonances (formants) that often last for 100 ms or more, a relatively long time for speech sounds. The most important acoustic cues to the perception of vowels lie in the frequencies and patterning of the speaker's formants. In the early 1950s, Delattre et al., at Haskins Laboratories, produced synthetic vowels with steady-state formants on a speech synthesizer

called the Pattern Playback (see below; also see Chapter 12). They systematically varied the frequencies of the formants to determine which patterns elicited the highest level of listener identifications for each vowel (Fig. 10.1). Listeners usually required only the first and second formants to identify a vowel. The experimenters also found that although both $F_1$ and $F_2$ were required for the identification of front vowels, a single formant, intermediate in frequency to $F_1$ and $F_2$, was sufficient for the identification of the back vowels. Swedish experimenters found that the most highly identifiable two-formant synthetic vowels differ systematically from natural vowels. For /i/, the second formant must be very high, close to the natural third formant, whereas for the rest of the front vowels, the second formant was best placed between the $F_2$ and $F_3$ frequencies of natural speech. Back vowels were best synthesized with the second formant close to a natural $F_2$. Apparently, $F_3$ is more important for the perception of front vowels than for the perception of back vowels.

We must be careful not to assume that steady-state formant frequencies are the only cues that listeners use to identify vowels. This cannot be so for a number of reasons. The first is the variety of vocal tract sizes producing the formants. We know from the Peterson and Barney study cited in Chapter 5 that men, women, and children produce the same vowel with different ranges of formant frequencies. In addition, there is a good deal of variation in formant frequency within the adult male, adult female, and child age group. The second reason that steady-state formant frequencies cannot be the only cues to vowel identification is that they are affected by context and rate of articulation. Thus, a single speaker will, for example, produce somewhat different formant frequencies for the vowel /ɑ/ in the word "father" than in the word "clock." The same is true of the formant frequencies for /ɑ/ in the word "father" said at two different rates or with different degrees of linguistic stress. With increased rate of speaking, vowels are often

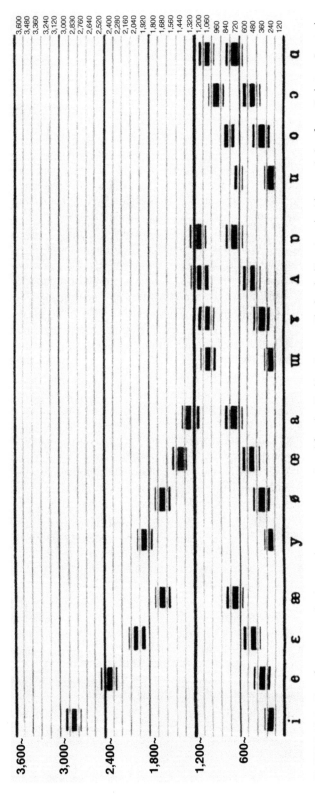

**FIGURE 10.1** Two-formant synthetic vowels as patterns painted for the Haskins Pattern Playback. (Reprinted with permission from Delattre, P., et al., An Experimental Study of the Acoustic Determinants of Vowel Color: Observations on One- and Two-Formant Vowels Synthesized From Spectrographic Patterns. *Word 8*, 1952, 195–210.)

neutralized, becoming more like schwa. Lindblom (1963) has shown that when vowels are weakly stressed, they become more similar to each other and to schwa ([ə]). The third reason, perhaps the most important one, is that one rarely finds steady-state formants in the acoustic signal when speech is articulated at normal conversational rates: Because the articulators are in virtually continual motion, the vocal tract shapes and therefore the peaks of resonance are continually changing.

If absolute formant frequency values are not reliable cues to vowel identification, how do listeners identify vowels? One possibility is that they use the patterns rather than the actual values of formant frequencies. No matter what the difference between the size of two speakers' vocal tracts, if each says the English vowel /i/, each will produce a sound with a first formant that is very low in frequency and a second formant that is very high in frequency, higher than for any other vowel they produce. Even though those formant frequencies will be different from one speaker to another, neither speaker will produce any other vowel sound displaying a greater frequency gap between $F_1$ and $F_2$. Analogous arguments can be constructed for the formant frequency patterns of the other point vowels, /ɑ/ and /u/.

But what of the vowels that lie between the point vowels? Given that the overall pattern of formant frequencies is quite similar across speakers, several researchers have suggested that listeners use the point vowels as reference points to scale or normalize formant frequency values in order to identify vowels. Ladefoged and Broadbent (1957) demonstrated that some vowels of a given speaker could be used by listeners to normalize for different vocal tract lengths. In their study, a vowel in the context [b–t] was heard as [ɪ] or as [ɛ], depending on which of two different speakers uttered an accompanying carrier phrase.

This concept of normalization, however, presents a number of problems. In the first place, it appears that no simple scaling for-

mula works to allow the listener to normalize the frequencies. This is partly explained by the fact that besides the difference in length between male and female vocal tracts, there is also a sex-related difference between the proportional areas of the pharyngeal and oral resonating cavities. The second problem is that speakers may not need to normalize to identify vowels. Normalization presupposes familiarity with the point vowels, at least, so that they can be used as references for the scaling process. But studies by Verbrugge et al. (1976) have shown that listeners can identify a vowel spoken by an unknown speaker without having previously heard him say any other vowels. They also found that vowel identification is more accurate for (1) vowels in context than for isolated formants and (2) for vowels in CVC syllables cued only by formant transitions rather than by isolated formants. That is, when the formants in the middle of the vowels were deleted, leaving only the consonant-to-vowel (CV) and vowel-to consonant (VC) transitions, listeners were more accurate in identifying the vowels than when they heard the isolated vowel formants with no transitions. Experimenters also report finding that listeners can use information from $F_3$ and from the fundamental frequency ($f_o$) to identify vowels. In recent years, normalization researchers have used this additional information and used scales other than linear frequency scales to reduce error rates in vowel identification studies.

Thus, although most researchers agree that formant frequencies, patterns of formant frequencies, and formant transitions play roles in vowel identification, it is unclear exactly how the listener extracts the information needed for vowel identification from these acoustic cues. One suggestion is that the information about the articulation is somehow coded directly into the acoustic signal and that because articulation across speakers is analogous, the listener can decode the articulatory information and recover the identity of the vowel. In fact, as we shall see in the next chapter, this type of theoretical construct works for all classes of speech sounds, but the details of the encoding and decoding processes are not completely understood at this time.

## Diphthongs

In Chapter 5, we described diphthongs as vowel sounds of changing resonance, so it is not surprising to find that relatively rapid changes in the formants of synthetic vowels are sufficient cues to diphthong perception. Gay (1970) systematically varied the duration of the $F_2$ frequency change and found that the rate of change was a more important cue to the identification of a diphthong than the exact formant frequencies at the end of the diphthongs /ɔɪ/, /aɪ/, and /aʊ/. It appears, then, that the phonetic transcriptions of these sounds are only approximations to the actual sounds they contain and that listeners depend more on the acoustic result of the tongue moving rapidly in a particular direction than on the attainment of a particular articulatory or acoustic targets for the beginning or ending of a diphthong.

## Semivowels

The semivowels /w/, /j/, /r/, and /l/, as in "wet," "yet," "red," and "led," like vowels and diphthongs, are classified as voiced and are characterized by changing formant frequencies called *transitions*. Formant transitions occur when a vowel precedes or follows a consonant, reflecting changes in resonance as the vocal tract shape changes to or from the more constricted consonant position. The formant transitions that characterize diphthongs and semivowels are internal to the sounds themselves and provide critical acoustic cues to their identification. Especially important to the perception of semivowels are the frequency changes in $F_2$ and, in some cases, $F_3$. Semivowels are distinguished from diphthongs by the greater rapidity of their formant transitions, which make them more consonant-like.

O'Connor et al. (1957) found that they could synthesize perceptually acceptable syllable-initial /w/ and /j/ with only two formants. This finding is not surprising when we recall that /w/ begins with a formant pattern similar to that of /u/ and /j/ begins with one similar to that of /i/. This means that it is the second formant that distinguishes /w/ from /j/, as the first formant for both these sounds is low, as it is for /u/ and /i/.

In contrast, three formants are usually required for the perception of /r/ and /l/, and it is the third formant that distinguishes them from each other. For /r/, $F_3$ is lower than for /l/; therefore, when /r/ precedes a vowel, $F_3$ must rise from its frequency for /r/ to that of the vowel. For /l/, $F_3$ is higher and in most vowel contexts does not vary significantly in frequency.

Figure 10.2 shows the formant patterns of most consistently perceived intervocalic semivowels in the context of the point vowels as Lisker (1957) synthesized them on the Pattern Playback. Note that the percent of identification of /l/ is generally somewhat lower than for the other semivowels, suggesting that additional cues must be needed for the unambiguous identification of this lateral consonant. The $F_2$ by $F_3$ chart (Fig. 10.3) summarizes the formant relationships listeners use to identify the semivowels.

## Nasal Consonants

Perception of nasals requires two decisions: whether a segment is nasal or not, and if nasal, whether it is labial /m/, alveolar /n/, or palatal–velar /ŋ/. By segmenting natural speech, Mermelstein (1977) found that the formant transitions of the vowels preceding and following nasals were effective cues to the identity of the nasals as a class. The obvious change in the spectrum from an orally produced vowel to a nasal includes two important features. The first is a weakening of intensity, especially in the upper formants, because of antiresonances. Listeners use this general decrease in intensity as a cue to nasal manner. The second spectral feature is the addition of a resonance below 500 Hz (often about 250 Hz) that is called the *nasal murmur*.

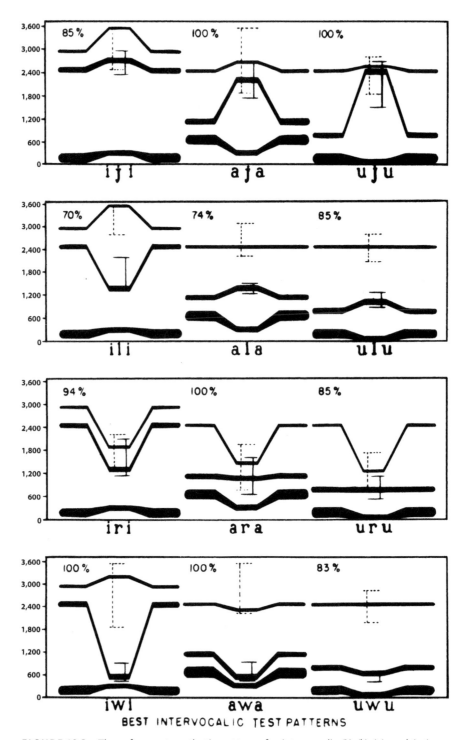

**FIGURE 10.2** Three-formant synthetic patterns for intervocalic /j/, /l/, /r/, and /w/ with the vowels /i/, /a/, and /u/. Listeners were asked to identify each of a series of patterns as one of the four stimuli. These patterns were most consistently identified. (Reprinted with permission from Lisker, L., *Word 13*, 1957, 256–257.)

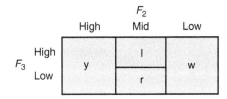

**FIGURE 10.3** The formant relationships among /y/, /w/, /r/, and /l/. (Adapted with permission from Lisker, L., *Word 13*, 1957, 256–267.)

This low-frequency nasal murmur has been shown to be a sufficient cue to nasal manner in synthetic speech stimuli from which upper formants were omitted.

Nasal manner can be cued in syllable-final nasals by the preceding vowel. In a tape-splicing study, Ali et al. (1971) found that listeners could perceive developing nasality during a vowel even when the vowel–consonant (VC) transitions and the following nasal had been deleted from the acoustic signal. The nasalization of vowels is, of course, the acoustic effect of coarticulation in sequences of vowel plus nasal. It is especially easy for listeners to perceive low vowels as being nasal. This is because low vowels lack a low-frequency resonance unless produced with nasality. High vowels, such as /i/ and /u/, normally have a low-frequency resonance ($F_1$) and therefore are acoustically more like nasals to begin with.

Perception of the place of nasal articulation is cued mainly by the direction of the formant transition (particularly of $F_2$) to or from an adjacent vowel. Cooper et al. (1952) found that the nasals /m,n,ŋ/ could be synthesized on the Pattern Playback with the same formant transitions used to synthesize /p,b/, /t,d/, and /k,g/, respectively. By tape-splicing natural speech, Malécot (1956) found that although listeners used the frequency of the nasal murmur itself as a cue for the place of articulation of the nasal, the formant transitions were a more powerful cue. After removing the transitions between the vowel formants and the nasal murmur, he found listeners much less able to report

which nasal they were hearing. There are both frequency and durational cues in the transitions. The formant transitions to and from /m/ are the lowest in frequency and the shortest in duration; those to and from /n/ are higher in frequency and a bit longer in duration; and those to and from /ŋ/ are the highest and most variable in frequency and the longest in duration. The difference in transition duration between /n/ and /ŋ/ probably occurs because the back of the tongue is slower to move than the tongue tip. It is not known how well listeners are able to trade off transition and nasal murmur cues for one another.

## Stops

The stop consonants /p, b, t, d, k, g/ have been studied more than any other class of speech sounds. The stops are interesting for three reasons: First, they demonstrate discontinuities (nonlinearities) in perception of synthesized speech or speech-like sounds. We will elaborate further on the nonlinear perception of speech in the section on categorical perception in Chapter 11. Second, stops, more than any other class of speech sounds, demonstrate the redundancy of acoustic cues. Third, stop perception provides the best example of how listeners use the acoustic overlapping of phonemes in the speech stream to perceive speech: The acoustic cues for the stops overlap the acoustic cues to neighboring vowels and consonants. As result of this overlap, listeners perceive stops and the sounds adjacent to them on the basis of their acoustic relationship to one another.

There are two obvious differences between stops and all other classes of sounds (except the affricates). First, there is a complete occlusion of the vocal tract (caused by simultaneous oral and velopharyngeal closures) and thus a momentary cessation of airflow emission that may be heard either as silence in the voiceless stops /p, t, k/ or as a brief attenuation of sound in the voiced stops /b, d, g/. Second, the stopped air is usually released as a transient burst of noise. Both the

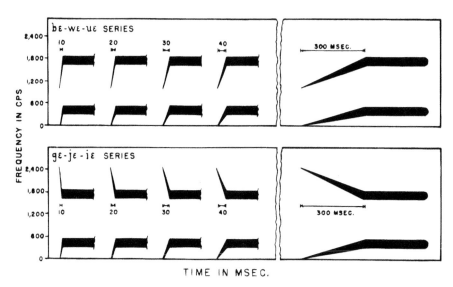

**FIGURE 10.4** Spectrographic patterns with varying durations of transition. The first four patterns in each row show how the tempo of the transitions varied. At the extreme right of each row is a complete stimulus pattern, that is, transition plus steady-state vowel, for the longest duration of transition tested. The patterns at the extreme left and right of the top row are judged as /be/ and /ue/, respectively. The corresponding patterns in the bottom row are judged as /ge/ and /ie/. (Modified with permission from Liberman, A. M., et al., Tempo of Frequency Change as a Cue for Distinguishing Classes of Speech Sounds. *J. Exp. Psychol. 52*, 1956, 127–137.)

(relative) silence and the presence of a release burst are acoustic cues to stop manner.

The stops are also marked by rapid changes in the formant frequencies of neighboring vowels. These formant frequency changes (transitions) occur between the release of a stop occlusion and a following vowel and between a preceding vowel and the onset of a stop occlusion. These rapid formant transitions are caused by the sudden change in vocal tract shape as the articulators move from the position for a stop consonant to that for a vowel or vice versa. The transitions occur before or after the articulators form the closures, oral and velopharyngeal, that mark the articulation of all stops. Such transitions are found in many other classes of consonant sounds but not in the semivowels, which display formant transitions of relatively long duration during the semivowel articulation. The Haskins group found that they could synthesize /be/ and /ge/ on the Pattern Playback (without including release bursts) simply by initiating the vowel with very brief formant transitions of less than 40 ms (Fig. 10.4). When they extended the duration of the transitions to 40 or 50 ms, listeners reported hearing the semivowel glides at the start of the syllables: /wε/ and /jε/. When the transitions were extended to 150 ms or more, listeners perceived a sequence of vowel sounds: /uε/ and /iε/.

These acoustic cues to the manner of articulation for stops—the (relative) silence, the presence of a release burst, and the short transitions to or from a neighboring vowel—are apparently more resistant to the masking effects of noise than are the acoustic cues to the place of articulation, which distinguish the labials, /p,b/, from the alveolars, /t,d/, from the palatal–velars, /k,g/. Miller and Nicely (1955) analyzed perceptual confusions of English consonants in the presence of noise and found that listeners can identify the manner of production even when place cues are masked.

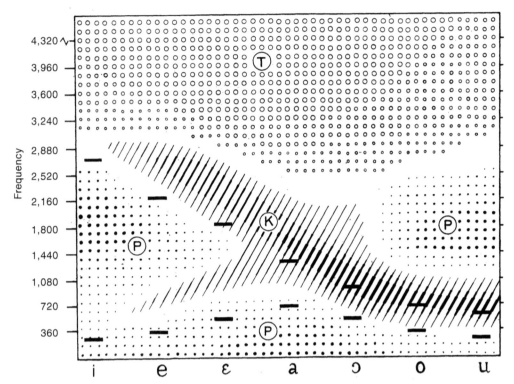

**FIGURE 10.5** Center frequency of burst perceived as a given voiceless stop, with various vowels. The filled dots indicate the frequency of bursts perceived as /p/, the open circles as /t/, and the slashes as /k/. The bolder face symbols in the grid indicate greater listener agreement. The two-formant pattern with which each burst was paired was appropriate for each of the indicated vowels. (Reprinted with permission from Liberman, A. M., et al., The Role of Selected Stimulus-Variables in the Perception of the Unvoiced Stop Consonants. *Am. J. Psychol. 65*, 1952, 497–516.)

Several cues indicate the place of articulation of a stop. Early experiments, using synthetic stimuli based on spectrograms of naturally produced speech, isolated two place cues as separate but sufficient: the frequency of the most intense portion of the burst and the $F_2$ transition to or from a neighboring vowel. High-frequency bursts preceding seven different two-formant synthetic vowels were all perceived as /t/. Low-frequency bursts preceding the vowels were perceived as /p/. Bursts perceived as /k/ were slightly above the frequency of $F_2$ of the following vowel (Fig. 10.5). Thus, /k/ percepts were reported for high-frequency bursts before front vowels with high $F_2$ frequencies and for low-frequency bursts before back vowels with low $F_2$ frequencies.

Further experiments indicated that stop place of articulation could also be cued by the rapid $F_2$ transitions between the stop consonants and the steady-state portions of the following vowels. The experimenters synthesized a series of stimuli that consisted of 11 two-formant C (consonant) plus /ɑ/ syllables (Fig. 10.6). The stimuli began with formant transitions only (no release bursts were synthesized). The first formant transition and the steady-state formant frequencies of the following /ɑ/ were held constant throughout the series. The independent variable was the slope of the $F_2$ transition, which varied systematically from sharply rising to sharply falling in 10 steps. Listeners identified all of the stimuli with the rising $F_2$ transitions as labial, /p,b/, but divided the stimuli with

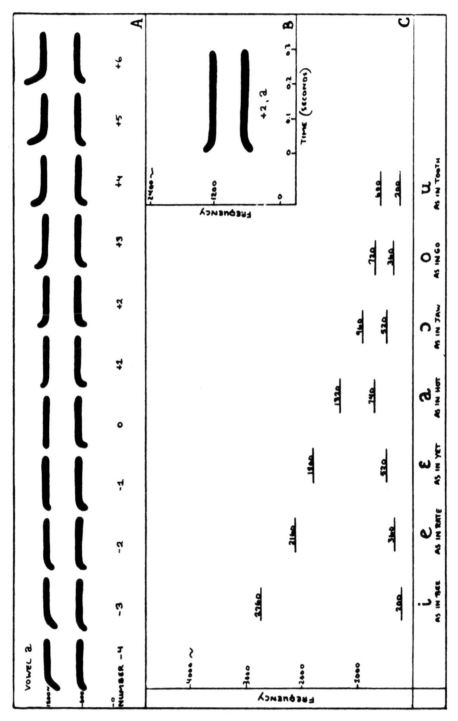

**FIGURE 10.6**   Two-formant synthetic pattern for the voiced stops. *A*. The vowel /a/ with a full range of transitions. *B*. A single pattern. *C*. The two-formant synthetic patterns for various vowels, combined with the range of transitions shown in *A*. (Reprinted with permission from Liberman, A. M., et al., The Role of Consonant-Vowel Transitions in the Perception of the Stop and Nasal Consonants. *Psychol. Monogr.: Gen. Appl. 68,* 1954, 1–13.)

falling $F_2$ transitions into two groups: Alveolar /t,d/ were reported when the slopes of the transitions were slightly falling, whereas the palatal–velar stops /k,g/ were reported when the slopes of the $F_2$ transitions fell sharply in frequency.

It is important to recognize that the patterns of $F_2$ transitions described above are limited to the context of the vowel /ɑ/, which has a low- to mid-range second formant frequency (around 1,300 Hz). If the stops are synthesized before a vowel with a high second formant, such as /i/, the $F_2$ transitions cueing the labials rise much more steeply than before /ɑ/, those cueing the alveolars rise rather than fall slightly, and the transitions cueing the velar stops fall less sharply than in the /ɑ/ context. Before a vowel with a low second formant, such as /u/, the transitions cueing both the alveolar and velar stops fall in frequency (more sharply in the case of the velars), and the transitions cueing the labials rise in frequency but less sharply than before /ɑ/ or /i/. In short, each combination of the stops with a different vowel yields a pattern of frequency change in the $F_2$ transition that is more or less different from every other combination.

The disparity in the patterns of formant transitions led investigators to search for some unifying principle that could interrelate the differing transitions for each place of articulation. A study by Delattre, Liberman, and Cooper (1955) resulted in the theory that an acoustic locus exists for each place of articulation. To explain the concept, we must return to a consideration of stop consonant production. When a stop consonant occlusion is released, the vocal tract shape will be associated with particular formant resonances that change as the vocal tract shape changes toward the following vowel. Because the place of occlusion for any given stop is essentially the same whatever the vowel precedes or follows it, there should be a systematic relationship between consonant–vowel combinations and the starting frequency of the $F_2$ transition. It is this articulatory relationship that underlies the findings of the locus experiment.

To test the locus theory, two-formant CV patterns were synthesized with some stop-like characteristics followed by a steady-state $F_2$. The best /g/ sound was perceived when the flat $F_2$ was at 3,000 Hz, the best /d/ when it was at 1,800 Hz, and the best /b/ when $F_2$ was at 720 Hz. The stimuli were synthesized with the same $F_1$ transitions but with $F_2$ transitions ranging from sharply rising to sharply falling. The experimenters found that if the $F_2$ transitions all pointed to a particular locus (one of the three best frequencies listed above), listeners identified the place of articulation on the basis of the acoustic locus, but only if the first half of each transition was removed (Fig. 10.7B). The results were different if the transitions originated at the locus frequencies, that is, if the first half of the transition had not been deleted. Under that condition, listeners seemed to perceive the place of articulation on a different and less systematic basis (Fig. 10.7A). There was some difficulty in identifying a particular $F_2$ transition or locus for palatal–velar stops. This difficulty results partly from the articulatory fact that these consonants are not restricted to one place of articulation and partly from the acoustic fact that as the place of constriction moves back in the oral cavity, the consonant resonance may change its allegiance from one formant to another. Thus, the transition of the third formant also plays a role in cueing the place of articulation of stops (as well as of other consonants).

Stops differ in voicing as well as place of articulation. For each oral place of articulation, there is a voiced and a voiceless stop. Cues to voicing class include the presence or absence of a fundamental frequency (phonation) during the period of stop closure (displayed on wideband spectrograms as a low-frequency voice bar composed of regularly spaced vertical striations), the presence or absence of noise (aspiration) after stop release, and variation in onset time of phonation and $F_1$ after the release of prevocalic stops. The Haskins group studied the effects on perception of progressively "cutting back" the first formant transition in a series of stimuli. The first stimulus had a voice bar and an $F_1$

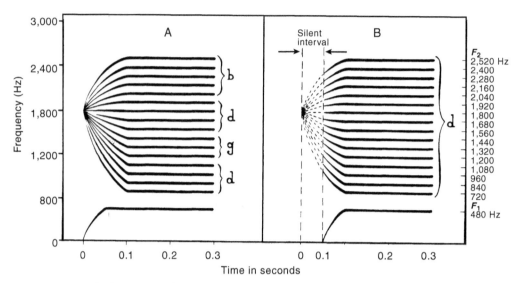

**FIGURE 10.7** The locus principle. *A.* The varying perceived identity of two-formant patterns with a rising first formant and a second formant with the origin at 1,800 Hz. If the first 50 ms of the pattern is erased, as in *B*, the patterns will all be heard as /d/, with a varying vowel. (Modified with permission from Delattre, P., et al., Acoustic Loci and Transitional Cues for Consonants. *J. Acoust. Soc. Am. 27*, 1955, 769–773.)

transition rising from the baseline. The voice bar was deleted in the second stimulus and in successive stimuli, 10 ms was removed from the $F_1$ transition (Fig. 10.8). The resulting delay of $F_1$ relative to $F_2$ onset was called $F_1$ cutback. Listeners reported hearing voiced stops for the first three stimuli in the series and, in most instances, voiceless stops for the last three stimuli with $F_1$ cutbacks of 30 ms or more. Further research indicated that the voiced versus voiceless distinction depended more on the amount of delay than on the starting frequency of $F_1$, which increased as the amount of cutback increased (Fig. 10.8).

Aspiration was not a sufficient cue to voiceless stops by itself, but when noise was added to the upper formants of stimuli with an $F_1$ cutback, listeners reported a stronger impression of voicelessness than they did with the $F_1$ cutback alone.

The experiments on $F_1$ cutback prefigured Lisker and Abramson's (1968) work on voice onset time (VOT), which we have discussed in Chapter 6. The timing of the $F_1$ onset in the synthetic stimuli corresponds to

the timing of the onset of phonation in natural speech. Moreover, the differences between the amount of cutback required for listeners to report hearing a voiceless (word initial) stop at the various places of articulation was in general mirrored in Lisker and Abramson's acoustic analysis of VOT in initial stops: Both $F_1$ cutback and VOT are greater for the velar stops than for the labials or alveolars. This finding has held for the voiced stops as well, although, as we would expect, the VOT values for /b d g/ are much smaller—closer to zero—than the VOT values for /p t k/.

The presence of (relative) silence has been mentioned as an acoustic cue to stop manner. Inserting silence between segments, such as the /s/ and /l/ of "slit," causes the word to be heard as "split." Differences in the duration of silence sometimes contribute to the cueing of the voiced–voiceless distinction for medial stops. For example, if the closure duration of the stop in the word "rabid" is increased to more than 70 ms, listeners report hearing "rapid," but only when the periodicity generated by phonation has been

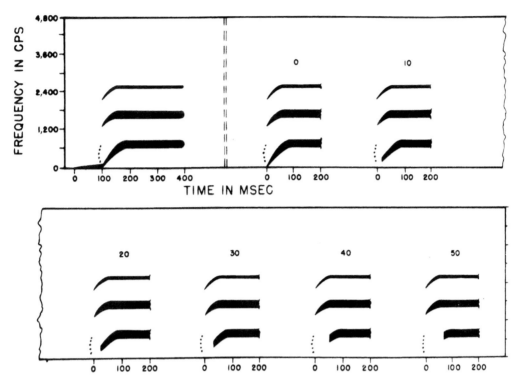

**FIGURE 10.8**  Synthetic patterns varying in $F_1$ cutback. The pattern at the top left corner has a voice bar. In the "0" pattern, $F_1$, $F_2$, and $F_3$ begin simultaneously. In successive patterns, $F_1$ onset is delayed in milliseconds by the time indicated above the pattern. After a certain degree of $F$ cutback, listeners reported hearing [pa] instead of [ba]. (Reprinted with permission from Liberman, A. M., et al., *Lang. Speech 1*, 1958.)

removed from the stop closure. The duration of vowels preceding syllable-final stops can also contribute to their classification as voiced or voiceless. Raphael, in experiments using both synthetic and natural speech stimuli, found that stops are most likely to be perceived as voiceless when preceded by vowels of shorter duration and as voiced when preceded by vowels of longer duration. The normally redundant vowel duration cue can help to disambiguate syllable-final stops when they are unreleased, as they occasionally are in American English.

In summary, listeners use several acoustic cues to determine the manner, place, and voicing classes of stop consonants. The presence of silence, the presence of a release burst, and relatively rapid formant transitions can all serve as cues to the stop manner of articulation. The acoustic cues for the place of articulation of stops are the frequency of the burst relative to the vowel and the formant transitions, especially of $F_2$, to or from a neighboring vowel. To recognize the voiced–voiceless contrast, listeners use several cues, depending on the context of the stop: the presence or absence of phonation and aspiration, $F_1$ delay, the duration of the silence marking the stop closure, and the duration of a preceding vowel. It is important to note that a single articulatory behavior can give rise to a number of different, redundant acoustic cues. For example, the timing of the onset of phonation relative to stop release accounts for VOT, for the presence or absence of aspiration, for the degree of $F_1$ cutback, and for other acoustic features that signal the voiced–voiceless opposition. This redundancy is useful for speech perception, which must be exact at rates of phoneme

## *C*LINICAL NOTE

There are at least two reasons why the nature of the acoustic cues to the perception of segmental phonemes are important for clinicians who are continually concerned with the evaluation and treatment of speech disorders. One of those reasons concerns the redundancy of the cues: The identity of the place, manner, or voicing classification of a particular sound may be conveyed in more than one way. There are indications that some listeners give more weight to certain perceptual cues than other listeners do, whether or not they present with perceptual disorders. In the case of a speaker who does evidence a disorder of phoneme perception, knowing which cues are not being processed efficiently can suggest treatment protocols that are client-specific and thus potentially more effective. A second, related, reason why understanding acoustic cues is important to the clinician is that the redundant cues often enter into trading relationships. That is, increasing the magnitude of certain cues while decreasing the magnitude of others may generate the same percept. Knowing which cues enhance perception may enable other speakers to communicate more effectively with a client. This is particularly true for those speakers, such as family members or teachers, who frequently engage the client in conversation or instruction. Understanding the nature of the acoustic cues to the perception of suprasegmental features of speech (discussed in the next section of this chapter) is also important, and for much the same reasons. You will note, for example, that the cues to syllable stress are, like the cues to many segmental phonemes, redundant.

transmission that can, on occasion, exceed 20 phonemes per second.

## Fricatives

The nature of fricative articulation gives rise to a relatively extended period of noise (frication) that is the principal acoustic cue to the perception of fricative manner. Although other acoustic features are associated with fricatives, none is as important as the presence of the noise generated by the turbulent airstream as it passes through the articulatory constriction required for the formation of this class of sounds.

Two of the acoustic cues to place of articulation are also a function of the noise generated by fricative articulation. These cues reside in the spectrum and intensity of the frication. Listeners distinguish the fricatives with relatively steep, high-frequency spectral peaks (the sibilants /s, z, ʃ, ʒ/) from those with relatively flat spectra (the nonsibilants /f, v, θ, ð/). This spectral distinction thus divides the fricatives into two general categories of place: posterior (sibilant) and an-

terior (nonsibilant). The posteriorly articulated sibilant fricatives can further be distinguished as being alveolar or postalveolar on the basis of the location of their lowest spectral peaks: in men, around 4 kHz for /s, z/ and 2.5 kHz for /ʃ, ʒ/. (Higher frequencies, of course, will be found for the smaller average vocal tract lengths of women and children.) The anteriorly articulated nonsibilant fricatives, labiodental /θ, ð/ and linguadental /f, v/, however, are not as reliably distinguished from each other because the dental constriction that characterizes them causes their spectra to be very similar. Miller and Nicely found /v/ and /ð/ to be among the most confusable of speech sounds to listeners when noise was added to the stimuli. Indeed, the dental fricatives are highly confusable in natural speech, and, in some dialects of English, one set (usually the labiodentals) is often substituted generally for the other (the linguadentals).

The intensity differences among the fricatives cue place of articulation just as the spectral differences do. That is, the sibilant fricatives are marked by relatively high-intensity levels, in contrast to the low-intensity levels of the nonsibilant fricatives. The absence of an appreciable resonating cavity in front of the dental constrictions of /θ, ð, f, v/ accounts for their generally low level of intensity. Listeners do not seem to use intensity cues to distinguish further among the places of articulation of fricatives. This has little importance with regard to the sibilant fricatives, which can be distinguished from each other on the basis of frequency cues, but it adds another source of confusion to the identification of the place of articulation of the nonsibilants, /f, v, θ, ð/.

The place of articulation of fricatives is also cued by the second and third formant transitions of the resonant sounds preceding and following them. The transition cues appear to be less important for the identification of place of articulation for fricatives than for stops. This is not surprising, considering the salience of the spectral cues to fricative place of articulation, especially for the sibilants. Once again, however, the greater articulatory difference between the constriction locations of the sibilant fricatives and between the sibilant and dental fricatives provides a more powerful formant transition cue than does the more similar constriction location of the dental nonsibilants. The similarity of the transitional cues of the nonsibilants provides yet another potential source of confusion among /f, v, θ, ð/.

To assess the relative importance of the spectral and transitional cues in fricative perception, Harris (1958) used recordings of fricative–vowel syllables in which each of the voiceless fricatives was combined with each of the vowels /i, e, o/ and /u/. The fricative noise in each syllable was separated from the vocalic portion. Each noise segment was then combined with each vocalic segment (which contained the formant transitions appropriate to the consonant that originally preceded it). A similar test was constructed for the voiced fricatives. Regardless of the vowel in any stimulus, whenever the noise segment for /s, z/ or /ʃ, ʒ/ was paired with any vocalic portion, listeners reported that they heard

/s, z/ or /ʃ, ʒ/, respectively. Listener judgments of /f, v/ or /θ, ð/, however, depended on the formant transitions in the vocalic segments, much as in the case of the nasal murmurs, which are also minimally distinctive and of relatively low intensity.

The presence or absence of phonation during the articulation of the sound is a salient perceptual cue to the voicing class of fricatives. Even without this cue, however, listeners can make reliable judgments about the voicing class of a syllable-final fricative based on its duration relative to the duration of the vowel preceding it. Denes (1955) used tape-splicing techniques to interchange the final fricatives in the noun "use" /jus/ and the verb "use" /juz/. In making the exchange, he shortened the normally longer /s/ and lengthened the /z/. The /s/ from /jus/ was heard as /z/ when spliced on the end of the /ju/ of /juz/ because the greater duration of the /u/ was appropriate to that of a vowel preceding a voiced consonant. Conversely, the /z/ from /juz/ was heard as /s/ when spliced after the shorter /u/. Denes showed that it is not the vowel duration alone that listeners use as the cue to final fricative voicing but, rather, the relative durations of the vowel and the fricative. It is also possible that listeners use intensity differences between the frication of voiced and voiceless fricatives to distinguish between the members of such cognate pairs as /s/ and /z/: Because the pulsing of the vocal folds interrupts the airflow during the production of a voiced fricative, the volume of air forced through the oral constriction is less for voiced than for voiceless fricatives, reducing the intensity of the frication generated at the point of articulatory constriction.

The experimental data suggest a possible perceptual strategy for fricative identification. First, listeners identify a fricative because they hear a noisy, aperiodic component of relatively long duration. They then seem to place the fricative into one of two groups, based on relative intensity: posteriorly articulated sibilants of higher intensity, /s, z, ʃ, ʒ/, or anteriorly articulated nonsibilant fricatives of low intensity, /θ, ð, f, v/.

The sibilants are then further distinguished according to the place of articulation on the basis of spectral cues, the alveolar fricatives /s/ and /z/ having a first spectral peak at about 4 kHz, and the alveolar-palatal fricatives /ʃ/ and /ʒ/ having a first spectral peak at about 2.5 kHz. The study by Harris indicates that listeners need to use both the spectral cues of the frication and those of the formant transitions from and to neighboring vowels to distinguish the linguadental from the labiodental fricatives. Decisions about voicing class are based on the presence versus absence of phonation during frication, the relative durations of vocalic and noise segments, and the relative intensity differences between voiced and voiceless fricatives (or some combination of these cues).

## Affricates

Because affricates are stops with a fricative release, they contain the acoustic cues to perception that are found in both stops and fricatives. The silence, the release burst, the rapid rise time, the frication, and the formant transitions in adjacent sounds are all presumably used by listeners in identifying affricates. Raphael, Dorman, and Isenberg varied duration of frication and closure and rise time of the noise in utterances such as "ditch" /dɪtʃ/ and "dish" /dɪʃ/, and they found that a trading relationship exists among the cues. For example, inserting an appropriate duration of silence between the /ɪ/ and /ʃ/ of "dish" will cause the stimulus to be heard as "ditch." Increasing the duration of the frication of /ʃ/, however, will cause the percept to revert to "dish." Listeners are, apparently, sensitive to the relative durational values of the acoustic cues in stimuli of this type.

## Cues for Manner, Place, and Voicing

To summarize the wealth of information on the acoustic cues to the perception of speech segments, it may be helpful to divide the cues into those important to the perception of (1) manner, (2) place, and (3) voicing distinctions. To identify the manner of articulation of a speech sound, listeners determine whether the sound is harmonically structured with no noise (which signals vowels, semivowels, or nasals) or contains an aperiodic component (which signals stops, fricatives, or affricates). The periodic, harmonically structured classes possess acoustic cues that are relatively low in frequency. In contrast, the aperiodic, noisy classes of speech sounds are cued by relatively high frequencies.

How do listeners further separate the harmonically structured vowels, nasals, and semivowels? The main manner cues available are the relative intensities of formants and the changes in formant frequency. The nasal consonants have weak formants that contrast strongly with the relatively high intensity of neighboring vowels and semivowels. In addition, the nasals have a distinctive low-frequency resonance, the nasal murmur. Semivowels display formants that change rapidly from one frequency to another compared with the relatively more steady-state formants of the vowels and nasals. The formants for some diphthongs change in frequency as much as those of any semivowel, but the changes are generally slower than those for semivowels.

One cue to the manner classes of sounds with an aperiodic component is the duration of the noise, which is briefest in the case of stops but which lasts longer for affricates and longest for fricatives. Figure 10.9 shows that all of the parameters of sound are important: Manner contrasts are conveyed by differences in frequency, intensity, and timing.

The acoustic cues for the place of articulation (Fig. 10.10) depend more on the single parameter of sound frequency. For vowels and semivowels, the formant relationships indicate tongue placement, mouth opening, and vocal tract length. Vowel articulation is reflected in the $F_1$ to $F_2$ acoustic space, with $F_1$ frequency indicating tongue height or mouth opening and $F_2$ frequency indicating the location of the constriction formed between the tongue and the palate. Semivowel production is mainly reflected in the frequency changes in $F_2$. The semivowel /j/ begins with the highest $F_2$; $F_2$ for /r/ and /l/

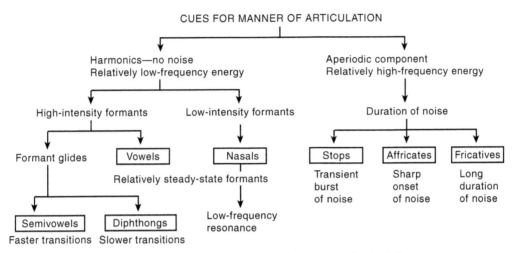

**FIGURE 10.9** Summary of the cues for manner of articulation.

originates in the middle frequencies; /w/ displays an $F_2$ with a relatively low frequency onset. $F_3$ serves to contrast the acoustic results of differing tongue tip placements for /r/ and /l/.

For stops, fricatives, and affricates, two prominent acoustic cues to the place of articulation are the $F_2$ transitions to and from neighboring vowels and the frequency of the noise components. In general, a second formant transition with a low-frequency locus cues the perception of a labial sound;

one with a higher locus cues the perception of an alveolar sound; and a variable, vowel-dependent locus cues a palatal or velar sound. The $F_2$ transition is also used to cue the difference between the labiodental and linguadental fricatives, although not very effectively.

The frequency of the noise component of a consonant cues the place of articulation. The high-frequency spectral peak for the noise in alveolar /s/ and /z/ is often at or above 4 kHz, whereas for the more retracted

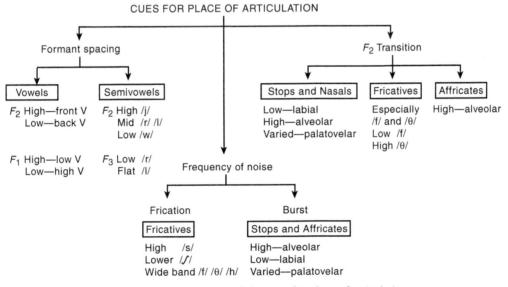

**FIGURE 10.10** Summary of the cues for place of articulation.

alveolar-palatal /ʃ/ and /ʒ/, it is more often closer to 2.5 kHz. If the frication covers a wide band of frequencies, has no prominent spectral peak, and has lower intensity than the neighboring vowel or vowels, it is more likely to be identified as /f, v/, or /θ, ð/. The spectrum of the noise component cues the place of articulation even when the noise is extremely brief, as in stop or affricate release bursts, with low-frequency spectral peaks cueing the perception of labial sounds, high-frequency peaks cueing the perception of alveolar sounds, and vowel-dependent mid-frequency range peaks cueing the perception of palatal and velar sounds.

Finally, the acoustic cues for consonant voicing (Fig. 10.11) depend more on relative durations and timing of events than on frequency or intensity differences. There is an exception: the presence or absence of phonation (glottal pulsing). The periodicity of voicing itself is important, but the fact that a speaker can whisper "The tie is blue" and "The dye is blue" and a listener can perceive the difference between "tie" and "dye" in the absence of phonation indicates that timing is an important cue to the perception of the voiced–voiceless distinction in conso-

nants. The timing differences used to signal the voiced–voiceless contrast have been measured in different ways. Longer VOTs, extended periods of aspiration, and longer closure durations cue /p, t, k/, the voiceless stops. Short VOTs, little or no aspiration, and short closure duration cue the voiced stops, /b, d, g/.

Fricatives and affricates are perceived as voiceless when the frication is of relatively long duration and, in the case of affricates, when the closure duration is also relatively long. Finally, the duration of a vowel can cue the voicing class of a following consonant: A voiced consonant may be perceived when the preceding vowel is relatively long in duration, and a voiceless consonant may be perceived when the duration of the preceding vowel is relatively short.

## Prosodic Features

The prosodic features of speech, including intonation, stress, and juncture, are perceived by listeners in terms of variations and contrasts in pitch, loudness, and length. As we mentioned in Chapter 7, the physical features of fundamental frequency, amplitude,

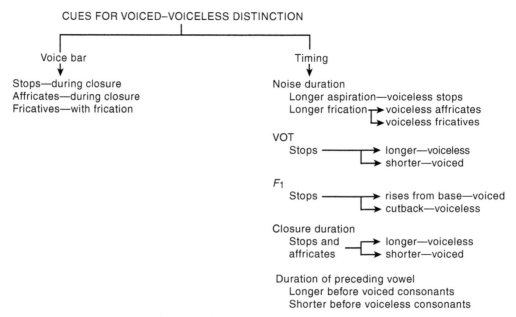

**FIGURE 10.11**   Summary of the cues for the voiced–voiceless distinction. VOT, voice onset time.

and duration are the principal determinants of the perceptual qualities. Fundamental frequency is the principal determinant of pitch; amplitude is the principal determinant of loudness; and duration is the principal determinant of length. It is important to maintain the distinctions between the perceptual qualities and the physical acoustic features that underlie them, because linguistic percepts such as stress and intonation do not have simple and direct representations in the acoustic signal. One cannot, for example, assume that because the second syllable in a word has greater duration than the first, it will be perceived as having greater linguistic stress than the first. Similarly, a rise in fundamental frequency at the end of a sentence is not a certain indication that the listener will perceive that there was a rise in pitch or that a yes–no question had been asked. Such percepts often depend on the extent of the physical changes, the covariation of a number of acoustic variables, and the degree of contrast between the values of the acoustic variables over a number of syllables.

The perception of intonation requires the ability to track pitch changes. This ability is one of the first skills that infants acquire. The tracking process is not well understood. Clearly, it allows listeners to detect changes in the direction of pitch and the extent of those changes. For instance, experiments by have shown that, given ambiguous speech material, a rising intonation pattern is perceived by listeners as a question, and a falling intonation pattern is perceived as a statement. The process must also enable listeners to locate the peaks of pitch in the intonation pattern with some precision. This ability is important in the perception of stress.

Any syllable may be spoken with a greater or lesser degree of stress, depending on the meaning demanded by context. For example, the first syllable in the noun "PERmit" is perceived as carrying more stress than the first syllable of the verb "per-MIT" if the speaker is following the usual convention. The reverse, of course, is true of the second syllables in these words. As we saw in Chapter 7, certain acoustic fea-

tures characterize a stressed syllable. Thus, the first syllable of the noun "'PERmit" is likely to have a higher fundamental frequency and greater duration and amplitude than the "same" syllable in the verb "per-MIT." We would expect, therefore, that listeners perceive the more stressed version of the syllable as higher in pitch and greater in length and loudness. In fact, untrained listeners may be quite poor at making explicit judgments of pitch, length, and loudness or even at specifying the location of a stressed syllable. Still, they must be capable of using the perceptual information if they understand and produce speech in a normal manner. Listeners thus do far better at identifying "'PERmit" as a noun than at identifying the first syllable in the word as having higher pitch or greater length, loudness, or stress.

Although fundamental frequency, duration, and amplitude all contribute to the perception of stress, they do not do so equally. Experiments by Fry, Bolinger, and others have shown that fundamental frequency is the most powerful cue to stress, followed by duration and amplitude. This finding runs counter to the intuitions of many speakers who indicate that when they wish to emphasize a syllable or word, they simply say it louder. It may be that this intention, which requires extra energy, accounts for the greater duration and higher $f_0$ that often mark stressed syllables: you will recall that an increase in subglottal pressure can raise $f_0$.

The prosodic feature of internal juncture (marking the difference between "a name" and "an aim" or between "why choose" and "white shoes") can be cued by a number of acoustic features, such as silence, vowel lengthening, and the presence or absence of phonation or aspiration. We like an example that Darwin cited from Shakespeare's *Troilus and Cressida*. The crowd shouts "the Troyans' trumpet!" which, if the juncture is misplaced by lengthening the frication of the /s/ in "Troyans" and decreasing the aspiration of the initial /t/ of "trumpet," sounds as if the crowd were announcing a prominent prostitute (Fig. 10.12).

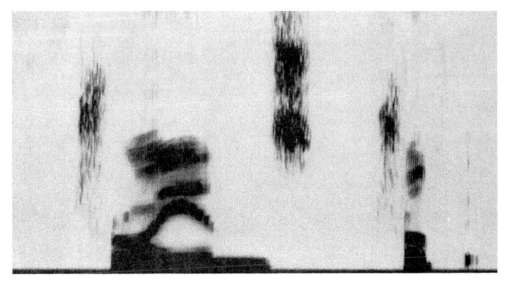

t   r o y a      n      's ——— t rumpe t

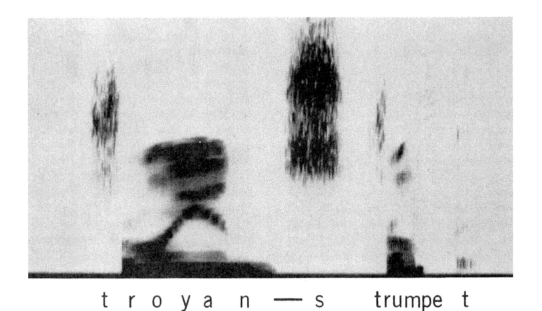

t    r  o  y  a   n  —— s       trumpe  t

**FIGURE 10.12**   Spectrograms of "Troyans' trumpet" and "Troyan strumpet." Notice the acoustic results of the change in juncture. The fricative is lengthened when in word-initial position, as is the aspiration for the /t/ in "trumpet".

## The Context of Acoustic Cues

The importance of context to speech perception is apparent in the recovery of both segmental and prosodic (suprasegmental) information. One word that we find ourselves writing repeatedly in this chapter is "relative." The importance of $f_o$ to the perception of stress is that it tends to be higher on a stressed syllable or word than it is on surrounding syllables or words. That is, the actual values of $f_0$ on the syllables in a word or sentence are irrelevant; the relative values are what matters. Similarly, formants need not be of particular frequencies to be recognized as particular vowels, but they must bear a certain general relation to one another, and further, may sometimes be perceived in relation to the frequencies of some other bit of speech produced by the same vocal tract.

Machines can be made to read print much more easily than they can be made to recognize speech, because the letters in printing or writing are discrete items that can be identified individually and then identified as a word. The letters "T,A,P" are segments and do not vary. "T" may appear as "t" or change size, but it is always a nearly vertical line with a nearly horizontal line crossing it at or near the top. In contrast, it is much more difficult to make a machine that can reliably recognize speech because the acoustic signal for [tæp] changes so continuously that it cannot be segmented the way the written word "TAP" can. One of the important acoustic cues to the /t/ is in the initial second formant transition to the vowel /æ/. The second formant transition at the end of the /æ/ supplies the listener with information about the /p/ to follow. That is, some of the information needed to identify the consonants is contained in the vowel between them. Therefore, attempts to identify the consonants are likely to fail if they rely only on the acoustic information within the limited period of time that the sounds are articulated. We can see, then, that to perceive speech, humans must behave very differently from the type of print- or speech-recognizing machine designed to act on a segment-by-segment basis.

## BIBLIOGRAPHY

### General Readings

Darwin, C. J., The Perception of Speech. In *Handbook of Perception, Vol. 7: Language and Speech*. E. C. Carterette and M. P. Friedman (Eds.). New York: Academic Press, 1976, pp. 175–226.

Denes, P., and Pinson, E. N., *The Speech Chain,* 2nd ed. New York: W. H. Freeman & Co., 1963.

Fant, G., Descriptive Analysis of the Acoustic Aspects of Speech. *Logos 5,* 1962, 3–17.

Kent, R. D., Atal, B. S., and Miller, J. L. (Eds.), *Papers in Speech Communication: Speech Production.* Woodbury, NY: Acoustical Society of America, 1991.

Liberman, A. M., *Speech: A Special Code.* Cambridge, MA: MIT Press, 1996.

Miller, J. L., Kent, R. D., and Atal, B. S. (Eds.), *Papers in Speech Communication: Speech Perception.* Woodbury, NY: Acoustical Society of America, 1991.

Pickett, J. M., *The Acoustics of Speech Communication.* Boston: Allyn and Bacon, 1999.

Raphael, L. J., Acoustic Cues to the Perception of Segmental Phonemes. In *The Handbook of Speech Perception.* D. B. Pisoni and R. E. Remez (Eds.). Malden, MA: Blackwell, 2005, pp. 182–206.

## Acoustic Cues

### Vowels, Diphthongs, and Semivowels

Delattre, P., Liberman, A. M., Cooper, F. S., and Gerstman, L. J., An Experimental Study of the Acoustic Determinants of Vowel Color: Observations on One- and Two-Formant Vowels Synthesized From Spectrographic Patterns. *Word 8,* 1952, 195–210.

Fry, D. B., Abramson, A. S., Eimas, P. D., and Liberman, A. M., The Identification and Discrimination of Synthetic Vowels. *Lang. Speech 5,* 1962, 171–189.

Gay, T., A Perceptual Study of American English Diphthongs. *Lang. Speech 13,* 1970, 65–88.

Gerstman, L. J., Classification of Self-Normalized Vowels. *IEEE Trans. Aud. Electroacoust. AU-16,* 1968, 78–80.

Halberstam, B., and Raphael, L. J., Vowel Normalization: The Role of Fundamental Frequency and Upper Formants. *J. Phonet. 32,* 2004, 423–434.

Ladefoged, P., and Broadbent, D. E., Information Conveyed by Vowels. *J. Acoust. Soc. Am. 39,* 1957, 98–104. Reprinted in Miller et al. 1991, 493–499.

Lindblom, B. E. F. Spectrographic Study of Vowel Production. *J. Acoust. Soc. Am. 36,* 1963, 1773–1781.

Lisker, L., Minimal Cues for Separating /w,r,l,y/ in Intervocalic Position. *Word 13,* 1957, 256–267.

Nordstrom, P. E., and Lindblom, B., A Normalization Procedure for Vowel Formant Data. Paper Presented at 8th International Congress of Phonetic Sciences, Leeds, England, Aug. 1975.

O'Connor, J. D., Gerstman, L. J., Liberman, A. M., Delattre, P. C., and Cooper, F. S., Acoustic Cues for the Perception of Initial /w,j,r,l/ in English. *Word 13,* 1957, 22–43.

Strange, W. Perception of Vowels. In *The Acoustics of Speech Communication.* Picket, J. M. (Ed.). Boston: Allyn & Bacon, 1999, pp. 153–165.

Strange, W., Verbrugge, R. R., Shankweiler, D. P., and Edman, T. R., Consonant Environment Specifies Vowel Identity. *J. Acoust. Soc. Am. 60,* 1976, 213–221.

Verbrugge, R. R., Strange, W., Shankweiler, D. P., and Edman, T. R., What Information Enables a Listener to Map a Talker's Vowel Space? *J. Acoust. Soc. Am. 60,* 1976, 198–212.

## Nasals, Stops, Fricatives, and Affricates

Ali, L., Gallagher, T., Goldstein, J., and Daniloff, R., Perception of Coarticulated Nasality. *J. Acoust. Soc. Am. 49,* 1971, 538–540.

Cooper, F. S., Delattre, P. C., Liberman, A. M., Borst, J. M., and Gerstman, L. J., Some Experiments on the Perception of Synthetic Speech Sounds. *J. Acoust. Soc. Am. 24,* 1952, 597–606.

Delattre, P. C., Liberman, A. M., and Cooper, F. S., Acoustic Loci and Transitional Cues for Consonants. *J. Acoust. Soc. Am. 27,* 1955, 769–773.

Denes, P., Effect of Duration on the Perception of Voicing. *J. Acoust. Soc. Am. 27,* 1955, 761–764.

Fruchter, D., and Sussman, H. M., The Perceptual Relevance of Locus Equations. *J. Acoust. Soc. Am. 102,* 1997, 2997–3008.

Harris, K. S., Cues for the Discrimination of American English Fricatives in Spoken Syllables. *Lang. Speech 1,* 1958, 1–7.

Kuhn, G. M., On the Front Cavity Resonance and Its Possible Role in Speech Perception. *J. Acoust. Soc. Am. 58,* 1975, 428–433.

Liberman, A. M., Delattre, P. C., and Cooper, F. S., The Role of Selected Stimulus-Variables in the Perception of the Unvoiced Stop Consonants. *Am. J. Psychol. 65,* 1952, 497–516.

Liberman, A. M., Delattre, P. C., and Cooper, F. S., Some Rules for the Distinction Between Voiced and Voiceless Stops in Initial Position. *Lang. Speech 1,* 1958, 153–167.

Liberman, A. M., Delattre, P. C., Cooper, F. S., and Gerstman, L. J., The Role of Consonant-Vowel Transitions in the Perception of the Stop and Nasal Consonants. *Psychol. Monogr.: Gen. Appl. 68,* 1954, 1–13.

Liberman, A. M., Delattre, P. C., Gerstman, L. J., and Cooper, F. S., Tempo of Frequency Change as a Cue for Distinguishing Classes of Speech Sounds. *J. Exp. Psychol. 52,* 1956, 127–137.

Lisker, L., "Voicing" in English: A Catalogue of Acoustic Features Signaling /b/ vs. /p/ in Trochees. *Lang. Speech, 29,* 1986, 3–11.

Lisker, L., and Abramson, A. S., The Voicing Dimension: Some Experiments in Comparative Phonetics. In *Proceedings of the Sixth International Congress of Phonetic Sciences, Prague, 1967.* Prague, Czech Republic: Academia Publishing House of the Czechoslovak Academy of Sciences, 1968, 563–567.

Malécot, A., Acoustic Cues for Nasal Consonants. *Language 32,* 1956, 274–278.

Mermelstein, P., On Detecting Nasals in Continuous Speech. *J. Acoust. Soc. Am. 61,* 1977, 581–587.

Miller, G. A., and Nicely, P. E., An Analysis of Perceptual Confusions Among Some English Consonants. *J. Acoust. Soc. Am. 27,* 1955, 338–352. Reprinted in Miller et al. 1991, 623–637.

Raphael, L. J., Durations and Contexts as Cues to Word-Final Cognate Opposition in English. *Phonetica 38,* 1981, 126–147.

Raphael, L. J., Preceding Vowel Duration as a Cue to the Perception of the Voicing Characteristic of Word-Final Consonants in American English. *J. Acoust. Soc. Am. 51,* 1972, 1296–1303.

Raphael, L. J., and Dorman, M. F., Acoustic Cues for a Fricative-Affricate Contrast in Word-Final Position. *J. Phonet. 8,* 1980, 397–405.

Repp, B. H. Perception of the [m]–[n] Distinction in CV Syllables. *J. Acoust. Soc. Am. 72,* 1986, 1987–1999.

## Prosodic Features

Bolinger, D. W., and Gerstman, L. J., Disjuncture as a Cue to Constructs. *Word 13,* 1957, 246–255.

Bolinger, D. L., A Theory of Pitch Accent in English. *Word 14,* 1958, 109–149.

Crystal, T. H. and House, A. S., Articulation Rate and the Duration of Syllables and Stress Groups in Connected Speech. *J. Acoust. Soc. Am. 88,* 1990, 101–112.

Fry, D. B., Experiments in the Perception of Stress. *Lang. Speech 1,* 1958, 126–152.

Fry, D. B., Prosodic Phenomena. In *Manual of Phonetics.* B. Malmberg (Ed.). Amsterdam, The Netherlands: North-Holland, 1968, pp. 365–410.

Hadding-Koch, K., and Studdert-Kennedy, M., An Experimental Study of Some Intonation Contours. *Phonetica 11,* 1964, 175–185.

Hermes, D. J. and Rump, H. H., Perception of Prominence in Speech Intonation Induced by Rising and Falling Pitch Movements. *J. Acoust. Soc. Am. 96,* 1994, 83–92.

Lehiste, I., *Suprasegmentals.* Cambridge, MA: MIT Press, 1970.

Mattys, S. L., The Perception of Primary and Secondary Stress in English. *Percept. Psychophys. 62,* 2000, 253–265.

Turk, A. E. and Sawusch, J. R., The Processing of Duration and Intensity Cues to Prominence. *J. Acoust. Soc. Am. 99,* 1996, 3782–3789.

# Strategies and Models

## 11

*The intellect pierces the form, overleaps the wall, detects intrinsic likeness between remote things and reduces all things into a few principles.*

–Ralph Waldo Emerson, *Intellect*, 1841

## CATEGORICAL PERCEPTION

In searching for the acoustic features of speech that are particularly important to perception, investigators found that constant changes in the $F_2$ transitions of synthetic two-formant consonant–vowel (CV) syllables resulted in the perception of three phonemes: /b/, /d/, and /g/ (Fig. 11.1). Subjects perceived /b/ for stimuli having the most sharply rising $F_2$ transitions. Then, as the transitions rose less and then began to fall slightly in frequency, their percepts shifted abruptly to a different category: /d/. Stimuli near the end of the continuum, those with $F_2$ transitions that fell more steeply, evoked another abrupt change in perception to /g/. When listeners were asked to discriminate stimuli drawn from the continuum, they could do so only if they had labeled them differently. This phenomenon, the ability to discriminate stimuli only as well as one can identify them, is called categorical perception. We shall present the details of one study of categorical perception as an example of how such studies were usually conducted.

A study by Liberman et al. (1957) has served as the model for many studies of categorical perception. The stimuli (Fig. 11.1) were synthesized on the Pattern Playback for precise control of frequency, intensity, and duration. The 14 two-formant CV patterns differed only in the direction and extent of the $F_2$ transition. The rapidly and sharply rising $F_2$ transition necessary for perception of an exemplary /b/ was the first stimulus of the continuum, and the rapidly, sharply falling $F_2$ transition necessary for perception of an exemplary /g/ was the fourteenth and last stimulus. The stimuli in between were constructed by raising the starting frequency of the $F_2$ transition in equal steps of 120 Hz.

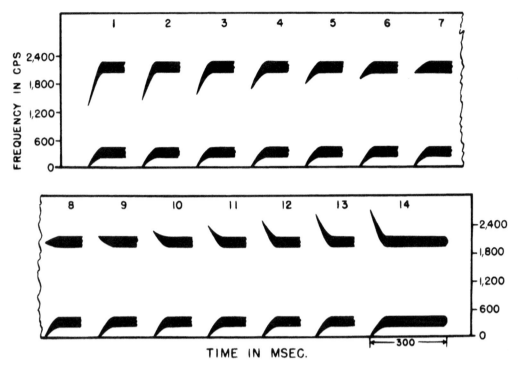

**FIGURE 11.1** Two-formant synthetic CV pattern series: the stimuli for /ba/, /da/, and /ga/. (Reprinted with permission from Liberman, A. M., et al., The Discrimination of Speech Sounds Within and Across Phoneme Boundaries. *J. Exp. Psychol. 54,* 1957, 358–368.)

Each stimulus was recorded several times. The recorded stimuli were randomized and presented to listeners in an *identification test*. In this type of test, listeners hear one stimulus at a time and are told to identify or label it and to guess if they are not sure which sound they have heard. When the subjects are instructed to use a restricted set of responses (e.g., /b/, /d/, or /g/), the test is called a *forced-choice test*. An *open response set* is used if the experimenters want to allow the subjects to label the stimuli in any way they choose. The forced-choice format has been used more frequently than the open response set.

The stimuli were also arranged in a second type of perceptual test, a *discrimination test*. The task of a subject in a discrimination test is simply to indicate whether two stimuli are the same or different, on any basis whatsoever, without overtly labeling them. It is important to note that there are no correct or incorrect answers in a labeling-identification

test: if you ask listeners what they perceived and they tell you, they can't be wrong, even if other listeners report hearing something different. Labeling tests, therefore, are never scored in terms of percent correct but rather in terms of percent recognition of a certain sound. Discrimination tests, on the other hand, do have correct or incorrect responses because the experimenter has control over the stimuli and can verify that they are the same or different. If they are different and if a listener says they are the same, then the listener is wrong; if the stimuli are identical and if a listener says they are different, then, again, the listener is wrong.

There are a number of discrimination paradigms, but the one that has been most frequently used is the *ABX format*. In each ABX set, listeners hear 1 of the 14 stimuli (A), followed by a different stimulus (B), and then followed by a third stimulus (X), which is the same as one of the first two. The subjects are told that A and B are different. The task of the subjects is to determine whether X was identical to A or to B and to guess if they were uncertain. The percentage of correct matching of X with the identical stimulus of the AB pair is the measure of discrimination in this test. If the subjects are guessing because they cannot discriminate A from B, their correct responses will be at chance level: 50%. The A and B are sometimes adjacent stimuli on the test continuum (a one-step test), and sometimes separated from each other by one or two stimuli (two- and three-step tests).

In the experiment by Liberman et al., the labeling and discrimination tests were presented in counterbalanced order to different subject groups. Results were equivalent regardless of the order of test presentation. In addition, subjects responded in the same way (1) whether or not they were told at the outset that the stimuli were synthetic speech sounds and (2) when their response choices on the labeling test were forced or drawn from an open set.

Figure 11.2 shows the results of the identification test and a two-step discrimination test for one subject. The subject identified the first three stimuli as /b/ between 90%

and 100% of the time. Stimulus 4 was identified more often as /d/ than as /b/, and stimuli 5 through 8 were always perceived as /d/. More than 80% of the presentations of stimulus 9 were labeled as /d/. A shift in perception to /g/ occurred for stimulus 10, and the remaining stimuli, 11 through 14, were reported to be /g/ almost all of the time. Two sharply defined perceptual shifts are evident in this identification function. The first, the *phoneme boundary* separating /b/ from /d/, occurs between stimuli 3 and 4, and the other, separating /d/ from /g/, occurs between stimuli 9 and 10.

The discrimination function for the same subject, shown by the solid line at the right side of Figure 11.2, represents the percentage of correct responses to the 42 ABX triads in which A and B were two steps apart in the stimulus series. Judgments at the 50% correct level indicate a failure to discriminate A from B: when a subject cannot perceive a difference between the first two stimuli, he must guess which one of them is the same as X. Because he has two choices, there is a 50% chance of selecting the correct answer. Note the two 100% peaks in the discrimination function. The first peak, occurring at point 3 on the abscissa, represents responses by this

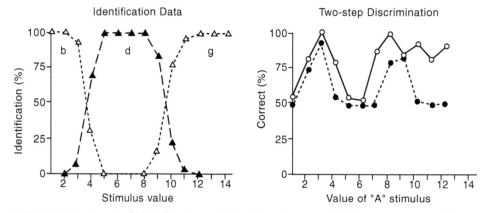

**FIGURE 11.2**   Result of identification and discrimination tests. *Left*: The percentage of the time each stimulus was identified as /b/, /d/, or /g/. *Right*: The result of the two-step discrimination test, compared with predictions derived from the identification test, using the technique described in the text of the article. (Modified with permission from Liberman, A. M., et al., The Discrimination of Speech Sounds Within and Across Phoneme Boundaries. *J. Exp. Psychol., 54,* 1957, 358–368.)

subject to ABX triads in which A and B were stimuli 3 and 5. Recall that the phoneme boundary between /b/ and /d/ for this subject was between stimuli 3 and 4, which is just the part of the stimulus series that this subject discriminates most accurately. The phoneme boundary between /d/ and /g/ was between stimuli 9 and 10 for this subject. Again, discrimination was perfect between stimuli 8 and 10. Thus, this subject discriminates best at phoneme boundaries, where the A and B stimuli belong to different phoneme categories, and less well between stimuli that belong to the same phoneme category.

The experimenters next tested the assumption that this subject (and each of the others) could discriminate the stimuli no better than he could label them as belonging to different phoneme categories—that is, that his perception was categorical. They used his labeling data as a basis to predict what his discrimination function ought to be, given the truth of the assumption. The predicted discrimination function is shown by the dashed line at the right side of Figure 11.2. The obtained discrimination function (the solid line) was higher than the predicted function, although the two were highly correlated. The fact that this subject (as well as the other subjects) could discriminate the stimuli somewhat better than if his perceptions were determined only by his labeling ability indicates that he might have been able to use some acoustic information to augment his phonemically based discrimination judgments.

It was surprising to find that people listening to synthetic speech sounds that change in equal steps in some acoustic dimension discriminate among them little better than they can label them. It is a well-known fact of psychoacoustics that in judging the relative pitch of pure tones, people can discriminate as many as 3,500 frequency steps but can label only a few pitches. Pitch perception is not linear with frequency change, because listeners can discriminate between low-frequency tones differing by only 3 or 4 Hz, whereas the discrimination of higher frequencies can require a difference of more than 20 Hz. Al-

though pitch perception is not linear, it is a continuous function. There are no sudden changes in the ability to detect pitch differences cued by frequency change as there are for differences among speech sounds cued by frequency change. One possible explanation for the discontinuities in the perception of speech stimuli has been provided by Stevens's (1989) *Quantal Theory.*

The quantal theory maintains that certain relatively large changes in articulator position cause little change in the acoustic signal, whereas other relatively small changes in articulator placement cause large changes in the acoustic signal. The extent of the acoustic change that occurs appears to be related to the particular region of the vocal tract where the articulation is located. In certain critical regions, a slight change in articulatory placement causes a large (quantal) change in sound. You can create an example of this sort of acoustic discontinuity by advancing the lingua-palatal constriction for [ʃ] very slowly forward until the sound becomes a lingua-alveolar [s]. You will hear very little change in the sound before the constriction reaches the alveolar ridge, but once it arrives at the ridge, there will be an almost immediate and substantial change in the frequency band of the frication. That is, there will be a quantal change from [ʃ] to [s]. Stevens has shown discontinuity for the acoustic effects of pharyngeal and velar consonant constrictions. He suggests that human languages use places of constriction located in those regions of the vocal tract where the acoustic output is stable. If this is so, speakers would be able to make many sounds acceptably without being overly precise in their articulation. In other words, the effects of coarticulation and assimilation could be easily accommodated by both the productive and perceptual mechanisms.

We must keep in mind that the discontinuities that Stevens describes are acoustic, not perceptual. In the speech perception study discussed earlier, the synthesizer produced a continuum of stimuli that changed in equal acoustic steps (something that a human speaker cannot do because of the acoustic discontinuities generated by the architecture of the vocal tract), yet the listeners perceived them categorically because of the inherently quantal nature of articulatory place. This fact has led some investigators to view quantal theory as supporting evidence for theories of speech perception that relate perception to articulation, on the grounds that the human auditory system is especially sensitive to quantal acoustic changes that the human articulatory system produces.

Because of the differences between the way listeners perceive nonspeech stimuli (such as tones) and speech stimuli, and because of the quantal nature of place of articulation, the categorical discontinuities found in speech perception have proven extremely interesting and have given rise to several questions that have been addressed in speech perception research: Do people perceive speech quite differently from the way they perceive nonspeech? Does the learning of a language sharpen some perceptions and dull others? Is categorical perception innate or learned? The first study reporting the categorical perception of speech did not answer these questions. It did, however, make the phenomenon explicit and sparked interest in looking further for the relative auditory and linguistic contributions to the effect.

## Within-Language and Cross-Language Studies of Categorical Perception in Adults

As we have just seen, the phenomenon of categorical perception was first demonstrated for place of articulation contrasts among stop consonants that were cued by formant transitions. We shall look at another such contrast, this time for liquids, and then go on to review some of the experimentation that has demonstrated categorical perception for manner of articulation and voicing contrasts.

In Chapter 6, we saw that differences in $F_3$ characterized the contrast between /r/ and /l/. It is, in fact, possible to construct a continuum of synthetic speech stimuli, beginning with /r/ and ending with /l/, by varying the transitions of $F_2$ and $F_3$. At Haskins Laboratories, Borden (1984) synthesized an /rɑ/ to /lɑ/ continuum (Fig. 11.3). The third-formant transition was graded from a relatively low

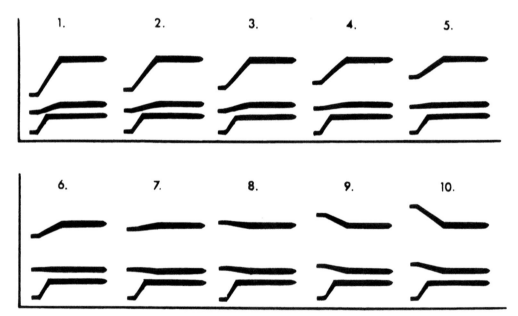

**FIGURE 11.3** A continuum of synthetic stimuli perceived as /rɑ/ or /lɑ/. Frequency is represented on the ordinate and time on the abscissa.

IDENTIFICATION TEST

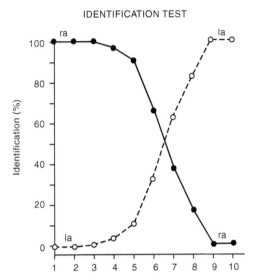

FIGURE 11.4 Identification functions for /ra/ and /la/. The 10 stimuli are on the abscissa and the percentage of listener judgments is on the ordinate. The boundary between /r/ and /l/ judgments lies between stimuli 6 and 7.

DISCRIMINATION TEST

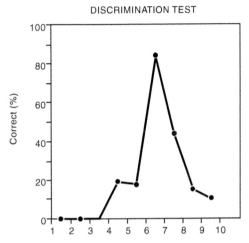

FIGURE 11.5 Discrimination function for pairs of stimuli separated by one step shown in Figure 11.3.

to a relatively high starting frequency, and the second formant transition was similarly varied but to a lesser extent. Listeners heard each stimulus 10 times in two randomized blocks of 50 stimuli. In this identification test, each stimulus followed a precursor phrase in natural speech: "Does this sound more like rock or lock?" Figure 11.4 shows typical identification functions. The first five stimuli were perceived almost unanimously as /ra/. Stimuli 6 and 7 were ambiguous, and the consonants in stimuli 8 through 10 were perceived as /la/. The phoneme boundary between /r/ and /l/ for these listeners occurred between stimuli 6 and 7.

Stimuli from the same continuum were paired in a discrimination test using one-, two-, and three-step differences. Once again a precursor sentence was used: each pair of items followed the question "Do these sound the same or not the same?" Subjects responded by checking either the column marked "same" or the column marked "not the same." The one-step discrimination function plotted in Figure 11.5 shows a peak in discrimination between stimuli 6 and 7, ex-

actly at the phoneme boundary in the identification test. Thus, the subjects discriminated the members of a pair of stimuli better when each was drawn from a different phoneme category than when they were drawn from the same phoneme category. In other words, their perception of the /r/–/l/ distinction was largely categorical.

Perception of the acoustic cues to manner of articulation has also been found to be categorical. For instance, increasing the duration of the transitions in such CV syllables as /ba/ and /ga/ shifts listeners' perceptions categorically, first from stop to semivowel (/wa, ja/) and then to sequences of vowels (/ua, ia/). Similarly, variations in the rise time of the intensity of frication from slow to rapid causes listeners to change their perception of /ʃ/ (as in "shop") to /tʃ/ (as in "chop") in a categorical manner.

Voicing contrasts may also be perceived categorically. Abramson and Lisker (1970) varied voice onset time (VOT) for syllable-initial stops in equal steps from −150 ms to +150 ms and found that listeners' percepts shifted categorically from the voiced to the voiceless categories. For example, English speakers located the /t/–/d/ phoneme boundary at about +25 ms VOT. The listeners were again good at discriminating stimuli drawn from opposite sides of the phoneme boundary. For pairs of stimuli within the same voicing category, however, listeners discriminated VOT differences relatively poorly.

The results of tests of vowel perception differ somewhat from those of consonant perception. Fry et al. (1962) synthesized a continuum of isolated steady-state vowels ranging from /ɪ/ to /ɛ/ to /æ/ by varying formant frequencies. The slopes of subjects' labeling functions were much less steep than those for stop consonants. More important, the peaks in the discrimination functions at the phoneme boundaries were lower and the percent correct discrimination of stimuli within each phoneme category was higher than for stop consonants. It would appear, then, that the perception of isolated vowels of relatively great duration is less categorical than the perception of stop (and some other) consonants. Stevens reports, however, that when the vowels are shorter in duration and embedded in consonant–vowel–consonant (CVC) contexts (with appropriately rapid formant transitions), the discrimination–identification relationship is more like that for consonants. That is, perception is more categorical than for the isolated vowels of relatively great duration.

Because steady-state vowels of long duration and nonspeech tones are perceived less categorically, whereas shorter vowels in CVC contexts and consonants are perceived more categorically, it seems that listeners perceive stimuli containing rapidly changing frequencies differently than they do stimuli that are more steady state in nature. And, of course, a rapidly changing spectrum is a defining characteristic of speech at normal rates.

An important aspect of categorical perception is the influence that linguistic knowledge can have on the perceived categories. The reason the /ra/–/la/ stimuli were prefaced with questions spoken in English is that Elman, Diehl, and Buchwald (1978) found that the language "set" that listeners have when making decisions about speech sound identity may change the boundary

between categories. Bilingual subjects divide such stimuli according to the phonemic contrasts of the particular language they are using immediately before each stimulus.

Strange and Jenkins (1978) have reviewed many studies of both monolingual and bilingual speakers. These studies offer evidence that the language experience of adults can influence their perception. For example, Spanish, French, and Thai speakers use different VOT criteria for voicing contrasts than do English speakers. Japanese speakers, who do not contrast /r/ and /l/, perceive equal changes in $F_3$ in an /ra/ to /la/ continuum differently from the two-category manner in which it is perceived by speakers of English. It is well known that English /r/ and /l/ are not so well discriminated or produced by native speakers of Japanese who may have learned little English, and often substitute one for the other.

Best, McRoberts, and Sithole (1988) has proposed a theory designed to account for which contrasts in phones are well perceived by listeners to a language not their own, and which are wholly or partially confused: the perceptual assimilation model (PAM). The basic premise of the PAM is that what naïve listeners perceive when they hear an unfamiliar language are the similarities and dissimilarities between its patterns and the familiar patterns of their native language. Therefore, when a sound is not in the listeners' native language, they assimilate it to the closest native sound or, in the extreme case, cannot classify it as a speech sound at all. The various PAM categories are shown in Table 11.1. Obviously, discrimination is poor in the single-category (SC) case, in which both sounds are assimilated to the same sound in the listener's native language, as is the case when Japanese listeners deal with American English /r/ and /l/.

Perhaps the most surprising PAM category (Table 11.1) is the nonassimilable (NA) category. It is easy to forget that the human vocal tract is capable of making some sounds that are not generally considered speech. For example, babies are often fond of making "raspberries," and there are a number

**TABLE 11.1** Assimilation Effects on Discrimination of Nonnative Contrasts

| Contrast Assimilation Type | Discrimination Effect |
| --- | --- |
| Two-Category (TC) | **Excellent discrimination** each nonnative sound is assimilated to a different native category |
| Category-Goodness Difference (CG) | **Moderate to very good discrimination** both nonnative sounds assimilated to the same native "ideal" (e.g., one is acceptable and the other is deviant) *can vary in degree of difference as members of some native category* |
| Single-Category (SC) | **Poor discrimination** both nonnative sounds assimilated to the same native category, but are equal in fit to the native "ideal" *better discrimination for pairs with poor fit (equally poor) to native category than pairs with good fit (equally good)* |
| Both Uncategorizable (UU) | **Poor to moderate discrimination** both nonnative sounds fall within unfamiliar phonetic space *can vary in their discriminability as uncategorizable speech sounds* |
| Uncategorized vs. Categorized (UC) | **Very good discrimination** one nonnative sound assimilated to a native category, the other falls in unfamiliar phonetic space, outside native categories |
| Nonassimilable (NA) | Good to very good discrimination both nonnative categories fall outside of speech domain and are heard as nonspeech sounds *can vary in their discriminability as nonspeech sounds* |

(From Best, C. T., Learning to Perceive the Sound Pattern of English. In *Advances in Infancy Research*. C. Rovee-Collier and L. Lipsitt (Eds.). Hillsdale, NJ: Ablex, 1994, pp. 217–304.)

of vocal party tricks, like imitating the sound of horses' hooves: Neither of these sound productions is considered speech by American listeners. Some sounds, however, are speech for the native speakers of some African languages, but not used at all by speakers of western European languages. Particularly interesting examples of this are the click sounds of the African Bantu languages. Although these sounds are part of very few of the world's languages, they can occur frequently in those few. According to Ladefoged and Traill (1984), Zulu has 15 clicks! All the clicks are produced on an ingressive airstream, in contrast to the sounds of English, which are produced only on an egressive pulmonary airstream. Clicks are made by creating a suction in the oral cavity followed by an abrupt release of the negative pressure, at one of several places in the vocal tract (apicovelar, palatovelar, and lateral alveolar), with various voicing conditions. Best et al. (1988) tested the PAM model by assessing the ability of speakers

of American English and Bantu to discriminate 18 minimal pair click contrasts, using an ABX paradigm. Although there was a small difference in percent correct discrimination between groups (78% correct for American listeners and 87% correct for Bantus), the results support the PAM model, even though the Americans had no experience with click languages.

Because adult listeners appear to sort phones into phonological categories differently depending on their native languages, investigators were surprised to find that creatures with little or no language ability (infants and animals) discriminate speech-like stimuli in a way similar to that of adults when they perceive speech categorically.

## Studies of Infant Speech Perception

The classic report on infant perception of speech-like stimuli was published in *Science* in 1971, by Eimas et al. They monitored infants sucking a pacifier wired to a transducer that

## *C*LINICAL NOTE

This chapter has presented a number of points of view and evidence concerning the roles of auditory and phonetic analysis in speech perception, the potential link between speech production and perception, and theories of speech perception. The position a clinician takes with regard to these and related issues can have a profound effect on the choice of testing and treatment protocols that should be provided. For instance, favoring a theoretical stance that projects speech perception as part of a general auditory ability to process sound will support the use of nonspeech materials in evaluating and treating a client. For instance, if a clinician assumes that a client's perceptual problems stem from inadequate processing of rapid frequency changes, there would be no reason not to use any auditory stimulus, pure tones, for example, to test for or to treat those problems. On the other hand, the assumption that speech perception is mediated by a specialized phonetic processor would lead a clinician to use speech for testing and treatment, or, at the very least, sounds acoustically like speech.

Much the same line of reasoning applies to assumptions concerning the relationship between speech production and speech perception. If a clinician believes that the productive and perceptual mechanisms are separate and independent, there would be no reason to incorporate measures of articulation in evaluating or treating perceptual problems, or to test perceptual acuity in evaluating or treating articulatory problems. In contrast, the assumption that the two mechanisms, articulatory and perceptual, are closely related would demand the use of both articulatory and perceptual materials.

In short, each decision the clinician makes about theoretical issues concerning speech perception (or to speech production) will lead to real consequences in the clinic with regard to what should happen there and why it should happen.

---

recorded sucking responses. A continuum of synthetic stop-plus-vowel syllables differing by 20-ms increments of VOT was synthesized. Infants as young as 1 month of age reacted to any new stimulus with a change in sucking rate. The investigators recorded the baseline rate of sucks per minute for each baby and then presented each auditory stimulus at an intensity that depended on the rate of sucking. As long as the baby maintained a high rate of sucking, the sound continued at high intensity. As the rate of sucking decreased, so did the loudness of the sound. Typically, when a new stimulus was introduced, the babies responded by increasing their rate of sucking. After a few minutes, as the novelty of the stimulus wore off, the sucking rate gradually decreased. This decrease in response rate, known as habituation, was allowed to proceed for 2 minutes, and then a different VOT stimulus was presented for several minutes and the observers

noted whether there was an increase in sucking rate, indicating that the infant was able to discriminate the new stimulus from the previous stimulus.

Figure 11.6 displays the mean responses of the 4-month-olds. The *dots* at the far *left* of each of the three graphs represent the baseline rate of sucking. With auditory reinforcement for sucking, the rate of responses increased, as can be seen by the sucking rates plotted to the left of the broken vertical line, those representing 5, 4, and 3 minutes before a change of stimulus. As the infants became habituated to the stimulus, the sucking rate decreased. The graph at the left represents what happened when the first stimulus, a /bɑ/-like stimulus with a VOT of +20 ms, was changed to a /pɑ/-like stimulus with a VOT of +40 ms. The sucking rate increased dramatically, indicating that the infants heard this shift as something new. The middle graph reveals no such increase in

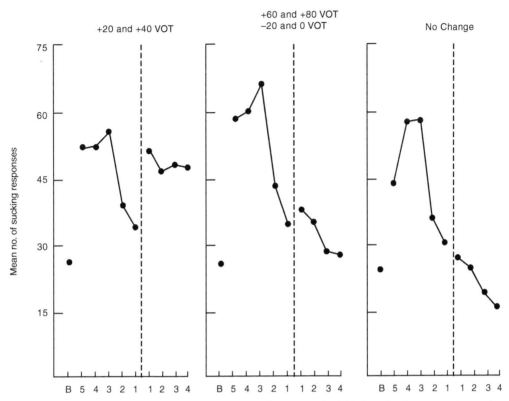

**FIGURE 11.6**  Mean number of sucking responses for 4-month-old infants in three experimental conditions. B is the baseline before presentation of a stimulus. Each panel shows sucking as a function of time with a change of stimulus at the point shown by the broken line, or in the right-hand panel, at the time the change would have occurred. In the left-hand panel, the stimuli straddle the /b/–/p/ category boundary for adults. In the middle panel, contrasting stimuli are within one category. (Adapted with permission from Eimas, P., et al., Speech Perception in Infants. *Science 171*, 1971, 303–306.)

sucking responses, even though the stimuli also differed by 20 ms VOT. In this condition, the VOT of the first stimulus was +60 ms and that of the second was +80 ms (both perceived by adults as /pɑ/) or the VOT of the first stimulus was −20 ms and that of the second was zero (both perceived by adults as /bɑ/). The infants did not respond to these changes with a significant increase in the sucking rate. The authors infer from these results that the infants perceive the +20 and +40 ms VOT stimuli as different but do not perceive the +60 and +80 ms or the −20 and 0 ms VOT stimuli as different. Again, this mirrors the phonemic grouping of stimuli found in adults.

The data for the control condition are shown in the graph on the right of the figure. When there is no change in the stimulus, habituation continues and the sucking rate continues to decrease in much the same way as when the stimuli were drawn from the same adult phonemic class. Eimas and his colleagues concluded that infants as young as 1 month old seem to discriminate acoustic changes in this speech continuum in the same way as do adults. That is, the infants' discrimination is best at about the same location where adults locate a phoneme boundary. We should point out that this is not an instance of categorical perception on the part of the infants because there are, of necessity, no labeling data to which the discrimination data can be related. This and other infant studies, however, do present the possibility that the ability to categorize speech sounds is innate. We will return to this issue later.

There have been many studies of infant speech perception since this original study. Techniques for assessing infants' discrimination of speech sounds have changed. Researchers find they may get more reliable results by conditioning infants, those who are old enough, to turn and look at a dancing bear or a moving toy as a reinforcer. (Infants younger than 6 months, however, are generally too immature motorically for head-turning.) The infant is conditioned to look at the toy only in response to a certain sound. Sounds that are acoustically similar or different can be delivered to see whether the infant perceives them as the same or different from the conditioned stimulus. Kuhl (1992) has reported that 6-month-old babies tested with this technique discriminate vowels and consonants even when stimuli vary in pitch, talker, and phonetic context. Jusczyk (1977, 1997) found that infants can perceive consonant contrasts in word-initial, -medial, or -final position, and in multisyllabic stimuli as well as in monosyllables. There are some preliminary indications that infants can discriminate stress contrasts, although more research is necessary to determine the validity of this finding.

The question that results from the increasing evidence of infant perceptual abilities is whether infants are innately equipped to detect linguistically significant contrasts or whether the distinctions they perceive are a result of characteristics of the auditory system without reference to language. The infants are obviously making auditory distinctions, but we do not know at what age they begin to make phonetic distinctions. In a series of experiments using 6-month-old children in the United States and in Sweden, Kuhl and others found that the subjects showed demonstrable effects of exposure to their native language. The experimenters used two synthetic vowels belonging to a single phonemic category in each language: /i/ (English) and /y/, a front, lip-rounded Swedish vowel. One vowel was judged by listeners to be the best exemplar of the /i/ or /y/ category in their language; the other was rated as a poor exemplar. The infants in each country performed two discrimination tasks for the vowels in their ambient language. In one task they discriminated the best exemplar from vowels that were more or less similar to it. They also performed the same task for the poor exemplar. Both Swedish and American children did less well in discriminating the best exemplar from similar stimuli. When each group was tested with the prototype from the other language, they were better able to discriminate it from other vowels than the prototype from their ambient language.

Kuhl has termed the discrimination results for the best exemplar the "magnet effect." She posits that the prototypical vowel has attracted similar vowels to it, perceptually. Thus, by at least 6 months of age, exposure to what will be their native language has rendered the children less able to make intraphonemic distinctions among sounds that are near the core of a phonemic category. It is as though the more prototypical allophones of the phoneme coalesce around the best exemplar, whereas the less prototypical allophones remain discriminable from each other. This change in the ability to discriminate is presumably overlaid on the innate ability to discriminate different phonemic categories. How early in development does the change occur? The influence of language experience (or lack of it) is evident in adults' categorization and discrimination of phonetic distinctions that do not contrast in their own language. Yet given that infants learn whatever language is used in their own homes in their first years, they must, at some time during that period, be able to perceive the contrasts between the phonetic classes used in any language spoken anywhere. As we indicated, this ability has been shown for infants in a number of language communities. More recently, a few studies have addressed the question of the development of language effects on speech perception during the first year of life.

A problem with the studies of speech perception in infants is that several different techniques have been used (e.g., nonnutritive sucking rate, measures of heart rate, head-turning paradigms), techniques that are not equally easy to use with children in their first year of life. A technique other than those described above, called visual fixation habituation, has been developed by Best and her coworkers, and has been used to evaluate the PAM (see above). An infant, seated in his mother's lap, looks at a checkerboard pattern on a screen while a recording of one member of a pair of stimuli is played. The infant's gaze time is recorded, up to the time the infant looks away. The gaze time is the score for the trial. Over a series of trials, the gaze time decreases, or habituates. When the gaze time has decreased to 50% of the time of the preceding two trials, the stimulus is changed to the other member of the pair. The measure of discrimination is the change of duration of fixation for the first two trials after the change of the stimulus.

In the study by Best and co-workers, three phonetic contrasts were examined for two groups of infants from monolingual

English-speaking households. Each group comprised 12 children. The age range of one group was from 6 to 8 months, and the age range of the other was from 10 to 12 months. The contrasts studied were the /ba–da/ contrast in English, a contrast between a pair of Zulu clicks, previously shown to be discriminable by American adults and infants, and a third contrast between a pair of Nthlakampx ejectives, which are both assimilated to /k/ in English-speaking adults. (Nthlakampx is an American Indian language.) According to the PAM hypothesis, the younger group of infants should have been able to distinguish all three pairs, but the older group should have lost this ability because of the effects of increasing familiarity with their native language, English.

The results are shown in Figure 11.7: the height of the bars shows the mean duration of gaze after habituation, for each of the three contrasts, for the two age groups. Although the English and Zulu contrasts are significantly well distinguished in both groups, the older group can no longer distinguish the /k/-like ejectives.

It should be noted that the earlier Eimas study of 4-month-old infants has been interpreted by some as indicating that speech sound boundaries are perceptually innate.

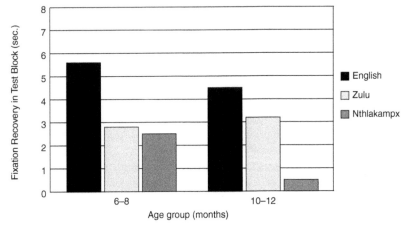

**FIGURE 11.7**  Recovery of fixation responses displayed as difference scores (preshift test block minus postshift test block). (Adapted from Best, C. T. et al., Divergent Developmental Patterns of Two Non-native Contrasts. *Infant Behav Dev. 18*, 1995, 339–350.)

The present study shows clearly that by about a year, when a spurt in language acquisition usually begins in most infants, the effects of speech experience are associated with a loss of discriminability for some consonant pairs.

## Studies of Animal Speech Perception

Is the ability of infants to discriminate speech sounds based on purely auditory ability or on innate mechanisms of phonetic processing? Some light is shed on this question by the finding that nonhumans discriminate acoustic differences in speech-like continua in what may be described as a categorical manner. Morse and Snowdon (1975) monitored heart rate of rhesus monkeys in response to changes in $F_2$ and $F_3$ that mark distinctions in places of articulation for humans. Waters and Wilson (1976) trained rhesus monkeys to avoid shock associated with a particular synthetic speech sound and thus measured the monkeys' perception of VOT changes. Kuhl and Miller (1975) used shock avoidance to study VOT contrast in the chinchilla. Results show that these nonhuman listeners display enhanced discrimination at the phonemic category boundaries of adult humans. The responses of chinchillas resemble those of people more than those of rhesus monkeys, perhaps because the auditory systems of humans and chinchillas are very similar.

It may be that the categorical perception of speech continua for adult speakers, which we know to be highly influenced by linguistic experience, is based on specific sensitivities of the auditory system to acoustic features. These sensitivities are found in the auditory systems of human infants and some other mammals. That is, the location of some phoneme boundaries in a language may be determined, in part, by innate auditory sensitivities that render certain acoustic differences maximally discriminable. Deviations from the category boundaries based on auditory sensitivity could be accounted for by the historical development of the sound systems of particular languages and could require the type of phonetic processing that adults seem to display when they identify speech sounds. We shall consider next some theories about how these auditory and phonetic levels of processing interact in speech perception.

## Auditory and Phonetic Analysis

We know that a specified complex acoustic event can result in a listener reporting that she heard the syllable /bɑ/. Furthermore, the listener can report that the initial consonant was /b/. Because the acoustic cues for /b/ are overlaid on those for /ɑ/, the listener must be analyzing the event on an auditory level to identify the /bɑ/ (the listener has to hear it) and on a phonetic level to extract the /b/ (the listener has to segment it). The question that remains is how the transformation from auditory to phonetic percept is made. How are phonemes individually recovered? Are features detected, and if so, are the features acoustic or phonetic? Is the syllable or some larger unit processed as a whole and then segmented, or is it first segmented and then recombined in a sort of perceptual synthesis?

We have seen that phonetic processing can influence categorical perception in that boundaries between phonemes vary among languages. On the other hand, the results with infants and animals seem more likely to be determined by auditory than by phonetic factors. Another approach to the attempt to separate auditory and phonetic factors in speech perception is to examine acoustic signals that can be perceived as speech or as nonspeech, depending on the "set" of the listener.

Several researchers have experimented with sine-wave analogs of the speech signal. In the stimuli they synthesized, three sine waves replaced the first three formants. This is equivalent to synthesizing formants with bandwidths of 1 Hz. The acoustic signal generated in this way contains almost none of the usual acoustic cues for speech. One aspect of the sine-wave stimuli that especially interested the researchers was that some listeners recognized them immediately as speech, whereas other listeners did not, hearing them as nonspeech electronic beeps, chimes, and tones. The results of experiments indicated that listeners' perception of the acoustic signal depended on whether they heard it as speech or as nonspeech. Evidently, hearing the sine-wave stimuli as speech allowed (or perhaps forced) the listeners to process the signal phonetically; hearing them as nonspeech allowed them to access auditory information that was unavailable to the "phonetic" listeners. For example, the sort of trading relationships between durations of silence and spectral characteristics reported by Raphael, Dorman, and Isenberg (see "Acoustic Cues to Affricates," Chapter 10) were found for listeners hearing the sine-wave stimuli as speech but not for listeners hearing the stimuli as nonspeech. "Auditory" listeners can usually be prompted to hear the sine-wave stimuli as speech. Once they have been converted to "phonetic" listeners, it appears that they can no longer access the auditory information in the sine-wave stimuli. Phonetic listeners, on the other hand, cannot be converted to hearing the sine-wave stimuli in an auditory mode, that is, as nonspeech.

Pisoni (1974) has proposed that the procedures used in testing listeners can themselves favor either phonetic or auditory processing of the stimuli because some methods put a greater load on memory than others. Historically, the most common method used to test discrimination has been the ABX paradigm, which we have already described. Another discrimination paradigm is the "oddity" or "oddball" method, in which subjects hear a triad of stimuli in which one stimulus differs from the other two. The task is to pick out the "different" stimulus. Pisoni and Lazarus (1974) questioned whether these discrimination paradigms placed an undue load on short-term memory for acoustic information. They used a four-interval forced choice (4IAX) paradigm in which listeners hear two pairs of stimuli. The members of one pair are identical (AA); the members of the other pair are different (AB).

The listeners were asked which pair was composed of different stimuli, that is, which was the AB pair. In this paradigm, as each pair was heard, the listener labeled it as "same" or "different." The linguistic label ("same" or "different") was then stored in memory, relieving the listener of the need to store the acoustic information for later comparison. The experimenters found that the 4IAX discrimination format resulted in better discrimination—that is, auditory processing of the speech stimuli.

Another group of experiments that bears on the distinction between auditory and phonetic levels of speech processing is based on *adaptation*.

## Adaptation Studies

If a listener repeatedly hears the stimulus at one end of a synthetic VOT speech continuum, /da/ for example, and is then presented with the usual randomized /da/ to /ta/ continuum for identification, the boundary between phonemes that would normally result is shifted toward the /da/ end of the continuum. That is, after exposure to so many prototypical /da/-like sounds, the listener identifies more of the stimuli as /ta/. Thus, VOT perception is adapted; the listener, having heard many tokens of the "voiced" end of the continuum, will perceive a smaller increase in VOT as a change to the "voiceless" category.

These results were originally explained by a theory positing the existence of phonetic feature detectors. If the nervous system contains neurons especially tuned to detect contrastive linguistic features, then the particular detectors responsive to small VOT values (corresponding to "voiced" stops, for example) might be fatigued by multiple presentations of /da/. With the detector for "voicing" fatigued, subjects would identify more "voiceless" items in the continuum.

Many studies on adaptation followed the original report by Eimas and Corbit in 1973. Darwin has reviewed the studies in detail. As the data accumulate, it is becoming clear that interpretations other than the idea of a feature detector are plausible. Adaptation studies do show, however, that auditory factors can have a measurable effect on categorical perception, just as cross-language studies show the importance of phonetic factors.

## Categorical Perception and Learning

We have described cross-language studies that show the influence of a particular language on perception of phoneme boundaries. We can infer from these studies that learning contributes to categorical perception. In addition, there are several more direct ways in which researchers have studied the effects of learning on categorical perception: by direct training in the laboratory, by studying perception in children receiving speech therapy for an articulation disorder, and by testing second-language learners. The conclusions of the studies are tentative. Strange (1972) succeeded in training English speakers to improve intraphonemic discrimination in a VOT continuum of labial stops but found that the training did not generalize to apical VOT stimuli. Carney and Widin (1976) found that training produced considerable improvement in subjects' discrimination. Several different labial VOT stimuli were used as standards. Subjects were successfully trained to hear differences between each standard and other VOT stimuli presented in AX pairs, with immediate feedback. It appears, then, that listeners can be trained to become more sensitive to differences among stimuli within a phonemic category.

Developmental studies are difficult to compare because few have used synthetic stimuli that could have been precisely described and few have tested intraphonemic discrimination. The research on infants' speech perception shows that they discriminate stimuli in a similar fashion, regardless of the speech or language community into which they have been born. For example, they can discriminate stimuli of +20 ms VOT and +60 ms VOT and stimuli of

−20 ms VOT and −60 ms VOT. They do not, however, discriminate stimuli of −20 ms VOT and +20 ms VOT. The reason may be that ±20 ms VOT sounds like the same event, whereas a longer time gap between a burst and voicing onset sounds like two events. Perception of speech seems to begin with an innate ability to make certain auditory distinctions. As a further indication that some distinctions may be natural to the auditory system, Stevens and Klatt (1974) point to the fact that adults divide a nonspeech continuum that is analogous to the VOT series with a boundary at approximately +20 ms VOT.

By at least 2 years of age, children perceive speech sounds categorically, and their phoneme boundaries are similar to those of adults. Zlatin and Koenigsknecht (1975) used voicing continua varying from "bees" to "peas" and from "dime" to "time" and found that although 2-year-olds perceived the stimuli with the same boundaries between categories as those of 6-year-olds and adults, the younger children's boundary areas were wider, indicating that they needed larger acoustic differences to mark the voiced–voiceless distinction. The longitudinal development of this perceptual ability has not yet been thoroughly studied; the difficulties in testing the abilities of very young children to label and to discriminate stimuli are considerable. There are indications, however, that identification and discrimination abilities may not develop at the same rate.

Although it is easier to study changes in perception in people learning a second language, because they are typically older and easier to test, we are not sure that the processes for learning to recognize the phonemes of a second language are the same as those for a first language. Williams (1974) found a slightly faster shift of phoneme boundaries toward the English voiced–voiceless boundary among younger (8 to 10 years) Spanish-speaking children learning English than among older children (14 to 16 years; Fig. 11.8). Again, longitudinal studies

| Age | Crossover Values by Exposure | | |
|---|---|---|---|
| | One | Two | Three |
| 14–16 | +2.0 | +5.7 | +8.7 |
| 8–10 | +4.7 | +7.5 | +12.0 |
| Difference | +2.7 | +1.8 | +3.3 |

**FIGURE 11.8** Differences (voice onset time [VOT] in milliseconds) in labeling crossover values for native Spanish-speaking children of two age groups. The children were also divided on the basis of exposure to English as measured by time in the United States: exposure one, 0–6 months; exposure two, 1.5–2 years; and exposure three, 3–3.5 years. (From Williams, L., *Speech Perception and Production as a Function of Exposure to a Second Language.* Unpublished doctoral dissertation, Harvard University, 1974.)

are needed to determine the progression. It would be particularly interesting to see more research in which production and perception are analyzed simultaneously.

## Production and Perception

Williams analyzed both production (by measuring spectrograms of the subjects' speech samples) and perception (by identification and discrimination tests) of the phoneme contrasts important in the second language (L2) being learned. Establishing the first language (L1) identification boundaries for /b/ and /p/ and the discrimination peaks for both English and Spanish adult speakers, she found that their production of /b/ and /p/ in word-initial position corresponded to their perception. The /b/–/p/ phoneme boundary for English speakers was located at +25 ms VOT, whereas Spanish speakers' boundary was at -4 ms VOT. Spanish speakers learning English varied more than monolinguals in the crossover points of their identification functions, and the discrimination peaks spanned both the monolingual English and Spanish boundaries. Thus, perception of the /b/–/p/ series for the adult bilingual native Spanish speakers represented a compromise.

For production, spectrograms showed that the L1 Spanish bilinguals produce /b/ with voicing lead in accordance with the Spanish system, even when uttering English words.

In a second study, Williams tracked changes in production and perception in young Puerto Rican Spanish-speaking children who were learning English. She found that the voiced–voiceless phoneme boundary gradually shifted toward the English boundary as exposure to English increased. Analogously, in production, the children's VOT values came closer to English values over time, both in English and Spanish words.

Turning again to adult learners, a study by Goto (1971) indicates that adult bilinguals are often quite insensitive to perceptual distinctions in their nonnative language, even if they can produce them. Japanese speakers judged by Americans to be making the English /r/–/l/ distinction appropriately as they produced words such as "lead," "read," "pray," and "play" nevertheless had difficulty perceiving the distinctions in word-initial position, both in recordings of their own speech or those of other speakers. Mochizuki (1981) obtained similar results. A more detailed analysis of /r/–/l/ perception by Japanese speakers by MacKain, Best, and Strange (1981) showed that a group of Japanese speakers with little experience of spoken English were virtually unable to discriminate stimuli straddling the English /r/–/l/ boundary. In contrast, Japanese speakers with more experience using English performed like American English speakers. Thus, we can be quite sure that experience modifies the perception of speech-like stimuli, but we have little information about what aspects of experience are important. More information is needed, but this brings us to the interesting question of how perception of one's own speech may relate to perception of the speech of others.

The anecdotal observation that some children may perceive distinctions in their own speech that adults fail to distinguish rests on experiences such as the following:

A child protests when others imitate a misarticulation: "I didn't say 'wabbit,' I said 'wabbit.'" This phenomenon can be interpreted as evidence that perception is ahead of production. Investigators have offered three possible explanations: When the child hears the adult say "wabbit," he perceives the mistake but is unable to produce an /r/ and fails to detect the mistake in his own speech. An alternative explanation is that the child perceives distinctions in his own speech in a different way than do adults. The child may make a perceptual distinction between his two /w/ sounds that the adult cannot make; that is, the phoneme category for the child's /r/ is wide enough to include some sounds that the adult would classify as /w/. A third explanation is that the child's perception is confused because he does not yet make the distinction productively. Thus, perception not only aids production, but the mastery of the production of speech sounds may aid the child in his efforts to discriminate and identify the sounds in the speech of others.

Aungst and Frick (1964) found that there was a low correlation between children's self-judgments of the correctness of /r/ production and their ability to identify errors in the speech of others: children with /r/ misarticulations had no problem perceiving the misarticulations of others but failed to detect their own errors. Kornfeld (1971) showed that children may produce /w/ sounds, saying [gwæs] for "glass" and for "grass," that seem the same to adult listeners. There are, however, spectrographic differences that may reflect the basis on which the children make distinctions. Goehl and Golden (1972) suggest that the child in this case has a phoneme representation differing from that of the adult /r/. The child's phoneme /r$^w$/ is directly represented phonetically as [r$^w$], whereas the adult phoneme /r/ does not include the [r$^w$] allophone. They found that children tend to recognize their own [r$^w$] as /r/ and are better at detecting it than other people are.

This phenomenon of children perceiving a difference between their misarticulation and the substitution as perceived by an adult

may not be as common as is supposed. Locke and Kutz (1975) found that of 75 children who said /wɪŋ/ in response to a picture of a ring, only about 20% of them pointed to the picture of a ring when they later heard their own misarticulation, whereas 80% pointed to a picture of a wing on hearing their misarticulation. McReynolds, Kohn, and Williams (1975) found that children with misarticulations are worse at recognizing the sounds they misarticulate than the sounds they produce correctly.

It may be that in learning phonemic contrasts, identification of phonemes in the speech of others develops before the ability to perceive one's own errors, with production and self-perception developing in parallel as motor maturity permits. The time course of perception–production interaction remains unclear, and children learning a first language or correcting misarticulations may evidence a quite different time course of perceptual and production interaction than do second-language learners.

## NEUROPHYSIOLOGY OF SPEECH PERCEPTION

Both sides of the brain are important for hearing. The auditory nerve reports to the temporal lobes of both cerebral hemispheres. However, further analysis of the sound patterns, such as those involved in the perception of speech, are to some extent lateralized to one cerebral hemisphere.

### Cerebral Lateralization

Evidence that one cerebral hemisphere, usually the left, is dominant during perception of speech comes from anatomic analyses, split-brain experiments, dichotic listening studies, and electroencephalographic (EEG) recordings. Wernicke (1874; see Chapter 3) was the first to implicate the left temporoparietal area surrounding the posterior portion of the Rolandic fissure in speech recognition and in linguistic expression. Not only did Wernicke find damage to the temporal portion of that area when he autopsied aphasic individuals, but Penfield and Roberts (1959) found that stimulation of the area interfered most severely with speech output in their patients.

Wernicke's area, as this part of the left cerebral cortex is called, is important for decoding the speech of others and for eliciting the acoustic model of what one intends to say. People who suffer a cerebral vascular accident (CVA) to the left temporoparietal area articulate distinctly despite some substitution of phonemes, and they speak fluently. Their conversation, however, often makes little sense. Goodglass and Geschwind (1976) describe the tendency of such patients to substitute a general pronoun, such as "it," for elusive nouns, or a general verb, such as "do," for missing verbs. These sorts of substitutions result in the following kind of response to a request to name something: "I know what it is, I use it to do my....I have one right here...." Here is another paragrammatical, fluent, but meaningless example from Goodglass and Geschwind: "The things I want to say...ah...the way I say things, but I understand mostly things, most of them and what the things are."

Along with the inability to recall the words necessary to convey an idea, there is often a decreased ability to recognize the meaning of something said aloud. A person with Wernicke's aphasia may recognize the class of a word but not its specific meaning. Thus, for the word "lamp," the person with such a comprehension disorder might point to a piece of furniture, but the wrong one.

If Wernicke's area itself is intact but the connections between the auditory centers of the temporal lobes and Wernicke's area are damaged or poorly functioning, a form of auditory agnosia results. The person may hear a word repeatedly with no comprehension at all and then suddenly understand it completely. This link between the centers for audition and the centers for comprehension may be what is manipulated and fatigued in people with normal perception who experience *verbal transformation* or *semantic sati-*

*ation.* When an utterance is repeated over and over, people report several changes in perception as they listen to the repetitions. For example, the nonword "flime" might be heard as "flying" for a while, then "climb," then "flank." Although we know nothing of the neural underpinnings of this phenomenon, it simulates a dysfunction in the link between hearing and perception.

Dramatic evidence of the role of the left hemisphere in language production and perception is found in the test responses of patients who have undergone surgical separation of the cerebral hemispheres to control severe epilepsy. This is done by severing the interhemispheric neural tissue of the corpus callosum. The patients do not seem impaired unless certain tests are conducted to present information to the hemispheres independently. Because the main connecting body between hemispheres is severed, the patient has functionally separated hemicerebrums. Sperry and Gazzaniga (1967), by testing one cerebrum at a time, have demonstrated that in split-brain patients, the left side does not know what the right side is doing and vice versa (Fig. 11.9). With a curtain in front of such a patient, visually masking objects such as a key, a fork, a letter, and a number, the patient can name an object touched with his right hand (the image being referred to the left hemisphere) or exposed to his left visual field, but cannot name it if the name of the object is relayed to his right visual hemisphere (via the right eye), although he can point to its picture or select it with his left hand. Research by Sperry and others has shown that the left hemisphere is dominant in most people for both spoken and written language expression. Despite the dominance of the left hemisphere, however, the right hemisphere displays some perceptual abilities relating to speech and language.

Zaidel (1973) designed special contact lenses used with prisms and mirrors to separate the left and right visual fields in one eye. Visual images were thus directed to only one cerebral hemisphere in people who had their corpus callosum severed and were

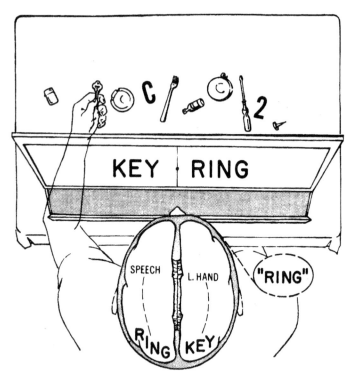

**FIGURE 11.9** A Sperry experiment with a split-brain patient. A subject reports on a visual stimulus (ring, in this case) presented to the left hemisphere. At the same time, the left hand correctly retrieves objects presented to the right hemisphere, although the subject denies knowledge of it. Asked to name an object the left hand selected, the subject names the stimulus presented to the left hemisphere. (Reprinted with permission from Sperry, R. W., *Hemispheric Specialization and Interaction.* B. Milner (Ed.). Cambridge, MA: MIT Press, 1975, 108–121.)

wearing a patch over one eye. Written sentences and phrases of various complexity were presented to each side of the brain independently. The results indicated that the left hemisphere is clearly more linguistically sophisticated than the right. Whole sentences could be processed by the left hemisphere, whereas only single words could be processed by the right hemisphere.

Lateralization of speech perception has been studied in normal subjects as well. A classic study in the neurophysiology of speech perception was Kimura's study of cerebral dominance by use of dichotic stimuli. You recall that in dichotic listening, one sound goes to one ear and another sound

to the opposite ear, both delivered simultaneously through earphones. Kimura (1961) used spoken digits as stimuli. When subjects were asked to report what they heard, they made mistakes because of the conflicting stimuli. Subjects made fewer mistakes in reporting stimuli delivered to the right ear than to the left ear. This effect is known as the *right ear advantage* (REA). Kimura's explanation of the REA was based on anatomic evidence that more neurons of the auditory nerve cross to the contralateral temporal lobe than course directly to the ipsilateral lobe. Thus, information sent along eighth cranial nerve fibers from the right cochlea would be strongly represented in the left cerebral hemisphere. Because the right ear demonstrates an advantage over the left in speech perception, she concluded that the left hemisphere is specialized for speech perception.

Shankweiler and Studdert-Kennedy (1967), in a series of studies, found a small but consistent REA for CV nonsense syllables, such as /ba/, /ta/, or /ga/, presented dichotically to right-handed listeners. The REA was obtained for stop–vowel syllables in both synthetic and natural speech. Steady-state vowels showed no consistent ear advantage.

Listeners appear to make fewer errors in identification when competing dichotic syllables share a phonemic feature. For example, presenting /da/ to one ear and /ta/ to the other is likely to result in correct identification of both consonants because they share the same place of articulation. A similar presentation of the syllables /da/ and /ka/ might result in more identification errors. When the competing syllables share the same voicing classification, /da/ and /ba/ for example, accuracy of identification is better than when the syllables /da/ and /pa/ are competing. Shared place of articulation yields greater accuracy than shared voicing class. There is no difference in ear advantage, however. Both ears are better when the dichotic pairs share features. Cutting (1973), and Day and Vigorito (1973) have shown the REA to be greatest for contrastive stops, less extreme for liquids, and smallest, if found at all, for vowels.

If, however, a dichotic test of vowel contrasts is made more difficult by shortening the vowels or placing them in CVC context, the REA is enhanced. The CV differences and similarities found in categorical perception studies are thus mirrored in dichotic studies. Isolated vowels of relatively long duration and high intensity are more accessible to auditory analysis and so can be held longer in auditory memory, are less categorically perceived, and yield a weak (or no) REA. Stop consonants and brief low-intensity vowels in CVC syllables that are less accessible to auditory analysis and so can be held only briefly in auditory memory, are categorized immediately, and yield a stronger REA. These results have been explained by positing a special speech processor in the left hemisphere or, alternatively, by suggestions that the left hemisphere is especially equipped to analyze stimuli that are brief, of low intensity, or marked by rapid spectral changes.

Experimenters have presented dichotic stimuli asynchronously. They found that listeners presented with a pair of dichotic stimuli having a *stimulus onset asynchrony* (SOA) estimated to be about 100 ms can identify the second stimulus with more accuracy than the first. This is called the *lag effect* because subjects are better at reporting the lagging syllable. The lag effect is an example of backward masking: the second syllable masks the first. If the syllables share voicing or other features, there is little backward masking or lag effect. Yet, as one might expect, the more acoustically similar the vowels of the syllables are to one another, the more pronounced is the backward masking, as Pisoni and McNabb (1974) have demonstrated. Thus, vowel similarity seems to produce a backward masking effect that can be explained on an auditory level, whereas consonant feature sharing seems to facilitate perception and might be explained on either a phonetic or an auditory level.

The final bit of evidence for cerebral lateralization of speech perception comes from a study of EEG recordings made from the surface of the heads of subjects who are listening to speech. Wood, Goff, and Day (1971) recorded evoked auditory responses from 10 right-handed subjects as they performed two identification tasks on a series of synthesized speech stimuli differing in $F_2$ transition and in fundamental frequency ($f_0$). Task 1 was considered to be linguistic, as subjects identified syllables as either /ba/ or /da/ by pressing an appropriate response key. Task 2 was considered to be nonlinguistic, as subjects identified /ba/ syllables to be either high or low in pitch. Recordings were made from both hemispheres at central locations and over the temporal areas during each task. Evoked potentials from the right hemisphere were identical for the linguistic and nonlinguistic tasks. The patterns from the left hemisphere for task 1, however, were significantly different from those for task 2. This result has been interpreted to mean that auditory processing occurs in both hemispheres but that phoneme identification is lateralized to the left hemisphere.

Something special is happening in the left hemisphere when we listen to speech, whether it is auditory analysis of transient, difficult stimuli or whether it is some form of linguistic analysis, such as the extraction of features or phoneme categorization. Because any analysis must involve short-term memory, let us consider the role of memory in speech perception.

## Memory and Speech Perception

When one knows a particular language, it must mean that one has stored the rules and the lexicon of the language in long-term memory. The rules include the phonological and articulatory rules for producing speech as well as the syntactic and semantic rules of the language. These rules are used as a reference not only for speech production but also for speech perception. We hear speech patterns, analyze them, and refer to our stored knowledge of the speech patterns in that particular language for recognition of what was said.

In addition to the long-term memory storage that plays a role in speech perception, it is assumed that there is also a short-term memory for auditory events, including speech sounds. Some research has presented the possibility of two forms of short-term auditory memory. The first is a brief echo of an auditory event lasting only a few milliseconds. This auditory image, which may present itself in the form of a neural spectrogram, is continuously being replaced by new information.

The second, a longer lasting auditory memory called *precategorical acoustic storage* (PAS) by Crowder and Morton (1969), is evidenced by the *recency effect*. When a list of

items (syllables, digits) is presented to subjects for recall, performance declines from the first item to the next to last item progressively, but the decline is reversed for the last item. Subjects tend to recall the most recent item in the list most accurately. The recency effect is stronger for lists of syllables in which the vowel changes than for lists in which the consonant changes. Lists made up of words that differ only in voiced consonants produce little or no recency effect. One interpretation of the effect is that the last item suffers no interference from a following item, so phonetic analysis can take place uninterrupted. Darwin and Baddeley (1974) suggest that because acoustically similar items like consonants are auditorily confusable, they show little recency effect, fading quickly in PAS. Items that are acoustically distinct, however, such as vowels, may remain longer in PAS and are available for finer auditory analysis, resulting in a recency effect.

When hearing natural speech, a listener is likely to be perceiving a stream of sounds that are acoustically more dissimilar than the /ba/, /da/, /ga/, or /ba/–/pa/ continua often synthesized in the laboratory. If this is true, PAS of speech material might operate on virtually all of the speech streams, allowing time for syllable and cross-syllable analysis. Studdert-Kennedy (1976) points out that another, longer term memory store of several seconds of auditory information is required for the recognition of relatively long prosodic patterns, intonation contours, and patterns of relative stress.

## Neurophysiologic Development and Perception

The auditory system of the human infant performs amazingly well, as we have discovered from studies of infants' sound discrimination that were described earlier. Infant auditory sensitivity seems to be especially tuned to the sounds distinctive in human speech.

The occurrence of babbling, although considered to be nonlinguistic, does signify that sensory–motor neural associations are being formed. The infant, who has already demonstrated auditory prowess, is slowly developing sound production abilities and so can make correlations between articulatory events and auditory results. During the babbling period, before speech has developed, the infant reveals sensitivity to intonation patterns of other speakers by mimicking them.

Whitaker (1976) theorizes that the connections between Wernicke's area and Broca's area are activated when babbling temporarily ceases. An auditory template of the language spoken in the infant's community may be registered at this stage. Thus, as the child starts to speak at approximately 1 year, he or she has been sensitized to the particular language and dialect of the community. If the connections between the child's perceptual and production centers for speech are not properly activated, language acquisition will be delayed. The child hears sound but fails to associate sound with speech and therefore has difficulty in learning to speak.

An important concept in the neurophysiology of speech perception is the *critical period* for learning speech. The critical period applies to both perception and production and especially to the ability to relate perception to production. Lenneberg (1967), and Penfield and Roberts have independently claimed that the critical period extends to puberty. It is easier to learn a language, especially the sounds of a language, before puberty than after. Cerebral lateralization, too, is generally thought to be complete by puberty, but there are some indications that the left hemisphere may be dominant for speech at an early age, perhaps at birth. Kimura found the REA for dichotically presented speech to be established in 4-year-olds. The critical period for language learning relates to a flexibility and plasticity of brain function that diminishes in adulthood. The younger the child, the more malleable the neural correlates of language learning. Thus, an acquired aphasia in a child is soon remedied by the other side of the brain assuming the functions of the damaged hemisphere. The neural flexibility during the youthful critical period allows children to compensate by establishing a linguistic center in an undamaged area of the brain, whereas the adult loses access to an already established linguistic store and has little neural flexibility left to establish a new one.

## THEORIES OF SPEECH PERCEPTION

Someone says "We beat you in soccer." How does a listener begin to extract the information necessary to understand that message? Disregarding the semantic and syntactic operations that must occur, how do listeners identify individual speech sounds from the continuous stream of sound at rates of transmission that normally exceed the powers of resolution of the hearing mechanism? Do they process the speech signal on a purely auditory basis, or do they extract phonetic information from it that informs them about the way the sounds were produced? Or do they do both? These are perhaps the most important questions that a theory of speech perception must answer, and, as yet, no theory has provided a completely satisfying answer to any of them.

Any theory of speech perception must account for certain generally accepted facts about the acoustic speech signal. Among them is the high degree of intraspeaker and interspeaker variability among signals that convey information about equivalent phonetic events. This variability, as we have seen, is caused by differences between the sizes of speakers' vocal tracts and the different phonetic contexts in which speech occurs. Theories must also account for the ability of speakers to resolve the stream of speech into linguistic units (phonemes), even when they are provided with an acoustic signal that contains no obvious discontinuities and that is delivered to them at rates as high as 20 to 25 sounds per second. The continuous nature of much of the acoustic signal for speech, as well as the high transmission rate of phonemes, derives from the ability of speakers to coarticulate sounds.

Because of coarticulation, any given portion of the acoustic signal can contain information about two or more phonemes.

The theories that seek to explain these facts may be divided into two general groups. One group views the process of speech perception as primarily auditory. Using the same hearing mechanism and perceptual processing used for any other types of sound, the listener simply identifies acoustic patterns or features and matches them directly to the learned and stored acoustic–phonetic features of the language. The other group of theories posits a link between speech perception and speech production. The listener must, according to such theories, extract information about articulation from the acoustic signal to cope adequately with the problems posed by variability, segmentation, and transmission rate. Because of the reference to articulation in the perception process, this type of theory is often called a *motor theory*. We shall discuss some motor theories first and then conclude with a discussion of auditory theories.

## Motor Theories

The first of the important motor theories that we shall consider is the *analysis-by-synthesis theory,* which Stevens and Halle developed at the Massachusetts Institute of Technology in the 1960s. According to this theory, the listener receives an auditory pattern and analyzes it by eliciting an auditory model of his own production of it. Assume, for example, that the listener hears [bitʃə] and hypothesizes that this represents "beat you." He rapidly generates a neural synthesis of the commands he would use to produce the utterance himself, and, if the patterns of projected output match those of the signal that was input, he accepts his perception as correct. An advantage of a theory such as this is that the listener can apply his knowledge of phonological rules when performing the rudimentary synthesis and thereby can normalize variations caused by the fast speaking rate and the context. In this way, the speaker is able to control for

the variability of phoneme representation in the acoustic signal.

As the authors of analysis-by-synthesis theory, especially Stevens, came to support auditory theories of speech perception, they ceased to develop it. By some time in the 1970s, it was more or less abandoned. Such was not the case for the motor theory of speech perception, proposed by Liberman and other researchers at Haskins Laboratories. Developed at about the same time as the Stevens and Halle theory, the motor theory of speech perception has been supported by ongoing research ever since and has been revised, both implicitly and explicitly, many times.

Motor theory starts with the premise that the sounds of speech are *encoded* in the acoustic signal rather than *enciphered* in it. Codes and ciphers differ in a number of ways. In the simpler forms of a cipher, the units to be enciphered, the *plaintext* units, are represented in an invariant one-to-one relation by units of the *ciphertext*. For example, suppose we encipher the letters of the alphabet by giving each a number:

| Plaintext Units | A | B | C | D | E | F | G... |
|---|---|---|---|---|---|---|---|
| Ciphertext Units | 1 | 2 | 3 | 4 | 5 | 6 | 7... |

Using such a cipher, we could represent the word "BAD" as "214," the word "DAB" as "412," "DEAD" as "4514," "FADED" as "61454," and so on. The critical point about this type of representation is that it is invariant. The number 4 always stands for the letter D, which must always be represented in the enciphered message by 4. We do not need to use another number or a different form of the number 4 depending on the context of the letter D in the plaintext; 4 will always do the job of representing D, no matter what its position in a word and no matter which letters precede or follow it. As we have seen, the representation of speech sounds in

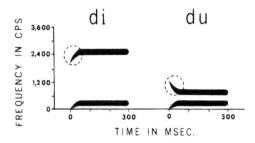

FIGURE 11.10 Synthetic patterns showing the syllables /di/ and /du/. Notice the difference in the direction of the $F_2$ transition. (Reprinted with permission from Liberman, A. M., The Grammars of Speech and Language. *Cogn. Psychol. 1*, 1970, 301–323.)

the acoustic signal is not of this nature. There is a *lack of invariance* in the way a particular phoneme is signaled acoustically. *Lack of invariance* is a characteristic of a code.

One often-cited example of the lack of invariance in the acoustic signal is the representation of /d/ in the syllables /di/ and /du/ (Fig. 11.10): A rising second formant transition in /di/ and a falling one in /du/ both serve as acoustic cues for /d/. This is analogous to representing the letter D with one number when it occurs before the letter A and with another number before the letter E. The acoustic signal for speech also contains examples of the sort of thing that would happen if it were possible to represent both B and D with the same number. In the study on the frequency of stop bursts as cues to the place of articulation, the experimenters found that the same burst, centered at 1,440 Hz, was heard as /p/ before /i/ and /u/, but as /k/ before /ɑ/. Schatz (1954), cross-splicing stop bursts with vowels, obtained similar results. The lack of correspondence between discrete acoustic events and separate phonemes, then, works both ways: different acoustic events can be perceived as the same phoneme, whereas the same acoustic event can be perceived as different phonemes in different contexts.

A second difference between codes and ciphers is implicit in the examples of the enciphered words above: A cipher text is seg-

mentable into units that correspond to units of the plaintext. If we see the ciphertext 214, even if we don't have the key, we will know that the plaintext is a word of three letters and that each number represents one of those letters. Moreover, the number 1 conveys no information about the letters that precede or follow A that it represents. This, as we have seen, is in direct contrast with the *non-segmentability* of the acoustic signal for speech. Nonsegmentability, another characteristic of a code, is accounted for in the speech signal by coarticulation, which distributes the acoustic features representing speech sounds to more than one place in the acoustic signal.

Liberman has used the word "bag" to exemplify the overlapping of acoustic features that is caused by coarticulation. In Figure 11.11, the acoustic cues for the /b/ overlap those for the /æ/, which, in turn, overlap those for the /g/. This "shingling" of the acoustic features that the listener receives results in a great deal of redundancy of cues to

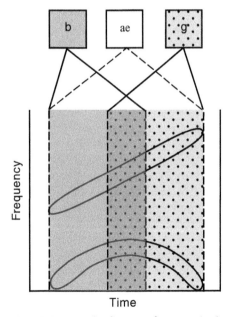

FIGURE 11.11 The first two formants in the word "bag," showing the overlap of acoustic cues to the speech sounds caused by coarticulation.

the phonemes encoded in the signal. It is this redundancy of cues that makes the speech signal extremely robust. On the phonemic level, perceptual cues to the manner of articulation of the phoneme /b/ in the word "bag" can be found in the silence before the release burst, in the presence of the release burst itself, in the rising $F_1$ transition to the following vowel, and in the rapid rise time after the release burst. Such multiple cues, frequently overlapping those to neighboring speech sounds, often make it impossible to segment the acoustic signal into phoneme-sized units.

A final difference between codes and ciphers relates to the relative efficiency with which they are capable of conveying information. In the simple cipher we have been using as an example, a separate lookup operation is required to recover each unit of the plaintext: four operations, one for each number-letter correspondence, are necessary to decipher 6135 as "face." A code might convey the same information by representing the entire word with a single symbol. One lookup operation for a code therefore yields more information faster. Listeners hearing a synthesized sentence such as "A bird in the hand is worth two in the bush" can accurately perceive more than 20 phonemes per second when pushed to the limits of their ability. This means that when they hear such an utterance and repeat it accurately or transcribe it in some fashion, they can correctly identify and order the 26 phonemes they have heard. But how well can they perform this task with enciphered nonspeech stimuli? Listeners hearing a sequence of 26 tones containing only three different tones (far fewer than the number of phonemes in a language) can identify and order them accurately only when they are presented at about the rate of one per second. When the tones are presented at the rate of 20 per second, all listeners report hearing is a blur of sound in which the individual tones are not even recognized as separate events.

A strong case, then, can be made that speech is encoded in the acoustic signal on the grounds of (1) lack of invariance between the acoustic signal and the speech sounds represented in it, (2) nonsegmentability of the acoustic signal, and (3) the relatively high efficiency of transmission of information by the acoustic signal. It then remains for motor theory to explain how the listener extracts speech sounds from the signal—that is, how decoding is accomplished.

It is, perhaps, a short step from acceptance of the fact that speech is an acoustic code generated by articulation to the incorporation of articulation into the process of perception. Early on, researchers noted that the discontinuities in labeling and discriminating speech sounds, revealed by studies of categorical perception, were coincidental with discontinuities in articulation. They argued, for instance, that just as there are no articulations intermediate to the labial and alveolar occlusions for stops, there are no percepts intermediate to, for example, /b/ and /d/; a listener will assign each stimulus of a smoothly varying acoustic continuum to one or the other category of stop sounds. Given the immense variability in absolute values of the acoustic cues that signal place of articulation, the listener must be able to relate those cues to the more or less invariant articulation that generated them. Further research, however, indicated that the articulations were, in fact, less, rather than more, invariant. Neither studies of muscle activity nor of articulator movement have revealed invariant gestures for particular speech sounds.

Motor theorists responded to this finding by positing more abstract representations of speech gestures, which they maintain are the actual objects of perception. The intended gesture for a particular sound is presumed to comprise many movements that do not occur simultaneously because of the effects of context. Coarticulation, then, is responsible for the temporal distribution of the component movements and of the resulting acoustic cues. Because the production and perception processes are linked together, biologically, listeners are able to perceive the intended gestures and recover the encoded phonemes they represent from the acoustic signal.

What is the nature of the biological link between speech production and speech perception? According to some motor theorists, humans possess a specialized perceptual *module* for the processing of speech. This module is one of several, such as those for sound localization and visual depth perception, which exist in humans and other animals. It consists of specialized neural structures that respond specifically to the acoustic signal for speech and relate the features of that signal to the intended gestures that produced it. In this view, listeners, because they understand the dynamics of vocal tract behavior, perceive the gestures directly and immediately.

Motor theorists point to a substantial body of experimental work that supports their point of view. Among the experiments purporting to demonstrate that listeners rely on their knowledge of vocal tract behavior to decode the acoustic speech signal are several that explore the effect of silence on speech perception. If an appropriate duration of silence is inserted between the /s/ and the /ɑ/ of the utterance /sɑ/, listeners report hearing /stɑ/. Moreover, the duration of silence must at least approximate the minimum needed for a speaker to articulate a stop consonant (about 50 ms). Listeners perceive stimuli containing between 10 and 50 ms of silence as /sɑ/ and cannot discriminate them from a /sɑ/ stimulus containing no silence. Motor theory argues that the speech module enables the listener to identify the silence as the stop gesture when its duration is appropriate to that gesture. Silent periods of lesser durations are not processed by the module because a vocal tract could not have produced them in the process of articulating speech. Motor theorists also point out that durations of silence well below 5 ms can be perceived when they occur in noise or in portions of the speech signal where they could not be articulated by a speaker (e.g., in the middle of a relatively steady-state vowel). The assumption might be that an auditory processor or mod-

ule, rather than a phonetic one, is responsible for perceiving such silences.

In related experiments, Dorman, Raphael, and Liberman (1979) found that when listeners perceive a sequence of stops in a disyllable such as /ɛbdɛ/, they process the cues for the /b–d/ closure and the /d/ release in a normal fashion. If, however, the duration of the closure period for the two stops is reduced to 0 ms, producing a stimulus that no single speaker could articulate, listeners do not perceive the first stop in the sequence. That is, they report hearing /ɛdɛ/. As the duration of closure lengthens, again to about the minimum time required for a speaker to articulate two stops, the /b/ is again heard, much as is the /t/ in the /sɑ–stɑ/ experiment. But there are two conditions in which both stops can be perceived in stimuli with no closure interval: Listeners report hearing /ɛbdɛ/ if each syllable is spoken by a different speaker or if each syllable, spoken by the same speaker, is delivered to a different ear via a headset. A motor theory interpretation of these results is that the speech module recognizes that two vocal tracts could produce the sequence of stops without an audible silent closure. Thus, both stops are perceived when the syllables are recognized as the outputs of two different vocal tracts, either because the voices sound different or because the 180° separation of the voices in the headset causes the listener to believe that they could not have been produced by the same speaker. In all cases, the listener's knowledge of what vocal tracts can and cannot do conditions perception.

Experimental support for the concept of modularity in general, and for existence of a speech module in particular, is found in the work of Liberman and others on *duplex* perception. In duplex perception a two- or three-formant stop + vowel synthetic syllable is split into two portions. One portion, containing only the transition of the second formant, is presented to one ear, and the rest of the stimulus, called the base, is presented to the other ear. Listeners report hearing both a complete stop + vowel syllable (in the ear to which the base is presented) and an isolated "chirp," a response to the $F_2$ transition, in the other ear. Evidently, the two parts of the stimuli fuse at some level, and the phonetic module then evokes the perception of the CV syllable. At about the same time, an auditory module processes the "chirp," accounting for the other part of the duplex percept. Moreover, changes in the frequency of the $F_2$ transition (the "chirp") that are detected by the auditory module are not detected by the phonetic module unless they cue a difference in the place of articulation of the stop. The relative independence of the parts of the duplex percept suggests, then, that separate processors are at work and that one of them is phonetic.

Motor theorists also point to the McGurk effect as evidence that speech production and perception are intimately related. In the McGurk effect experiments, subjects both hear and see a speaker repeating syllables such as /bɑ/, /vɑ/, /dɑ/, or /gɑ/. When the acoustic signal is mismatched with the visual signal, as for example when a speaker is shown producing a labiodental sound such as /vɑ/ while the acoustic signal carries the information that a bilabial /bɑ/ has been articulated, observers report perceiving /vɑ/. That is, their percept is derived from what they have seen, not from what they have heard. The effect can also produce a compromise percept, as when observers see a speaker articulate /gɑ/, hear the acoustic signal for /bɑ/, and report perceiving /dɑ/.

Evidence of a different sort pertaining to a link between speech perception and production was provided in an experiment performed by Bell-Berti et al. (1979). Using electromyography (EMG), they found that each of their 10 subjects used one of two discrete patterns of genioglossus activity to distinguish front tense vowels from front lax vowels. The subjects were then presented with two identification tests of a seven-stimulus five-formant synthetic vowel continuum, ranging from the tense vowel /i/ to the lax vowel /I/. In the first randomized test, each stimulus was presented 10 times.

A labeling function was plotted, and the phoneme boundary between /i/ and /I/ was determined. In the second randomized test, the first stimulus in the continuum, /i/, was heard 40 times, whereas each of the other six stimuli was again heard 10 times. The result of this type of test is much like that found in the selective adaptation experiments described earlier in this chapter: There is a shift in the phoneme boundary toward the stimulus that is heard more frequently than the others. Indeed, all of the subjects in the EMG experiment showed such a shift in their perceptual data, but again, they fell into two discrete groups based on the size of the boundary shift. The members of each group were the same as the members of the groups using the different production strategies to differentiate tense from lax vowels. The experimenters concluded that the differences in the perception data reflected the differences in production strategies, establishing a production–perception link, at least for the vowels and the muscle they investigated.

Finally, work by Chistovich, Klass, and Kuzmin (1962) in Russia points to the importance of the knowledge of speech production for the perception of speech. They conducted "shadowing" experiments, in which subjects repeated messages they had never heard before as quickly as possible. The shadowers started to produce consonants *before* hearing all of the relevant acoustic cues. This finding indicates that cues at the beginning of the syllable signal what is to come, and that listeners refer the incoming patterns immediately to monitor articulatory patterns, before they understand the message.

The general class of perceptual motor theory that we have been discussing has recently been extended to account for both production and perception. In Chapter 8, we mentioned *action theory* by referring to the work of Fowler, Turvey, and Kelso. This explicitly ecologic view of speech perception and production posits a direct connection between the coordinated actions of the speaker and the environment and a direct relationship between speech perception and the act of speaking. Although the similarity of action theory to the motor theory of Liberman and his colleagues is obvious, the two theories differ in several ways. Action theory is as much a theory of speech production as of speech perception. It suggests that both processes are relatively simple and straightforward. The complex interactions, coarticulations, and acoustic signals that we study result from the natural properties of the production mechanism. Action theory does not require that phonemes be extracted from the acoustic signal. The difficulties of segmentation are thus neutralized on the grounds that the listener perceives a larger, more abstract, more dynamic chunk of speech that is understood because of its direct relationship to the dynamic act of speaking. Because a person is both a producer and a perceiver of speech, no translation is necessary; according to this theory, the listener is not extracting phonetic features or phonemes but rather information on how to produce the speech. For example, if you heard someone say [lɪdlæmzidaɪvi], you could repeat it exactly even if you failed to grasp the message "little lambs eat ivy."

Michael Studdert-Kennedy points out that aspects of such an action theory are supported by research in speech perception and are in basic agreement with recent studies of speech and language acquisition: children can understand utterances such as /pinʌtbʌtɚndʒeli/, long before they know "peanut" and "jelly" as separate words or that /dʒ/ is distinctive in the language. The biological foundation of such a theory of action has not been specified, but many researchers believe that we are getting closer to a biology of language.

We could cite other theoretical variants and many more experiments that support the several aspects of a motor theory. As is often the case, however, the interpretations of experimental results often differ depending on the theoretical orientation of the interpreters. Those who favor auditory theories of speech perception interpret results differently from those who support a motor theory, and, of course, they offer contrary evidence of their own. We now turn to some of these alternative explanations and the data that support them.

## Auditory Theories

Auditory theories of speech perception emphasize the sensory, filtering mechanisms of the listener and relegate speech production knowledge to a minor, secondary role in which it is used only in difficult perceptual conditions.

Fant (1962) has modeled speech perception as primarily sensory. He maintains that the perceptual and production mechanisms share a pool of distinctive features (Fig. 11.12) but that the listener need not refer to production to perceive speech. Linguistic centers in the brain are common to both incoming and outgoing messages, but the centers responsible for peripheral subphonemic aspects of production and perception are viewed as independent. According to this auditory model (Fig. 11.12), speech perception proceeds along the route ABCDE, whereas for a motor model, the route would be ABCJFE. Fant's view is that listeners, having been exposed to language, are sensitive to the distinctive patterns of the speech wave and only need to refer to their own ability to speak when shadowing or listening under other unusual circumstances. Morton and Broadbent (1967) hold a similar theory. They concur with Fant in the belief that listeners can decode directly, although reference to production may be made when the perceptual task is difficult, as in transcribing speech phonetically.

Inherent in most auditory approaches to speech perception, including Fant's, is the idea of sensitivity to acoustic patterns or to particular acoustic features. Some theorists, those who support the notion that speech perception can be explained by sensitivity to acoustic patterns, have proposed a process of *template matching* as the basis for the recognition of speech sounds. The concept of an

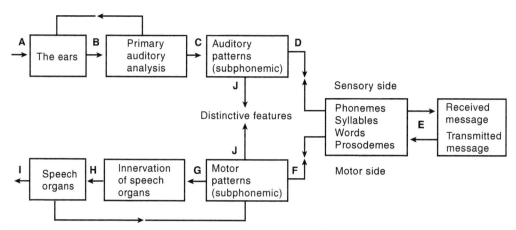

**FIGURE 11.12**  Fant's model of the brain mechanisms in speech perception and production. (Redrawn with permission from Fant, G., *Models for the Perception of Speech and Visual Form.* W. Wathen-Dunn (Ed.). Cambridge, MA: MIT Press, 1967, pp. 111–125.)

auditory template arises from experimental work on birdsong. Some birds are born with a rudimentary version of the song characteristic of their species. This template is further refined as the young birds hear the song of mature birds in the environment. Later, they sing themselves, matching their efforts to their stored templates. Marler (1970) suggests that human infants may proceed somewhat similarly when learning speech. A similar process has been proposed to explain speech perception. Adult speakers are presumed to have stored abstract patterns of speech: templates of phonemes or syllables. When they listen to speech, they match the incoming auditory patterns to the stored templates to identify the sounds.

Theorists who believe that the auditory system is sensitive to particular acoustic features have proposed a process of *feature detection* as the basis for speech perception. The concept of feature detection was borrowed from research on vision demonstrating that specific cortical nerve cells are sensitive to a particular aspect of an image. For example, there are special detectors for horizontal lines. By analogy, a feature detector for speech is thought to be sensitive to specific complex stimuli, such as $F_2$ transitions. Initially, adaptation studies were interpreted in terms of a feature detector theory. If repetition of a particular stimulus resulted in a shift

in phoneme identification, it was theorized that the shift occurred because the detector for that particular feature had been fatigued by overstimulation (the multiple repetitions of a stimulus from one end of a continuum). Studies of infants' speech perception were also interpreted in terms of feature detection: The ability of the infants to discriminate stimuli belonging to different linguistic categories was explained by their sensitivity to certain acoustic features. The theory connotes a nativist approach; humans are viewed as possessing an innate linguistic capacity in the form of special neural receptors tuned to universal distinctive features of speech.

In the view of some theorists, the processes of template matching and feature detection are incapable of resolving the problem of variability in the acoustic signal. They point to the multiplicity of acoustic patterns that can represent a particular speech sound and conclude that storage of all the possible patterns would place an unacceptable load on memory. Similarly, the number of feature detectors required to process all of the acoustic features conveying a single phonological feature (e.g., voicing) often appears to be inordinately large. One response to these objections has been to propose patterns or features that are more abstract than those found in the spectrographic representation of the speech signal.

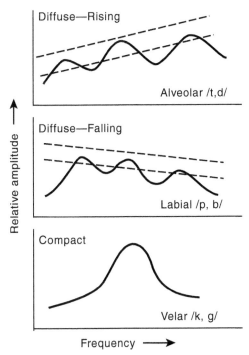

Relative amplitude →

Diffuse—Rising

Alveolar /t, d/

Diffuse—Falling

Labial /p, b/

Compact

Velar /k, g/

Frequency ⟶

**FIGURE 11.13**  Steven's and Blumstein's averaged short-term spectra, displaying distinctive and invariant patterns that distinguish stop place of articulation.

Stevens and Blumstein (1978), for example, have proposed that the place of articulation of stop consonants can be recognized from the shape of the spectrum averaged over the duration of the burst and the first few milliseconds after the burst. They describe what they call distinctive "spectral tilts" that characterize each place of stop articulation in an invariant fashion (Fig. 11.13): Alveolar stops display an average short-term spectrum that is called "diffuse-rising" because there is an increase in the relative amplitude of successive spectral peaks; labial stops display a "diffuse-falling" pattern, as the spectral peaks decrease in amplitude as they increase in frequency; and velar stops display a "compact" pattern, with a single spectral peak at a midrange frequency.

Cole and Scott (1974) have proposed a somewhat different approach to the problem of acoustic variability within the framework of an essentially auditory theory. They posit that perception of the syllable is ac-

complished by reference to both invariant and context-conditioned cues. For example, they would view [s] frication in the first syllable (/sɑ/ of "soccer" as an invariant cue), but would also recognize the existence of context-conditioned cues for both the [s] and the [k] in [sakɚ] inherent in the transitions to and from the relatively steady-state formants of [ɑ]. They agree with Liberman that transitions are important in providing the listener with the perception of the temporal order of sounds in a syllable. Cole and Scott suggest that the invariant and variable cues maintain their independence as cues and that listeners make use of both for syllable recognition. Evidence of their independence is provided by studies of the repeated presentation of a stimulus that gives rise to an effect known as "streaming." If, for example, a listener hears the syllable [sɑ] repeatedly, the percept separates into two discrete streams: a hiss, conditioned by the [s] frication and [dɑ], conditioned by the transition and steady state of the vocalic portion. In addition to invariant and context-conditioned cues, they propose a third cue, the waveform, which is processed over a longer time and gives rise to percepts of relative intensity, duration, and pitch.

Some theorists have attempted to combine the notions of auditory and phonetic feature detectors in a single model of speech perception. Pisoni and Sawusch (1975) have proposed a model that provides for the short-term storage of information elicited from the long-term store during the period of recognition. The recognized speech is then referred simultaneously for phonological, syntactic, and semantic analyses (Fig. 11.14). According to this theory, features detected by auditory property detectors are mapped onto a system of phonetic features as detected within a whole syllable and then combined into a rough feature matrix for further analysis. We should make it clear that although this sort of theory encompasses the detection of both auditory and phonetic features, it does not address the relationship between production and perception. It is, rather, a theory about the sensory stage common to both motor and auditory theories.

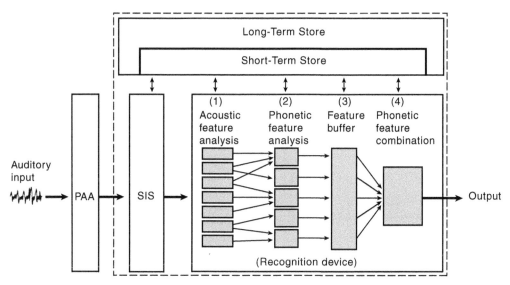

**FIGURE 11.14**  Pisoni and Sawusch's model of speech recognition. Phonetic and acoustic features are analyzed, and short-term memory figures specifically in the model. PAA, preliminary auditory analysis; SIS, sensory information store. (Modified with permission from Pisoni, D. B., and Sawusch, J. R., *Structure and Process in Speech Perception,* A. Cohen and S. G. Nooteboom (Eds.). Berlin, Germany: Springer-Verlag, 1975, pp. 16–34.)

The debate between the schools of thought supporting motor and auditory theories of speech perception will not soon end. A great deal of needed experimentation lies ahead, much of which will have to await the development of new technology. The outcome will reveal a great deal about the human ability to produce and perceive both speech and language: "If language is a window on the mind, speech is the thin end of an experimental wedge that will pry the window open."

# REFERENCES

## General Readings

Bartlett, F. C., *Remembering.* Cambridge, England: University Press, 1932. Reprinted in 1950.

Darwin, C. J., The Perception of Speech. In *Handbook of Perception,* Vol. 7. *Language and Speech.* E. C. Carterette and M. P. Friedman (Eds.). New York: Academic Press, 1976, pp. 175–226.

Denes, P., and Pinson, E. N., *The Speech Chain,* 2nd ed. New York: W. H. Freeman & Co., 1963.

Fant, G., Descriptive Analysis of the Acoustic Aspects of Speech. *Logos 5,* 1962, 3–17.

Kent, R. D., Atal, B. S., and Miller, J. L. (Eds.), *Papers in Speech Communication: Speech Production.* Woodbury, NY: Acoustical Society of America, 1991.

Liberman, A. M., *Speech: A Special Code.* Cambridge, MA: MIT Press, 1996.

Miller, J. L., Kent, R. D., and Atal, B. S. (Eds.), *Papers in Speech Communication: Speech Perception.* Woodbury, NY: Acoustical Society of America, 1991.

Pickett, J. M., *The Sounds of Speech Communication.* Baltimore: University Park Press, 1980.

Studdert-Kennedy, M., Speech Perception. In *Contemporary Issues in Experimental Phonetics.* N. J. Lass (Ed.). New York: Academic Press, 1976, pp. 243–293.

## Categorical Perception

### Adults

Abramson, A. S., and Lisker, L., Discriminability Along the Voicing Continuum: Cross-

Language Tests. In *Proceedings of the Sixth International Congress of Phonetic Sciences*. Prague, Czech Republic: Academia, Czechoslovak Academy of Sciences, 1970, pp. 569–573.

Best, C. T., McRoberts, G. W., and Sithole, N. M., Examination of Perceptual Reorganization for Nonnative Speech Contrasts: Zulu Click Discrimination by English-Speaking Adults and Children. *J. Exp. Psychol. Percept. Perform. 14,* 1988, 345–360.

Elman, L. L., Diehl, R. L. and Buchwald, S. E. Perceptual Switching in Bilinguals. *J. Acoust. Soc. Am., 62,* 1977, 991-994.

Fry, D., Abramson, A., Eimas, P., and Liberman, A. M., The Identification and Discrimination of Synthetic Vowels. *Lang. Speech 5,* 1962, 171–189.

Ladefoged, P., and Traill, A., Linguistic Phonetic Descriptions of Clicks. *Language 60,* 1984, 1–20.

Liberman, A. M., Harris, K. S., Hoffman, H. S., and Griffith, B. C., The Discrimination of Speech Sounds Within and Across Phoneme Boundaries. *J. Exp. Psychol. 54,* 1957, 358–368.

Lisker, L., and Abramson, A. S., A Cross-Language Study of Voicing in Initial Stops: Acoustical Measurements. *Word 20,* 1964, 384–422. Reprinted in Kent et al. 1991, 527–565.

Miyawaki, K., Strange, W., Verbrugge, R. R., Liberman, A. M., Jenkins, J. J., and Fujimura, O., An Effect of Linguistic Experience: The Discrimination of [r] and [l] by Native Speakers of Japanese and English. *Percept. Psychophys. 18,* 1975, 331–340. Reprinted in Miller et al. 1991, 405–414.

Repp, B. H., Categorical Perception: Issues, Methods, Findings. In *Speech and Language: Advances in Basic Research and Practice,* Vol. 10. N. J. Lass (Ed.). New York: Academic Press, 1984, pp. 243–335.

Stevens, K. N., Liberman, A. M., Studdert-Kennedy, M., and Öhman, S., Cross-Language Study of Vowel Perception. *Lang. Speech 12,* 1969, 1–23.

Stevens, K. N., On the Quantal Nature of Speech. *J. Phonet. 17,* 1989, 3–45.

Strange, W., and Jenkins, J. J., The Role of Linguistic Experience in the Perception of Speech. In *Perception and Experience.* R. D. Walk and H. L. Pick (Eds.). New York: Plenum Press, 1978, pp. 125–169.

## Infants and Animals

Best, C. T., Learning to Perceive the Sound Pattern of English. In *Advances in Infancy Research.* C. Rovee-Collier and L. Lipsitt (Eds.). Hillsdale, NJ: Ablex, 1994, pp. 217–304.

Best, C. T., McRoberts, G. W., LaFleur, R. L., and Silver-Isenstadt, J., Divergent Developmental Patterns for Infants' Perception of Two Nonnative Consonant Contrasts. *Infant Behav. Dev. 18,* 1995, 339–350.

Eimas, P. D., Speech Perception in Early Infancy. In *Infant Perception.* L. B. Cohen and P. Salapatek (Eds.). New York: Academic Press, 1975, pp. 193–231.

Eimas, P. D., Siqueland, E. R., Jusczyk, P., and Vigorito, J., Speech Perception in Infants. *Science 171,* 1971, 303–306. Reprinted in Miller et al. 1991, 681–684.

Houston, D. M., Speech Perception in Infants. In *The Handbook of Speech Perception.* D. B. Pisoni and R. E. Remez (Eds.). Malden, MA: Blackwell, 2005, pp. 417–448.

Jusczyk, P. W., *The Discovery of Spoken Language.* Cambridge, MA: MIT Press, 1997.

Jusczyk, P. W., Perception of Syllable-Final Stop Consonants by Two-Month-Old Infants. *Percept. Psychophys. 21,* 1977, 450–454.

Kuhl, P. K., and Miller, J. D., Speech Perception by the Chinchilla: Voiced–Voiceless Distinction in Alveolar Plosive Consonants. *Science 190,* 1975, 69–72.

Kuhl, P. K., Infants' Perception and Representation of Speech: Development of a New Theory. *Proc. 1992 Int. Conf. Spoken Lang. Process. 1,* 1992, pp. 449–456.

Morse, P. A., Speech Perception in the Human Infant and the Rhesus Monkey. Conference on Origins and Evolution of Language and Speech. *Ann. N.Y. Acad. Sci. 280,* 1976, 694–707.

Morse, P. A., and Snowdon, C. T., An Investigation of Categorical Speech Discrimination by Rhesus Monkeys. *Percept. Psychophys. 17,* 1975, 9–16.

Waters, R. S., and Wilson, W. A., Jr., Speech Perception by Rhesus Monkeys: The Voicing Distinction in Synthesized Labial and Velar Stop Consonants. *Percept. Psychophys. 19,* 1976, 285–289.

## Auditory and Phonetic Analysis

Best, C. T., Morrongielllo, B., and Robson, R., Perceptual Equivalence of Acoustic Cues in Speech and Nonspeech Perception. *Percept. Psychophys. 29,* 1981, 191–211.

Carney, A. E., and Widin, G. P., Acoustic Discrimination Within Phonetic Categories. *J. Acoust. Soc. Am. 59,* 1976, S25 (A).

Cutting, J., and Rosner, B. S., Categories and Boundaries in Speech and Music. *Percept. Psychophys. 16,* 1974, 564–570.

Eimas, P. D., and Corbit, J. D., Selective Adaptation of Linguistic Feature Detectors. *Cogn. Psychol. 4,* 1973, 99–109. Reprinted in Miller et al. 1991, 3–13.

Pisoni, D. B., and Lazarus, J. H., Categorical and Noncategorical Modes of Speech Perception Along the Voicing Continuum. *J. Acoust. Soc. Am. 55,* 1974, 328–333.

Remez, R. E., Rubin, P. E., Pisoni, D. B., and Carrell, T. D., Speech Perception Without Traditional Speech Cues. *Science 212,* 1981, 947–950.

Strange, W., *The Effects of Training on the Perception of Synthetic Speech Sounds: Voice Onset Time.* Unpublished doctoral dissertation, University of Minnesota, 1972.

## Perception and Learning

Stevens, K. N., and Klatt, D. H., Role of Formant Transitions in the Voiced–Voiceless Distinction for Stops. *J. Acoust. Soc. Am. 55,* 1974, 653–659.

Williams, L., *Speech Perception and Production as a Function of Exposure to a Second Language.* Unpublished doctoral dissertation, Harvard University, 1974.

Zlatin, M. A., and Koenigsknecht, R. A., Development of the Voicing Contrast: Perception of Stop Consonants. *J. Speech Hear. Res. 18,* 1975, 541–553.

## Production and Perception

Aungst, L. F., and Frick, I. V., Auditory Discriminability and Consistency of Articulation of /r/. *J. Speech Hear. Disord. 29,* 1964, 76–85.

Bell-Berti, F., Raphael, L. J., Pisoni, D. B., and Sawusch, J., Some Relationships Between Speech Production and Perception. *Phonetica 36,* 1979, 373–383.

Borden, G. J., Use of Feedback in Established and Developing Speech. In *Speech and Language: Advances in Basic Research and Practice,* Vol. 3. N. J. Lass (Ed.). New York: Academic Press, 1984, pp. 223–242.

Fowler, C. A., and Galantucci, B., The Relation of Speech Perception and Speech Production. In *The Handbook of Speech Perception.* D. B. Pisoni and R. E. Remez (Eds.). Malden, MA: Blackwell, 2005, pp. 633–652.

Goehl, H., and Golden, S., A Psycholinguistic Account of Why Children Do Not Detect Their Own Errors. Paper presented at ASHA meeting, Detroit, 1972.

Goto, H., Auditory Perception by Normal Japanese Adults of the Sounds "L" and "R." *Neuropsychologia 9,* 1971, 317–323.

Kornfeld, I. R., What Initial Clusters Tell Us About the Child's Speech Code. *Q. Prog. Rep. Res. Lab. Electron. M.I.T. 101,* 1971, 218–221.

Locke, J. L., and Kutz, K. J., Memory for Speech and Speech for Memory. *J. Speech Hear. Res. 18,* 1975, 176–191.

MacKain, K. S., Best, C. T., and Strange, W., Categorical Perception of English /r/ and /l/ by Japanese Bilinguals. *Appl. Psycholinguist. 2,* 1981, 369–390.

McReynolds, L. V., Kohn, J., and Williams, G. C., Articulatory-Defective Children's Discrimination of Their Production Errors. *J. Speech Hear. Disord. 40,* 1975, 327–338.

Menyuk, P., and Anderson, S., Children's Identification and Reproduction of /w/, /r/ and /l/. *J. Speech Hear. Res. 12,* 1969, 39–52.

Mochizuki, M., The Identification of /r/ and /l/ in Natural and Synthesized Speech. *J. Phonet. 9,* 1981, 293–303.

## Neurophysiology of Speech Perception

Berlin, C., Hemispheric Asymmetry in the Location of Auditory Tasks. In *Localization in the Nervous System.* S. Harnad, R. W. Doty, L. Goldstein, J. Jaynes, and G. Krautheimer (Eds.). New York: Academic Press, 1977, pp. 303–324.

Cole, R. A., Different Memory Functions for Consonants and Vowels. *Cogn. Psychol. 4,* 1973, 39–54.

Crowder, R. G., Visual and Auditory Memory. In *Language by Ear and Eye: The Relationships Between*

*Speech and Reading.* J. F. Kavanagh and I. G. Mattingly (Eds.). Cambridge, MA: MIT Press, 1972, pp. 251–275.

Crowder, R. G., and Morton, J., Precategorical Acoustic Storage (PAS). *Percept. Psychophys. 5,* 1969, 365–373.

Cutting, J. E., A Parallel Between Encodedness and the Ear Advantage: Evidence From an Ear-Monitoring Task. *J. Acoust. Soc. Am. 53,* 1973, 358 (A).

Darwin, C. J., Ear Differences in the Recall of Fricatives and Vowels. *Q. J. Exp. Psychol. 23,* 1971, 46–62.

Darwin, C. J., Dichotic Backward Masking of Complex Sounds. *Q. J. Exp. Psychol. 23,* 1971, 386–392.

Darwin, C. J., and Baddeley, A. D., Acoustic Memory and the Perception of Speech. *Cogn. Psychol. 6,* 1974, 41–60.

Day, R. S., and Vigorito, J. M., A Parallel Between Encodedness and the Ear Advantage: Evidence From a Temporal-Order Judgment Task. *J. Acoust. Soc. Am. 53,* 1973, 358 (A).

Gardner, H., *The Shattered Mind.* Westminster, MD: Knopf, 1975.

Gazzaniga, M. S., and Sperry, R. W., Language After Section of the Cerebral Commissures. *Brain 90,* 1967, 131–148.

Godfrey, J. J., Perceptual Difficulty and the Right Ear Advantage for Vowels. *Brain Lang. 4,* 1974, 323–336.

Goodglass, H., and Geschwind, N., Language Disorders (Aphasia). In *Handbook of Perception,* Vol. 7. *Language and Speech.* E. C. Carterette and M. P. Friedman (Eds.). New York: Academic Press, 1976, pp. 389–428.

Kimura, D., Cerebral Dominance and the Perception of Verbal Stimuli. *Can. J. Psychol. 15,* 1961, 166–171.

Kimura, D., Functional Asymmetry of the Brain in Dichotic Listening. *Cortex 3,* 1967, 163–178.

Lenneberg, E. H., *Biological Foundations of Language.* New York: Wiley & Sons, 1967.

Massaro, D. W., Preperceptual Images, Processing Time, and Perceptual Units in Auditory Perception. *Psychol. Rev. 79,* 1972, 124–145.

Milner, B. (Ed.), *Hemisphere Specialization and Interaction.* Cambridge, MA: MIT Press, 1975.

Norman, D. A., *Memory and Attention.* New York: Wiley & Sons, 1969.

Penfield, W. L., and Roberts, L., *Speech and Brain Mechanisms.* Princeton, NJ: Princeton University Press, 1959.

Pisoni, D. B., and McNabb, S. D., Dichotic Interactions of Speech Sounds and Phonetic Feature Processing. *Brain Lang. 4,* 1974, 351–362.

Shankweiler, D. P., and Studdert-Kennedy, M., Identification of Consonants and Vowels Presented to Left and Right Ears. *Q. J. Exp. Psychol. 19,* 1967, 59–63.

Sperry, R. W., and Gazzaniga, M. S., Language Following Surgical Disconnection of the Hemispheres. In *Brain Mechanisms Underlying Speech and Language.* C. H. Millikan and F. L. Darley (Eds.). New York: Grune & Stratton, 1967, pp. 108–121.

Studdert-Kennedy, M., and Shankweiler, D. P., Hemispheric Specialization for Speech Perception. *J. Acoust. Soc. Am. 48,* 1970, 579–594. Reprinted in Miller et al. 1991, 293–308.

Studdert-Kennedy, M., Shankweiler, D. P., and Schulman, S., Opposed Effects of a Delayed Channel on Perception of Dichotically and Monotically Presented CV Syllables. *J. Acoust. Soc. Am. 48,* 1970, 599–602.

Warren, R. M., Verbal Transformation Effect and Auditory Perceptual Mechanisms. *Psychol. Bull. 70,* 1968, 261–270.

Weiss, M., and House, A. S., Perception of Dichotically Presented Vowels. *J. Acoust. Soc. Am. 53,* 1973, 51–58.

Wernicke, C., *Der aphasische Symptomencomplex.* Breslau, Poland: Franck & Weigert, 1874.

Whitaker, H. A., Neurobiology of Language. In *Handbook of Speech Perception,* Vol. 7. *Language and Speech.* E. C. Carterette and M. P. Friedman (Eds.). New York: Academic Press, 1976, pp. 389–428.

Wood, C. C., Auditory and Phonetic Levels of Processing in Speech Perception: Neurophysiological and Information-Processing Analysis. *J. Exp. Psychol. (Hum. Percept.)* 104, 1975, 3–20.

Wood, C. C., Goff, W. R., and Day, R. S., Auditory Evoked Potentials During Speech Perception. *Science 173,* 1971, 1248–1251.

Zaidel, E., *Linguistic Competence and Related Functions in the Right Cerebral Hemisphere of Man.* Unpublished doctoral dissertation, California Institute of Technology, 1973.

## Theories of Speech Perception

Abbs, J. H., and Sussman, H. M., Neurophysiological Feature Detectors and Speech Perception: A Discussion of Theoretical Implications. *J. Speech Hear. Res. 14,* 1971, 23–36.

Ades, A. E., How Phonetic Is Selective Adaptation? Experiments on Syllable Position and Environment. *Percept. Psychophys. 16,* 1974, 61–66.

Bailey, P., Perceptual Adaptation for Acoustical Features in Speech. *Speech Perception Report on Speech Research in Progress,* Series 2. Belfast, UK: Psychology Department, The Queens University, 1973, pp. 29–34.

Bell-Berti, F., Raphael, L. J., Pisoni, D. B., and Sawusch, J. R., Some Relationships Between Speech Production and Perception. *Phonetica 36,* 1979, 373–383.

Chistovich, L. A., Klass, V. A., and Kuzmin, Y. I., The Process of Speech Sound Discrimination. *Vopr. Psikhol. 8,* 1962, 26–39.

Cole, R. A., and Scott, B., Toward a Theory of Speech Perception. *Psychol. Rev. 81,* 1974, 348–374.

Cooper, W. E., Adaptation of Phonetic Feature Analyzers for Place of Articulation. *J. Acoust. Soc. Am. 56,* 1974, 617–627.

Cooper, W. E., and Blumstein, S., A "Labial" Feature Analyzer in Speech Perception. *Percept. Psychophys. 15,* 1974, 591–600.

Dorman, M. F., Raphael, L. J., and Liberman, A. M., Some Experiments on the Sound of Silence in Phonetic Perception. *J. Acoust. Soc. Am. 65,* 1979, 1518–1532.

Fant, G., Auditory Patterns of Speech. In *Models for the Perception of Speech and Visual Form.* W. Wathen-Dunn (Ed.). Cambridge, MA: MIT Press, 1967, pp. 111–125.

Fowler, C. A., Brown, J., Sabadini, L. and Weihing, J., Rapid Access to Speech Gestures in Perception: Evidence From Choice and Simple Response Time Tasks. *J. Mem. Lang.* 49, 2003, 396–413.

Fowler, C. A., and Galantucci, B., The Relation of Speech Perception and Speech Production. In *The Handbook of Speech Perception.* D. B. Pisoni and R. E. Remez (Eds.). Malden, MA: Blackwell, 2005, pp. 633–652.

Green, K. P., The Use of Auditory and Visual Information During Phonetic Processing: Implications for Theories of Speech Perception.

In *Hearing by Eye II: Advances in the Psychology of Speechreading and Audiovisual Speech.* R. Campbell and B. Dodd (Eds.). Hove, UK: Psychology Press, 1998, pp. 3–25.

Lane, H. L., The Motor Theory of Speech Perception: A Critical Review. *Psychol. Rev. 72,* 1965, 275–309.

Liberman, A. M., The Grammars of Speech and Language. *Cogn. Psychol. 1,* 1970, 301–323.

Liberman, A. M., Cooper, F. S., Shankweiler, D. S., and Studdert-Kennedy, M., Perception of the Speech Code. *Psychol. Rev. 74,* 1967, 431–461. Reprinted in Miller et al. 1991, 75–105.

Liberman, A. M., Isenberg, D., and Rakerd, B., Duplex Perception of Cues for Stop Consonants: Evidence for a Phonetic Mode. *Percept. Psychophys. 30,* 1981, 133–143.

Liberman, A. M., and Mattingly, I. G., The Motor Theory of Speech Perception Revised. *Cognition 21,* 1985, 1–36. Reprinted in Miller et al. 1991, 107–142.

Marler, P., A Comparative Approach to Vocal Development: Song Learning in the White-Crowned Sparrow. *J. Comp. Physiol. Psychol. 71,* 1970, 1–25.

McGurk, H., and MacDonald, J. W., Hearing Lips and Seeing Voices. *Nature 264,* 1976, 746–748.

Morton, J., and Broadbent, D. E., Passive Versus Active Recognition Models or Is Your Homunculus Really Necessary? In *Models for the Perception of Speech and Visual Form.* W. Wathen-Dunn (Ed.). Cambridge, MA: MIT Press, 1967, pp. 103–110.

Pisoni, D. B., and Sawusch, J. R., Some Stages of Processing in Speech Perception. In *Structure and Process in Speech Perception.* A. Cohen and S. G. Nooteboom (Eds.). Berlin, Germany: Springer-Verlag, 1975, pp. 16–34.

Rosenblum, L. D., Primacy of Multimodal Speech Perception. In *The Handbook of Speech Perception.* D. B. Pisoni and R. E. Remez (Eds.). Malden, MA: Blackwell, 2005, pp. 51–78.

Schatz, C. D., The Role of Context in the Perception of Stops. *Language 30,* 1954, 47–56.

Stevens, K. N., The Quantal Nature of Speech: Evidence from Articulatory–Acoustic Data. In *Human Communication: A Unified View.* E. E. David, Jr., and P. B. Denes (Eds.). New York: McGraw-Hill, 1972, pp. 51–66.

Stevens, K. N., Further Theoretical and Experimental Bases for Quantal Places of Articulation for Consonants. *Q. Prog. Rep. Res. Lab. Electron. M.I.T. 108,* 1973, 248–252.

Stevens, K. N., and Halle, M., Remarks on Analysis by Synthesis and Distinctive Features. In *Models for the Perception of Speech and Visual Form.* W. Wathen-Dunn (Ed.). Cambridge, MA: MIT Press, 1967, pp. 88–102.

Stevens, K. N., and House, A. S., Speech Perception. In *Foundations of Modern Auditory Theory,* Vol. 2. J. Tobias (Ed.). New York: Academic Press, 1972, pp. 3–57.

Stevens, K. N., and Perkell, J. S., Speech Physiology and Phonetic Features. In *Dynamic Aspects of Speech Production.* M. Sawashima and F. S. Cooper (Eds.). Tokyo: University of Tokyo Press, 1977, pp. 323–341.

Stevens, K. N., and Blumstein, S. E., Invariant Cues for Place of Articulation in Stop Consonants. *J. Acoust. Soc. Am. 64,* 1978, 1358–1368. Reprinted in Miller et al. 1991, 281–291.

Studdert-Kennedy, M., The Emergence of Structure. *Cognition 10,* 1981, 301–306.

Studdert-Kennedy, M., Liberman, A. M., Harris, K. S., and Cooper, F. S., Motor Theory of Speech Perception: A Reply to Lane's Critical Review. *Psychol. Rev. 77,* 1970, 234–249.

Whitfield, I. C., and Evans, E. F., Responses of Auditory Cortical Neurons to Stimuli of Changing Frequency. *J. Neurophysiol. 28,* 1965, 655–672.

**SECTION V**  Instrumentation

# Pioneers in Speech Science

**12**

*History is the essence of innumerable biographies.*

−Thomas Carlyle, *On History*

The three chapters in the fifth and last section of this book deal, in one way or another, with instrumentation. The first of the chapters describes some of the accomplishments of the pioneers of speech science. These pioneers all either helped to develop instrumentation or used instrumentation innovatively to advance our understanding of the production and perception of speech. The other two chapters deal, respectively, with the instrumentation used to investigate the acoustic analysis and perception of speech and, finally, the physiology of speech production.

Why take up space retelling the stories of speech scientists? The easy answer to that question is to say that just as all physicists know about Newton and Einstein, and all naturalists know about Darwin, and all geneticists know who Crick and Watson were and what they did, so should speech scientists know about the important contributors to their field. But that answer, although basically true, does not fit the facts exactly because some of the speech scientists whose work we will discuss do not have the exalted reputations of Newton, Einstein, Darwin, and Crick and Watson. In fact, some of them are not primarily known as speech scientists (e.g., von Helmholtz and Alexander Graham Bell). But all of them have been important to the origins and development of speech science. So many people have been instrumental in the development of speech science that it would be more confusing than helpful to name them, even were we to limit ourselves to the most influential. Rather than attempting to provide a comprehensive outline of the history of speech science and scientists, we will demonstrate the diversity of approaches inherent in this discipline by describing the contributions of a selected few of the pioneers in different aspects of the field. You will see that those scientists whom we have called pioneers are not necessarily the most important historically, but is rather one of the first to use a given approach.

Speech science, as you are well aware by now, is the study of the articulation and physiology of speech production, the acoustical characteristics of speech, and the processes by which listeners perceive speech. It has attracted the interest of phoneticians, linguists, psychologists, engineers, and speech-language pathologists. The interests of phoneticians and linguists traditionally overlap. Phoneticians concentrate on describing the normal production of actual speech sounds (see Chapter 1) in terms of articulatory physiology and acoustics. Linguists tend to be more interested in describing sound systems (phonology) of languages, the rules under which those systems operate, and how those rules relate to the rules of syntax and semantics. The psychologists are primarily interested in psychoacoustics, the perceptual cues to speech, measurement of speech intelligibility, and the ways in which the human brain processes the speech signal. The engineers are primarily interested in the analysis of the sounds of speech, the transmission of speech in communication systems, the development of visual speech displays, and the development of speech synthesizers and machines that recognize speech and individual speakers. The speech-language pathologists are primarily interested in speech production and its disorders, including the inception of speech in the central nervous system, the mechanisms that control speech production, including muscle activity, articulatory movements, and the resulting changes in air pressure and sound. They also explore the connections between speech and language production in disordered populations. In practice, however, the phonetician, linguist, psychologist, engineer, physicist, and speech pathologist often share interests and work together on research projects.

## HERMANN VON HELMHOLTZ: ACOUSTICS OF SPEECH

The human ear was a valuable instrument in the study of the acoustics of speech long before the electronic age brought with it electrical frequency analyzers and computers. Hermann Ludwig Ferdinand von Helmholtz (1821–1894), born near Berlin of English, German, and French ancestry, used his ears extensively to study the acoustics of the human voice and the resonances of the vocal tract. A man of wide interests living before the age of specialization, he studied mathematics, physics, and medicine and contributed to physiology, optics, acoustics, mathematics, mechanics, and electricity through his university teaching and research. He published more than 200 papers and books. His father was a teacher of philology and philosophy. His mother was a descendant of William Penn, the founder of the State of Pennsylvania, on her father's side, and of French ancestry on her mother's side. A sickly child, Helmholtz had trouble with grammar, history, and vocabulary and had difficulty in distinguishing left from right, but he read widely and from an early age displayed curiosity about the physical and biologic sciences. After studying medicine at the University of Berlin and working as a surgeon in the army, he became a professor, first at Königsberg, then Bonn, and finally in Heidelberg and Berlin. Helmholtz always combined teaching with research. He thought it was important to experiment and to demonstrate to himself the principles to be taught in the lecture hall. He studied the physiology and sensation of hearing with regard to both pure and complex tones.

Helmholtz was a pioneer in developing the mathematics of resonance. He discovered that when he blew across the open necks of bottles with varying amounts of water in them, he could produce different sounds. For instance, he could make one bottle produce a vowel that resembled /u/ (as in shoe). When he blew across the necks of two bottles

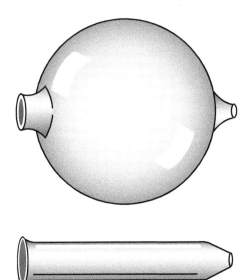

**FIGURE 12.1**  Helmholtz resonators.
(Adapted from *On the Sensations of Tone as a Physiological Basis for the Theory of Music*, 1863.)

simultaneously, he produced a vowel very much like /o/ (as in go).

Using hollow glass globes with two openings, later known as Helmholtz resonators (Fig. 12.1), he developed a technique to analyze the frequency components of complex tones. First he would coat the smaller nipple-shaped end with sealing wax and obtain an airtight fit into his ear canal. Each globe was tuned to a different tone, its natural frequency. Stopping up his other ear with more sealing wax, he would listen to complex (speech) sounds. The glass globes would resonate only to those frequencies that were the same as, or mathematically related to, their natural frequencies. He was thus able to identify the fundamental frequency and harmonics of a human voice and the major resonant frequencies of a vocal tract long before the invention of electronic devices that analyze sound.

To discover why a particular vowel has a distinctive quality whether said or sung and whether said by men, women, or children, Helmholtz held tuning forks of different fre-

quencies in front of his mouth and those of other people, having them shape their vocal tracts for a particular vowel. He found that different shapes produced different resonant frequencies (formants). In this way, Helmholtz determined what he thought were the absolute resonant frequencies of each vowel; later, however, the resonant frequencies were found to be determined by vocal tract size and thus to vary among speakers for any particular vowel. In 1863, he published his great work on acoustics of speech and on harmonic theory, *On the Sensations of Tone as a Physiological Basis for the Theory of Music*.

Helmholtz is described as a calm, reserved scholar. He liked to go mountain climbing and claimed that thoughts often came to him when he was hiking. Married twice, he had two children by his first wife, who died when he lived in Heidelberg. His daughter married the son of Werner von Siemens, the founder of the Physico-Technical Institute near Berlin. Helmholtz was the first director of the institute. One of his students was Heinrich Hertz, who later demonstrated electromagnetic waves and for whom the unit of frequency (Hz) has been named. Besides his scholarly activities, Helmholtz thought it was important to lecture on scientific subjects to the public, which was unusual in Germany at that time. Helmholtz would undoubtedly be surprised to know that today he is being hailed here as a pioneer in speech science, as his interests ranged much farther. For example, he invented the ophthalmoscope and provided mathematical proof of the conservation of energy. Nonetheless, Helmholtz helped us to understand some of the most important principles of the acoustics and physics of speech: that the puffs of air emitted between the vibrating vocal folds are the acoustic source of the voice, that the harmonics of the voice are resonated in the pharynx and oral cavities, and that vowels are recognized because of their distinctive resonances.

## HENRY SWEET: DESCRIPTIVE PHONETICS

When Henry Sweet (1845–1912) was born in England, Helmholtz was 24 years old and had already published his first paper on the connection between nerve cells and fibers. Sweet was to come to the study of speech by an entirely different route: an interest in languages and phonetics. He was a teacher of English pronunciation and served as the model for George Bernard Shaw's Henry Higgins in the play *Pygmalion,* later adapted as Lerner and Loewe's musical *My Fair Lady.* Sweet graduated from Balliol College at Oxford, but partly because he obtained a low grade in Greats (the examinations), he was never made a professor of philology and was better appreciated in Germany than in his own country. He was influenced by the German school of philology, by the impressive work in phonetics done in India, and by a phonetic transcription system called Visible Speech, which was developed by Alexander Melville Bell for educating the deaf. In 1877, Sweet wrote of his adaptation of Visible Speech (which he called Broad Romic) as follows: "I use . . . 'Broad Romic' as a kind of algebraic notation, each letter representing a group of similar sounds." This formulation of the phonemic principle, the idea that individual distinct sounds (allophones) can be identified as members of a single family of sounds (a phoneme), was new. (Although he may be said to have been the first to state the concept of the phoneme, the word itself was not coined by him.) Sweet's transcription system was a precursor of the International Phonetic Alphabet (see Appendix A). Sweet was one of the first speech scientists to use instruments to analyze speech and established one of the earliest laboratories devoted to the study of phonetics.

With the publication of his *Handbook of Phonetics* in 1877, he established England as the European birthplace of the science of phonetics. Despite his obvious preeminence in England in phonetics, Sweet was not ap-pointed in 1876 to the Chair of Comparative Philology at University College, London, and he was passed over again in 1885 as a candidate for the Merton Professorship of English Language and Literature at Oxford. The final blow came in 1901, when he was denied the Professorship of Comparative Philology at Oxford. Linguistics scholars in Europe were astonished at the lack of academic recognition given to Sweet in England. He was merely appointed a Reader in Phonetics at Oxford, a position that was, however, created especially for him.

Unlike the calm, reserved Helmholtz, Sweet was bitter and sarcastic. His scholarship and writings continued at full pace despite his disappointments, and he published *A History of English Sounds* in 1874, revised in 1888. In 1890, he brought out *A Primer of Phonetics,* containing detailed articulatory descriptions of speech sounds. He was an early member of the Philological Society in London; the society finally recognized his great contribution to the study of descriptive phonetics in the presidential address given by Christopher L. Wrenn in 1946, 34 years after Sweet's death.

## ALEXANDER GRAHAM BELL: TEACHING THE DEAF

Only 2 years after the birth of Henry Sweet in England, Alexander Graham Bell (1847–1922) was born in Edinburgh. Later to be world renowned as the inventor of the telephone, he always considered himself to be a scientist and inventor by avocation and a teacher of the deaf by vocation. His father, Alexander Melville Bell, was a speech teacher and elocutionist who lectured at the University of Edinburgh and wrote pamphlets and books on elocution. Bell senior's greatest achievement was the development of Visible Speech (Fig. 12.2), originally a system of symbols representing the articulation underlying each speech sound. The tongue was represented by a horseshoe-shaped

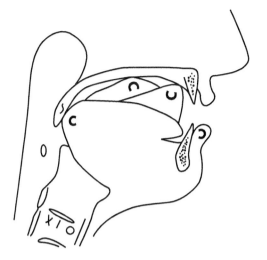

Ʒxɑʄʊ ɷɪ ɷɭƷ

I caught the thief

**FIGURE 12.2** Simple utterance as represented in Bell's visible speech with a schematic drawing of the parts of the vocal tract involved in various sounds. (Adapted from Bell, A. G., *English Visible Speech in Twelve Lessons*, 1895. Bell wrote this book to popularize his father's transcription system.)

symbol, its position indicating the most active part of the tongue. With additional symbols for lip activity and phonation, any speech sound could be represented visually. Alexander Graham Bell spent much of his life instructing teachers in the use of his father's system for describing speech production.

As a child, Bell junior was extremely musical and curious about nature but uninterested in formal studies. At 15, he went to London to live with his 70-year-old grandfather, a teacher of public speaking, who also instructed stutterers and those with other speech disorders. Under the guidance of his grandfather, Bell learned to apply himself to serious study, to be independent in the control of his own finances, to recite passages from Shakespeare's plays, and to dress "like a gentleman."

Back in Edinburgh a year later, he started a long career of teaching while he was still a student, first at Weston House at Elgin, then at Edinburgh University. Unaware that he was repeating the experiments of Helmholtz, Bell discovered the resonances of the vocal tract cavities by snapping his finger against his throat and cheeks as he assumed various vocal tract shapes. He also repeated the experiment of determining the frequencies of the resonators by vibrating tuning forks in front of his mouth as he positioned his articulators for different vowels.

After losing two other sons to illness, the family emigrated to Canada for Bell senior's retirement when Bell junior was 23. In Great Britain, Bell junior had gained a reputation as an outstanding teacher of speech to the deaf, using his father's Visible Speech method. In America, he continued teaching the deaf and trained teachers in schools for the deaf to use the Visible Speech system. He came into contact with the scientific community in Boston, started work on his many ideas for inventions, and in 1876 shouted the famous line—"Mr. Watson, come here; I want to see you"—that his assistant, Thomas Watson, heard and understood through the receiver of the first telephone, installed between Bell's laboratory and his bedroom down the hall.

In 1877, Bell married Mabel Hubbard, the deaf daughter of Gardiner Hubbard, one of his partners in the newly established Bell Telephone Company. They returned briefly to England to promote the telephone and Visible Speech for the deaf, but the family, which eventually included two daughters, settled in Washington during the winters and at their large estate in Nova Scotia during the summers. Although Bell made many profitable inventions, he always considered his work for the deaf to be paramount. He established the Volta Bureau, a center of information about deafness, developed the audiometer for testing hearing, and continued to promote Visible Speech. Throughout his life, he was sleepless most of the night, preferring to sleep late into the morning. By working at night, he could be alone and more productive during his most active years.

Basically a solitary man himself, Alexander Graham Bell helped other people to communicate with one another, even those who could not hear.

## R. H. STETSON: SPEECH PHYSIOLOGY

Raymond Herbert Stetson (1872–1950) provides an instructive example of a scientist whose current reputation is based more on his pioneering efforts in the development of methodology and instrumentation than on the acceptance of his research findings. Stetson was a broadly educated man whose knowledge spanned a number of sciences (psychology, zoology, chemistry) and the humanities. He received his undergraduate degree from Oberlin College in 1893 and his doctorate in 1901 from Harvard University. He returned to Oberlin in 1909 as the head of the psychology department and remained there until his death in 1950.

Stetson devoted much of his career to developing and refining objective methods for measuring the movements of the respiratory mechanism and the articulators in speech production. In the early 1920s, he visited France, where he worked and studied with L'Abbé Rousselot, often described as the father of modern experimental phonetics. On his return to the United States, Stetson did much to advance Rousselot's work with the kymograph, a device invented by Rousselot that was used to record airflow, air pressure, and articulatory movements. In later years, he adapted the oscillograph for use in making physiologic measurements of speech and, in fact, named his workplace at Oberlin College the Oscillograph Laboratory.

Rousselot's influence can also be found in Stetson's refinement of palatography, a technique used to specify and measure the points of contact between the tongue and the roof of the mouth in the articulation of speech sounds. He studied the acoustic and physiologic nature of vowels and consonants and the distinctions between them and conducted a number of important experiments on the physiologic basis underlying the distinction between voiced and voiceless consonants. His writings, which appeared in many of the important journals of his day, ranged from studies of metrics and poetics to phonology.

Stetson's best-known research concerned the nature of the syllable with regard to both its production and its structure. In his *Motor Phonetics* (1928, revised 1951, 1988), he posited the existence of a chest pulse as the basis for the production of syllables. Subsequent research has led to general rejection of his findings with regard to the chest pulse, and as this was generally considered his most significant formulation with regard to speech production, it left Stetson labeled the brilliant scientist who was wrong.

It is a pity that so much emphasis has been placed on the failure of Stetson's theory, for it has surely directed attention away from a great deal of research and writing in which he made significant contributions to our knowledge of the production of speech and language. Virtually, all of his research findings, right or wrong, were and are important because of the other important studies and instrumental advances they gave rise to. It is for this reason that Stetson is still respected as a speech scientist and remembered as the most important of the researchers who provided a modern scientific basis for the study of speech production in North America.

## HOMER W. DUDLEY: ELECTRONIC SYNTHESIS OF CONTINUOUS SPEECH

The science of speech has benefitted from the contribution of a psychophysicist in Helmholtz, a phonetician and linguist in Sweet, a speech pathologist in Bell, a physiologic psychologist in Stetson, and an electrical engineer in the person of Homer Dudley (1896–1987). Dudley was a pioneer in speech synthesis, making machines that could produce speech-like sounds. In the

18th and 19th centuries, speech was produced artificially by mechanical manipulation of artificial heads and mechanisms designed to simulate the lungs, the larynx, and the vocal tract of a speaker, but speech synthesis as we know it had to await the 20th century arrival of electronic circuits. It was Dudley's invention, called the Voder, built in 1937 and 1938 at Bell Laboratories, that first synthesized continuous speech by electric circuits.

Homer Dudley started his career in Pennsylvania, where his family moved from Virginia when he was a schoolboy. His father was a preacher, and on moving to Pennsylvania, his parents gave lessons to pupils who were interested in the classics, in other academic subjects, and in studying for the ministry. Dudley graduated from high school early. On his first teaching assignment, he taught the fifth through eighth grades in one room; his second position was as a high school teacher. Finding it difficult to keep discipline in the classroom, Dudley abandoned his plans to teach and started working his way through The Pennsylvania State University where electrical engineering courses were being introduced to the curriculum. Dudley joined the technical staff of Bell Laboratories, the engineering laboratory of Western Electric. He worked there for more than 40 years, much of that time in the telephone transmission division.

Later on, he worked with Robert Riesz and others on the development of the Vocoder. The purpose of the Vocoder was to filter speech into 10 bands in such a way that the information could be transmitted over narrower bandwidths than were previously possible. After transmission, the channel information, along with a noise (aperiodic source) circuit for consonant sounds and a buzz (periodic source) circuit for phonation, was used to synthesize speech that closely resembled the original, except for some loss in voice quality. The Vocoder was demonstrated at the tercentennial celebration at Harvard and led to the celebrated talking machine, the Voder, a Voice Operation Demon-

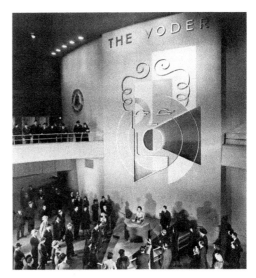

**FIGURE 12.3**  Bell Telephone demonstration of the Voder at the 1939 World's Fair. (Reprinted with permission of American Telephone and Telegraph Company.)

strator. The Voder synthesizer was shown at the 1939 and 1940 World's Fairs (Fig. 12.3). It made recognizable speech sounds, at least if listeners were cued to know the sort of utterances to expect. The operator pushed a pedal to control the periodic or aperiodic sources and pressed 10 keys to control the resonances. Special keys simulated the stop consonants such as /p/ or /t/. In the demonstrations, a dialog would be conducted between a person and the Voder, which was operated by a woman (seated behind the desk in Fig. 12.3). More than 20 telephone operators were trained to operate the machine during the World's Fair demonstrations. Unlike previous synthesizers, the Voder was based more closely on the acoustics of speech than on its articulation. In analogy with radio transmission, accomplished by modulating the frequency (FM) or amplitude (AM) of a carrier tone, Dudley conceived of speech as a carrier tone or sound source modulated by the movements of the vocal tract, that is, as a source–filter system (see Chapter 5).

Homer Dudley's most important contributions to speech science made explicit the carrier nature of speech and applied the carrier idea to specific principles for speech analysis and synthesis. These ideas underlie modern conceptualizations of the speech production process.

## FRANKLIN COOPER, ALVIN LIBERMAN, AND PIERRE DELATTRE: SPEECH PERCEPTION AND THE PATTERN PLAYBACK

Up to this point, our discussion has been limited to pioneers in the study of speech production and acoustics. Little systematic work in speech perception was possible until speech scientists knew enough about the acoustics of speech to control acoustic parameters individually when testing listeners. In the 1940s, Ralph Potter and his colleagues at Bell Laboratories developed the sound spectrograph, providing an instrument that let investigators conveniently analyze the frequencies represented in speech across time, producing a visual display called a spectrogram. With it came a sudden increase in information about the acoustics of speech. Important questions about speech perception, however, remained, such as: Which features of the complex acoustic pattern of speech are critical for the identification of speech sounds, and which features are less important? Answers to this question and many others were supplied by an engineer, a psychologist, and a linguist, who combined their talents at Haskins Laboratories.

Potter conceived of the reverse of the sound spectrograph as a machine that could convert visible acoustic patterns to sound. At Haskins Laboratories, Franklin Cooper (1908–1999) saw that the development of such a pattern playback would provide a powerful instrument for the study of speech perception. Cooper, born and educated in Illinois, received his doctorate in physics from the Massachusetts Institute of Technology in 1936. In 1939, after a few years with General Electric Research Laboratories, Cooper became associate research director of Haskins Laboratories, then its

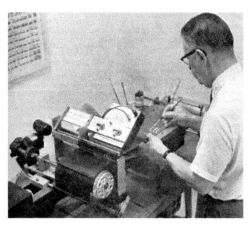

**FIGURE 12.4** F. S. Cooper painting a syllable on the Pattern Playback synthesizer. Speech was synthesized by converting patterns painted on acetate film loops to acoustic signals by a photoelectric system. (Reprinted with permission from Haskins Laboratories.)

president and director. As part of his efforts to develop a reading machine for the blind, Cooper constructed a speech synthesizer called the Pattern Playback (Fig. 12.4). The Playback was capable of converting machine-generated spectrograms and hand-painted copies of spectrograms to intelligible speech. By hand-painting selected portions of the spectrograms, Cooper and his colleagues were able to test the perceptual importance of individual acoustic features.

Alvin Liberman (1918–2000), a psychologist who received his bachelor and master of arts degrees at the University of Missouri and his doctorate at Yale, was a professor of psychology and linguistics at the University of Connecticut and at Yale. He joined Haskins Laboratories in 1944 and eventually succeeded Cooper as its president. Together with Cooper, he used the Pattern Playback to vary the acoustic parameters of speech systematically to determine the cues used in speech perception.

In 1950, at the invitation of Cooper and Liberman, Pierre Delattre (1903–1969), a Frenchman by birth, joined the Haskins experimental team working on speech perception. Delattre was an expert in French linguistics whose specialty was teaching

## CLINICAL NOTE

The work of the speech pioneers is relevant to the clinical concerns of speech-language pathologists and audiologists for at least three reasons. First, although most of the pioneers mentioned here studied normal speech production and perception, their findings have provided a basis for identifying the nature of speech and hearing disorders: It is not possible to describe a disorder or to plan a course of clinical treatment without knowing what speakers or listeners without that disorder do when producing or perceiving speech.

Second, the pioneers, along with the new ideas they generated, often were responsible for the development of instruments for studying speech and hearing. Many of these instruments would be considered "primitive" today, but they are the ancestors of contemporary devices, many of which are used in clinical settings. The following chapters on instrumentation in this book describe many of the instruments that can be found in clinical facilities.

Third, the pioneers continued the scientific tradition of disseminating the results of their research for the benefit of colleagues and students. That tradition is very much alive, and a great deal of research, much of it related to clinical concerns, becomes available virtually every day. The dissemination of research information is accomplished in two principal ways. One is by word of mouth—the presentation of papers—at the conventions and special meetings of professional organizations. Important forums for the presentation of studies of normal and disordered speech production and perception are the fall and spring meetings of the Acoustical Society of America (ASA). Equally as important for professional exchanges of ideas relevant to clinical applications of research is the annual convention of the American Speech-Language-Hearing Association (ASHA). Clinicians and speech scientists belong to many other regional, state, national, and international professional organizations that hold regularly scheduled meetings.

A second method for the exchange of ideas and research is found in the journals published by ASHA and ASA. ASA publishes the *Journal of the Acoustical Society of America,* usually called *JASA.* ASHA publishes one basic research journal, the *Journal of Speech-Language and Hearing Research,* and the more clinically oriented journals: the *American Journal of Speech-Language Pathology* and the *American Journal of Audiology: A Journal of Clinical Practice.* Many other journals include research on normal and disordered speech production, speech acoustics, and speech perception. The *Journal of Fluency Disorders, Journal of Phonetics, Ear & Hearing, Speech Communication, Brain and Language, Perception and Psychophysics, Phonetica, Clinical Linguistics and Phonetics,* and the *Journal of Voice* are but a few.

foreigners to master French phonetics. For 16 years, he directed the French phonetics program held during summers at Middlebury College in Vermont. During much of this time, he was a member of the faculty at the University of Pennsylvania. He was expert at painting playback patterns and in evaluating the sounds that the patterns produced. He helped to develop the rules for painting synthetic patterns without reference to actual spectrograms and even composed a piece of synthesized music that he called "Scotch Plaid."

The collaboration of Cooper, Liberman, and Delattre lasted until Delattre's death and produced most of the early work in speech perception. The value of the Pattern Playback as an instrument for speech perception remained unsurpassed until computer-controlled synthesizers became available. The experimenter could see at a glance the entire acoustic pattern, repeatedly hear how it sounded, and easily modify it. Systematically varying a single acoustic feature thought to be important to perception, the investigators had listeners label and discriminate the synthesized stimuli. By such means, the Haskins group, which included many other investigators, demonstrated the effects of linguistic experience on speech perception, identified specific acoustic features as cues to the perception of speech sounds, and formulated the earliest versions of the motor theory of speech perception. Although Haskins Laboratories pioneered the systematic study of speech perception, we cite it chiefly because it is a good example of the point we are trying to emphasize: that the roads to speech science are many and varied. At Haskins Laboratories today, as well as at other research institutions, engineers, phoneticians, linguists, speech pathologists, and psychologists are interested in experimental phonetics or speech science.

## SINCE THEN

In general, the experimental study of the acoustics of speech is ahead of the study of speech physiology. On the basis of spectrographic analysis and the systematic synthesis of speech, we now know a substantial amount about the acoustics of speech. This knowledge has made synthetic speech or talking machines possible. We know less about speech physiology from experimental studies, but work in this area is progressing rapidly through the efforts of many speech scientists at universities and laboratories throughout the United States and abroad. Speech perception research has diversified during the years, and has come to include, at least, infant and animal perception, the role of cerebral hemispheres in perception, the role of context and linguistic experience in perception, the role of memory and attention, and descriptions of the stages of processing involved in the perception of speech.

The future of speech science lies in work to investigate the ways speech production and speech perception may interact, in studies of how disordered speech differs from normal speech, and in work that will lead to automatic speech recognition as well as synthesis. In the following chapters, we survey some of the instruments and techniques that are being used to continue these investigations.

## REFERENCES

Bell, A. G., *The Mechanism of Speech*. New York: Funk & Wagnalls, 1908.

Bell, A. G., *English Visible Speech in Twelve Lessons*. Washington: Volta Bureau, 1895.

Bell, A. M., *Visible Speech: The Science of Universal Alphabetics; or Self-Interpreting Physiological Letters for the Printing and Writing of all Languages in One Alphabet; elucidated by Theoretical Explanations, Tables, Diagrams, and Examples*. London: Simpkin, Marshall, 1867.

Bronstein, A. J., Raphael, L. J., and Stevens, C. J. (Eds.), *Biographical Dictionary of the Phonetic Sciences*. New York: The Press of Lehman College, 1977.

Bruce, R. V., *Bell: Alexander Graham Bell and the Conquest of Solitude*. Boston: Little, Brown & Co., 1973.

Cooper, F. S., Liberman, A. M., and Borst, J. M., The Interconversion of Audible and Visible Patterns as a Basis for Research in the Perception of Speech. *Proc. Nat. Acad. Sci. U.S.A. 37*, 1951, 318–325.

Delattre, P. C., Liberman, A. M., Cooper, F. S., and Gerstman, L. J., An Experimental Study of Vowel Color; Observations on One- and Two-Formant Vowels Synthesized From Spectrographic Patterns. *Word 8*, 1952, 195–210.

Dudley, H., The Carrier Nature of Speech. *Bell Syst. Tech. J. 19*, 1940, 495–515. Reprinted in *Speech Synthesis: Benchmark Papers in Acoustics*. J. L. Flanagan and L. R. Rabiner (Eds.). Stroudsburg, PA: Dowden, Hutchinson & Ross, 1973, pp. 22–42.

Dudley, H., Riesz, R. R., and Watkins, S. A., A Synthetic Speaker. *J. Franklin Inst. 227*, 1939, 739–764.

Fowler, C., and Harris, K. S., Speech Research at Haskins Laboratories. In *A Guide to the History of the Phonetic Sciences in the United States*. J. J. Ohala, A. J. Bronstein, M. G. Busà, J. A. Lewis, and W. F. Weigel (Eds.). Berkeley: University of California at Berkeley, 1999, pp. 51–54.

Helmholtz, H. L. F., *Die Lehre von den Tonempfindungen als Physiologische Grundlage für die Theorie der Musik*. Braunschweig, Germany: F. Vieweg und Sohn, 1863. Translated by A. S. Ellis as *On the Sensations of Tone as a Physiological Basis for the Theory of Music*, 2nd English translation from the 4th German edition of 1877. New York: Dover Publications, 1954.

Koenig, W., Dunn, H. K., and Lacy, L. Y., The Sound Spectrograph. *J. Acoust. Soc. Am. 17*, 1946, 19–49.

Liberman, A. M., Delattre, P., and Cooper, F. S, The Role of Selected Stimulus Variables in the Perception of the Unvoiced Stop Consonants. *Am. J. Psychol. 65*, 1952, 497–516.

Liberman, A. M., Cooper, F. S., Shankweiler, D. P., and Studdert-Kennedy, M., Perception of the Speech Code. *Psychol. Rev. 74*, 1967, 431–461. Also in *Human Communication: A Unified View*. E. E. David, Jr., and P. B. Denes (Eds.). New York: McGraw-Hill, 1972, pp. 13–50.

McKendrick, J. G., *Hermann Ludwig Ferdinand von Helmholtz*. New York: Longmans, Green & Co., 1899.

Raphael, L. J., A Large Size in Stockings is Hard to Sell: Franklin Cooper and the Pattern Playback. *J. Acoust. Soc. Am. 107*, 2000, 2825 (A).

Stetson, R. H., *Motor Phonetics: A Study of Speech Movements in Action*. Amsterdam, The Netherlands: North Holland, 1951. Revised by S. Kelso and K. Munhall, San Diego: Singular Publishing Group, 1988.

Studdert-Kennedy, M., and Whalen, D. H., A Brief History of Speech Perception Research in the United States. In *A Guide to the History of the Phonetic Sciences in the United States*. J. J. Ohala, A. J. Bronstein, M. G. Busà, J. A. Lewis, and W. F. Weigel (Eds.). Berkeley: University of California at Berkeley, 1999, pp. 21–24.

Sweet, H., *Handbook of Phonetics*. Oxford: Clarendon Press, 1877.

Sweet H., *History of English Sounds*. Oxford: Clarendon Press, 1874 (revised 1888).

Sweet, H., *A Primer of Phonetics*. Oxford: Clarendon Press, 1890.

Wrenn, C. L., Henry Sweet: Presidential Address Delivered to the Philological Society on Friday, 10th May, 1946. Reprinted in *Portraits of Linguists*. T. A. Sebeok (Ed.). Bloomington, IN: Indiana University Press, 1966, pp. 512–532.

# Research Tools for the Study of Acoustic Analysis and Speech Perception

# 13

*To know that we know what we know, and that we do not know what we do not know, that is true knowledge.*

—Thoreau, *Walden* (quoting Confucius)

The purpose of research is to find answers to questions about ourselves and the world around us. This goal may never be perfectly attained, however, because the results of research attain meaning only through the interpretations of researchers. Because the interpretive process always includes a substantial subjective component, the significance of any single piece of research is often less clear-cut and more disputable than we would like. Nonetheless, the research process does, in the long run, allow us to analyze complex behavior into its components, and, in turn, better understand how those components are united to generate the behavior we are studying.

In this and in the following chapter, we will describe some of the instruments and techniques that are used to investigate the production and perception of speech. This chapter will focus on the tools used for acous-

tic analysis and perceptual testing. These tools are generally employed in what are loosely called "experiments." In fact, studies that are called experiments in common usage are, from the scientific point of view, often not experiments. Therefore, before we begin our survey, we must draw some fundamental distinctions between investigations that are truly experimental and those that are not.

## DESCRIPTIVE AND EXPERIMENTAL RESEARCH

When seeking the answers to research questions, the speech scientist usually proceeds in one of two ways: by carrying out a descriptive study or by carrying out an experimental study. In a descriptive study, the scientist simply observes and records behavioral events and then, in most instances, tries to systematize the relationships among them. In an experimental study, the scientist observes and records behavior under controlled conditions in which experimental variables are systematically changed by the experimenter.

Consider the following example of a descriptive study that uses only observation and the recording of data. Let us assume that a researcher is seeking to describe the physiologic factors that control fundamental frequency ($f_o$) in normal speech production. The researcher might ask the speakers who are serving as subjects to read a passage as naturally as possible at their normal rate and level of loudness. The researcher records the speech while simultaneously measuring $f_o$, the output of a number of laryngeal muscles, and the subglottal air pressure. The physiologic parameters could then be correlated with the subsequent analysis of the acoustic output. For instance, the researcher might determine the relation between cricothyroid muscle activity and $f_o$ of phonation (Atkinson, 1978). Because the researcher is only seeking to observe normal behavior and not to alter that behavior in any way, the research would be classified as descriptive. It is important to remember that no matter how much scientific equipment is used in recording or analyzing data, if the researcher has not tried to manipulate the normal, natural behavior of the subjects in the study, it is not, formally, an experiment.

It would, however, be possible to convert the study described above into an example of experimental research by introducing an experimental variable. If, for example, the researcher has the subjects do everything they did in the descriptive study, but, in addition, asks the subjects to repeat their reading under delayed auditory feedback (DAF), then the study would meet the requirements of an experiment. That is, by introducing an experimental variable, DAF, the researcher has altered (or attempted to alter) the behavior of the subjects and can describe the differences between the normal and altered behavior.

Another example of an experimental study that uses observation and the recording of data both before and after the application of an experimental variable would be one in which the researcher seeks to discover the role of tactile feedback in speech production. In carrying out such an experiment, the researcher would have subjects produce a given sample of speech, first normally (the control condition) and then after the application of an oral anesthetic (the experimental condition), to observe the effects of desensitization (Borden, 1979). In this example, the dependent variable (the parameter observed for any changes) is the speech, and the independent variable (the parameter that the investigator manipulates) is the presence versus absence of anesthetization.

Experimental studies are very common in studies of speech perception. The experimental variable might be the systematic change in some aspect of the formant pattern or the duration of synthetic speech stimuli (Raphael, 1972). The dependent variable is the effect of such changes on the perceptions of listeners. It is, of course, also possible to use natural speech stimuli in experimental studies of speech perception. The independent variable might be the insertion of clicks into a recording of natural speech, or the deletion of segments of the acoustic signal, or the general distortion of some aspect of the acoustic signal (Fodor and Bever, 1965). As in an experiment using synthetic speech stimuli, the dependent variable is the effect of these modifications of the acoustic signal on listeners' perceptions of speech sounds.

Often, when a research tool first becomes available to scientists, there is a period in which research tends to be mainly descriptive. The advent of the sound spectrograph, for example, fostered a large number of studies in which acoustic patterns were related to the features, phones, and syllables of speech. Later, with the introduction of electromyography (EMG; see Chapter 14) as a research technique, research focused on describing the relationships between muscle activity patterns in EMG recordings and other, more clearly understood aspects of speech production. Usually, the descriptive studies lead to the creation of theories or models that are later tested experimentally. As more information becomes available, the model or theory is modified and then retested in new experiments. In this way, descriptive and experimental research complement one another.

To carry out descriptive or experimental studies, the speech scientist must use a variety of research tools, both instruments and techniques. Some of these tools are used to generate the stimuli used to study speech perception, others are used for acoustic analysis of the speech signal, and still others are used for physiologic measurements of speech production. We will consider each of these types of instruments and techniques in turn.

## THE COMPUTER AS A RESEARCH TOOL

Among the "instruments" alluded to above, there is one, the computer, that has become pervasive in speech research, as in virtually all other fields of inquiry. The computer in itself, of course, is not a dedicated speech research tool. But the technology that it represents and uses has generated profound changes in the way research is conducted and in the way data are gathered and processed. Many of these devices, especially those constructed to perform acoustic analysis, have been replaced by software. Where once there was a machine or instrument of substantial bulk, there is now a central processing unit and a monitor. Where once there was a paper printout of a spectrogram from which the values of acoustic features were measured with a ruler and a pencil, there is now a mouse controlling a cursor and an instant digital readout of the measurements made by a researcher. In the previous chapter of this book, you read about the development of the first sound spectrograph at Bell Laboratories in the 1940s. That device produced the first sound spectrograms, the visible representation of the acoustic speech signal, of which

you have seen many examples in previous chapters. So the spectrogram is still with us, but for the most part the spectrograph as a specific instrument is gone. What we have in its place is a computer and the relevant software.

But the computer's uses are not limited to acoustic analysis. In the study of physiological phonetics, computers can transform any analog signal, for example, from devices that measure air pressure, articulator movement, brain waves, or muscle contraction, into graphic displays. They can display images generated by computed tomographic scans and magnetic resonance images. In the study of speech perception, they can be used to create stimuli by editing recordings of natural speech and by creating synthetic speech. They are used to average data, measure reaction times, and record frequencies of occurrence of observed events. And, of course, they provide a more or less permanent store of data and results that can be printed out or consulted online in the future.

As computers continue to become less expensive and more compact, powerful, and user-friendly, we should expect that the opportunity to use them to conduct research into both normal and disordered speech will be available to virtually all students.

## SPEECH PERCEPTION

The uses of computers are evident in the procedure and instrumentation array required for studying how listeners perceive speech (Fig. 13.1). The procedure depicted is one by which an investigator analyzes responses given by listeners to natural or synthetic speech stimuli.

### Creating Stimuli

#### *Waveform Editing*

The ability to digitize the speech signal and store it in computer memory has enabled speech scientists to perform complex editing tasks with speed and accuracy when preparing stimuli for perceptual testing. The stored

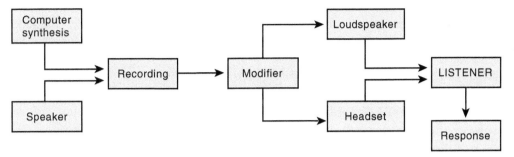

**FIGURE 13.1**   Instrumentation array used in speech perception studies.

speech is displayed as a waveform or a spectrogram on a computer monitor, and cursors are used to select the portions to be edited. Portions of the signal can be simply excised (and the gap of silence created by their removal can be closed) or stored and reinserted one or more times at any place in the stream of speech. In this way, the durations of naturally produced speech sounds or portions of those sounds, such as stop closures, can be decreased or increased in steps of any size.

One drawback of this sort of editing is that the experimenter is, for the most part, limited to making changes in the temporal domain (although adjustments to the spectrum and amplitude of the signal may also be made by filtering selected frequency regions or modifying the amplitude envelope). Source and resonance frequencies cannot be manipulated directly by waveform editing. On the other hand, the experimenter has the advantage of using stimuli that closely approximate naturally produced speech. (Synthetic speech stimuli, as we shall see, always contain simplifications and omissions of the features of natural speech.) Nonetheless, the experimenter using edited natural speech stimuli must always be aware of the acoustic structure of material being edited so that the effects of the editing on the stimuli can be specified and assessed when interpreting the perceptual judgments of listeners.

### Speech Synthesis

As we indicated in our discussion of waveform editing, the synthetic speech stimuli used in testing perception are never identical copies of natural speech. In spite of this, experimenters synthesize stimuli because they have the option of creating speech in which any or all of the acoustic features (frequency, amplitude, duration, source characteristics) can vary independently and can be specified exactly. For example, synthetic stimuli were essential in creating the experimental continua in which the frequencies of consonant–vowel formant transitions were systematically varied to discover the acoustic cues to place of articulation (see Chapter 10). The experimenters could be confident about their findings because all of the other potential variables in the stimuli were held at constant values. In theory, experimenters know everything about the acoustic content and structure of a synthesized stimulus because everything in it has been put there by them. Most of the perceptual experiments that we discussed in Chapters 10 and 11 used synthetic speech stimuli, some generated by the Pattern Playback (see Chapter 12) as many as 55 years ago, others produced by synthesizers of a more recent vintage.

There are, of course, substantial differences between the way the Pattern Playback operated and the way contemporary synthesizers generate speech. Most synthesizers in use today do not require a handmade graphic input that is optically scanned by mechanical means and then converted to sound. Rather, the input is typed into a computer in the form of numbers that represent frequencies, durations, amplitudes, bandwidths, and any other acoustic features under the control of the experimenter. The computer then converts the input to digital instructions to the synthesizer, which, in turn, generates the specified acoustic signal.

It is interesting to note that the computer programs controlling synthesis are virtually always capable of displaying the input as a schematic spectrogram of the type you have seen in Chapters 10 and 11 (e.g., Figs. 10.4, 10.8, and 11.3). Experimenters, evidently, are so used to the visual representation of the acoustic signal that they rely on it as confirmation of the appropriateness of their numerical input to the synthesizer. It is important to remember, however, that such visual displays do not confirm that the output of the synthesizer matches the input; they are only representations of the instructions that have been entered into the computer. If a synthesizer is not functioning properly, the experimenter will not find out by looking at a display of the intended input. The experienced and cautious user of a synthesizer analyzes its acoustic output to verify the identity of input with the input.

Acoustic speech synthesizers generally function in one of two ways. Parallel resonance synthesizers generate three (or, occasionally, four) formants (Fig. 13.2). The center frequencies and amplitudes of each formant are input by the experimenter, as are the choice of sound source (periodic/buzz, aperiodic/hiss, or both), the frequency range and amplitude of aperiodic resonances, and the presence, frequency, and amplitude of nasal resonances. In parallel resonance synthesis, the bandwidths of formants are fixed by the synthesizer.

Serial synthesizers generate five or more formants (Fig. 13.2). The experimenter selects the frequencies of the lowest three formants, but formants above the third have predetermined frequencies. In serial synthesis, the experimenter selects the bandwidths of all resonances, but their relative amplitudes are determined by the serial connection of the synthesizer and by subsequent spectral shaping. As in parallel resonance synthesis, the experimenter has a choice of sound source: periodic (buzz), aperiodic (hiss), or both. When the aperiodic source is selected, the spectrum of the sound is determined by a peak of resonance and an antiresonance that are paired by the synthesis program.

Serial synthesis sometimes sounds more natural than parallel resonance synthesis, but both, when carefully generated, are highly intelligible. Intelligibility is generally considered to be more important than naturalness in the preparation of synthetic speech stimuli. Both parallel resonance and serial synthesis have been used to replicate experiments that used unnatural-sounding (but intelligible) pattern playback stimuli, usually with equivalent results. In recent years, serial synthesis has been more widely used than parallel resonance synthesis because of its availability in software programs that can be used on personal computers.

It is also possible to synthesize speech according to articulatory rather than acoustic rules. X-ray, ultrasound, magnetometer, electropalatography (EPG), and other types of physiological data (see Chapter 14) have provided us with information about the positions and movements of the articulators and the changing shapes of the vocal tract. Because we know the rules for making vocal tract shape-to-acoustic-output conversions, we can program a computer-controlled synthesizer to use a schematic midsagittal drawing of a vocal tract as its input and to generate the appropriate acoustic signal. If we produce a sequence of schematic vocal tract shapes, in effect an animation, the computer will cause the synthesizer to generate the synthetic equivalent of articulated speech. Attainment of the predicted acoustic output can thus serve as a confirmation of physiological research and so help us to better understand speech production as well as speech perception.

## Perceptual Testing

Once the stimuli have been prepared, the experimenter must present them to listeners in identification or discrimination tasks (see Chapter 11). No special devices are

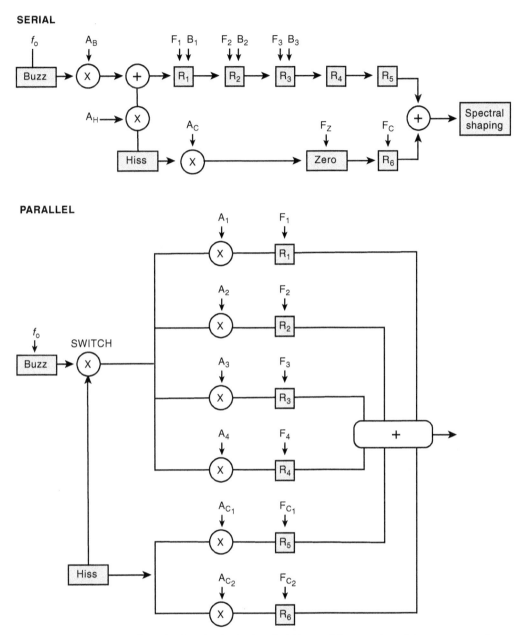

**FIGURE 13.2** In a serial synthesizer (top), the bandwidths and frequencies of the resonances for the voiced sound are set; the relative amplitude of the formants is fixed by the serial connection and the overall spectral shaping. When the hiss is connected, characteristics of the sound are a consequence of a spectral pole and zero pair. In the parallel synthesizer (bottom), a switch controls the generation of a buzz or hiss source. The frequency and amplitude of each resonance is adjusted individually. The output of the separate formants is added together.

actually required, but the arrangement of the equipment and the methods used to record responses must be carefully considered. It is convenient, for instance, to have a well-designed listening station for the testing of subjects. Ideally, a listening station should be a sound-treated room equipped to permit the simultaneous testing of several subjects, whether over headsets or in an open field using a high-quality loudspeaker equidistant from each subject.

More sophisticated listening stations have separate control rooms from which the experimenter administers the test, presenting stimuli generated directly from the synthesizer under computer control and allowing subjects to enter their responses directly into the computer for immediate processing. Aside from the speed, equivalent results can be obtained if the experimenter is in the room with the subjects and depresses a button to play the recording of the test stimuli while the subjects circle their responses on a prepared form that is later scored by hand.

## THE ACOUSTIC ANALYSIS OF SPEECH PRODUCTION

Whether the researcher carrying out perceptual studies uses edited natural speech stimuli or stimuli generated by a synthesizer, he or she must be able to describe those stimuli and specify the ways they resemble or differ from naturally produced, unedited speech. In other words, acoustic analysis must, at some level, underlie the creation of stimuli used to test speech perception.

The recording and analysis devices and programs used today vary widely in type and method of operation, but any of them is likely to generate a visual analog of some aspect or aspects of the acoustic signal. The essence of the acoustic analysis of speech is the conversion of sound waves to visual representations that can be inspected, measured in various ways, and related to the articulatory gestures that produced them. Certain types of analyses and their visual representa-

tions have proved more useful than others, and it is those types that we shall describe here. We shall not describe specific commercially available devices because they are numerous, various, and constantly undergoing change in response to technological innovations.

## Recording Speech

Before discussing the types of acoustic analyses and visual displays available to the speech scientist, we must consider the nature of the input to the analysis devices. Although it has become common recently to record speech samples directly into a computer or some other digital device where they can be saved for later analysis, some researchers and clinicians still use tape recordings of the speech sample(s) to be analyzed. Tape recorders may be analog or digital devices. Whichever kind of device is used, the way a scientist makes a recording can be as important as the way the acoustic analysis is carried out. A faulty recording may partially or completely invalidate an analysis. It is important, therefore, to take appropriate care during recording sessions.

The goal in recording is to capture a clear speech signal with little or no distortion and a low level of background noise. The location for making the recording is extremely important. An acoustically shielded booth with sound-absorbent walls in which the speaker sits in front of the microphone with the door closed is ideal. If an acoustically shielded booth is not available, it is often sufficient to record speech in a quiet room, one that has been acoustically treated with materials that damp extraneous sounds.

Microphones respond to pressure waves in the air and convert them to time-varying electrical signals. The choice of microphone is important. A unidirectional microphone several centimeters from the lips of the speaker transmits a higher signal-to-noise ratio than a microphone that is responsive equally to the speaker and to other sounds in the room.

## CLINICAL NOTE

The obvious value of acoustic analysis in the clinic is that it allows the clinician to infer many of the features of articulation that occur too quickly to be processed by the ear in real time. If we consider the fact that most speakers can easily produce from 7 to 12 phonemes per second (or even more, if they make the effort), and that each of those phonemes requires the movements of several articulators, we can understand why specifying articulatory details using only auditory input is not possible. By recording speakers and later subjecting their speech to analysis, clinicians can, in a relatively leisurely fashion, inspect the acoustic output and make reasoned decisions about when and where the articulators were moving. Moreover, having access to a digitized version of the speech signal allows the clinician to isolate specific syllables (or even smaller segments) that are particularly difficult to identify perceptually when they are heard in context. In other words, the auditory–perceptual analysis and the acoustic analysis complement each other, providing a more complete picture of the articulatory process.

Using acoustic analysis can provide very precise data concerning such facts as when the vocal folds are or are not vibrating, the absolute durations of acoustic segments such as the closures for stop consonants, changes in the fundamental and formant frequency, and so on. The clinician must bear in mind that deciding on the articulatory strategy that produced a particular acoustic feature is only an inference: It is possible to produce the same acoustic result using more than one set of articulatory gestures. Nonetheless, the relationship between articulation and acoustics is moderately well understood and is often used as the basis for the kinds of inferences that can be clinically useful.

Acoustic analysis is also valuable as a way of tracking the progress (or lack of progress) of those being treated for speech disorders. For example, if a patient is having difficulty producing voiceless aspirated stops, that fact can be documented at intake by making VOT measurements from wideband spectrograms. As therapy progresses, the VOT values, assuming therapy is successful, will grow and can be documented in the acoustic record. Even if the therapy is not successful, the acoustic analysis can verify the validity of the initial evaluation.

The benefits of even the best recording environment and microphone can be overridden if the speech is not recorded at an appropriate level of intensity. Most recording devices, including computers, come equipped with some sort of intensity-monitoring capability. Too much amplification (overloading) will result in a distorted signal because the high-amplitude peaks of the signal will be clipped. Underamplified recordings can be subsequently increased in intensity using computer-controlled programs, although experimenters must be careful not to introduce distortions.

Computer-driven digital recording devices automatically convert the acoustic signal to digital form and produce recordings that have a number of advantages over analog tape recordings. For one thing, digital recordings have greater fidelity than analog recordings. Second, they can be copied exactly with no loss of sound quality. Third, the signal-to-noise ratio and dynamic recording range is more advantageous in the digital format than in analog recordings. Finally, digital recordings are compatible with digital analysis devices; that is, their output signal can be fed into an analysis device without a digital-to-analog signal conversion.

A word of caution is in order for those who are still using tape recorders, whether analog or digital, that can be run on either batteries or line current: Such devices should be run only on line current. That is, under no circumstances should recordings be made on a unit of any sort that is powered by batteries.

Worn-down batteries can negatively affect the quality of recordings (especially on analog devices), and thus the measurements of frequency, duration, and amplitude will be rendered both invalid and unreliable. Although digital audiotape (DAT) recorders are less susceptible to this problem than analog recorders, it is still wiser to operate them only on line current. When batteries die, so do recording sessions.

## Waveform Analysis

One way to make sound waves visible for analysis is to generate a waveform, an amplitude-by-time display of the acoustic signal (Fig. 13.3). This is most frequently done using the software of an acoustic analysis program. The software for such analysis permits the investigator to generate waveforms and to measure them very rapidly by positioning cursors on the screen of the monitor. The computer-driven analysis software can immediately display the values of the measurements at or between cursors to units of time, frequency, or amplitude.

Waveforms are useful not only for making acoustic measurements but also for displaying and measuring the output of physiological devices (see Chapter 14). For example, variations in air pressure and flow (recorded within the oral and nasal cavities or at the lips), transduced movement of articulators, EMG signals, brain waves (EEG), or any time-varying signal that has been transformed into voltage variation by microphones, transducers, or electrodes can be displayed as waveforms on a computer monitor.

Although the fundamental frequency of complex periodic speech sounds can be established from a waveform, the other frequency components in such waves and the many frequency components in aperiodic speech signals are not easily measured from a waveform. This is because a waveform is an interference pattern. An interference pattern is the sum of many frequencies with different amplitudes and phase relations. It would be difficult and time-consuming to specify component frequencies from a waveform alone. Instead they can be determined using spectral analysis.

## Spectral Analysis

We have briefly discussed some forms of spectral analysis in Chapters 2, 3, and 5. Of these types of analysis, the one that has proven most interesting to speech scientists is the spectrogram. The value of the sound spectrogram rests in the fact that it can depict the rapid variations in the acoustic signal that characterize speech. Moreover, spectrograms provide an analysis of the frequency components of the acoustic signal in terms of either its harmonics or its peaks of resonance (formants). Standard spectrograms also convey some useful information about signal amplitude by rendering the more intense portions of the signal as darker than the less intense portions.

The instruments used to generate spectrograms, like those used to produce waveforms, have undergone change. The sound

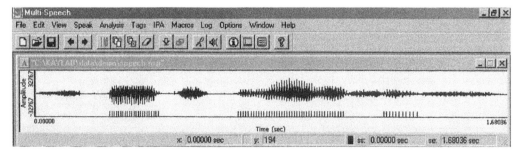

**FIGURE 13.3**  A computer software-generated waveform. (Courtesy of Kay Elemetrics Corporation.)

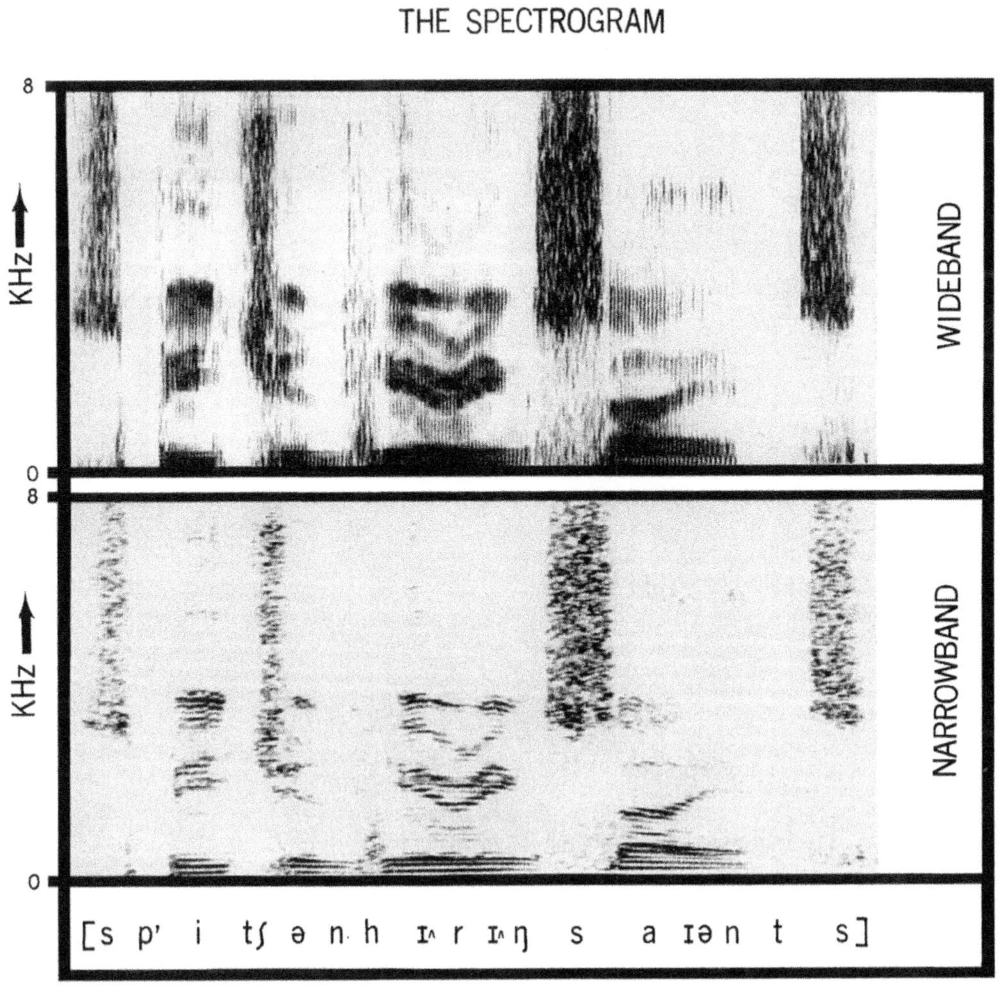

## THE SPECTROGRAM

**FIGURE 13.4**  Narrowband (bottom) and wideband (top) spectrograms of the utterance "speech and hearing science."

spectrograph, a free-standing device largely dedicated to producing hard-copy versions of spectrographic displays, has been largely replaced by commercial computer software that is available in several versions.

A researcher who wishes to analyze the acoustic speech signal by making spectrograms must decide what kind of information he or she wishes to see displayed. As we have seen, this is basically of two types: harmonic structure or resonance (formant) structure. Once the decision has been made, the researcher must select the appropriate filter bandwidth settings on the analysis device. In general, the choice is between a narrow

bandwidth setting and a wide bandwidth setting. A narrow bandwidth setting generates a display of harmonics on a narrowband spectrogram; a wide bandwidth setting produces a display of formants on a wideband spectrogram. Figure 13.4 shows a narrowband (at the bottom) and a wideband spectrogram (at the top) of the phrase "speech and hearing science." Let us first consider the information displayed in the narrowband spectrogram.

### The Narrowband Spectrogram

The most noticeable features of narrowband spectrograms are the more or less narrow horizontal bands, which represent the harmonics of the glottal source. The darker bands represent the harmonics closest to peaks of resonance in the vocal tract. The lighter bands represent harmonics whose frequencies are further from the resonance peaks. If harmonics are far enough from peaks of resonance, they may be too weak to be depicted on spectrograms; however, this depends to some extent on the settings used to generate the display. The relatively large horizontal blank spaces between the bands of harmonics in Figure 13.4 are at the frequencies of these most weakly resonated harmonics. The complete absence of harmonics at any frequency at various temporal locations in the spectrogram indicates that there is no periodic (harmonic) source exciting the vocal tract. When voiceless sounds such as [ʃʃ], [s], and [p] are being produced, there will be a total absence of harmonics throughout the frequency range of the spectrogram for some time. An obvious example can be seen at the top of the narrowband spectrogram in Figure 13.4 during the closures for the voiceless stops [p] and [t]. During the production of [s] and [ʃ], the spectrogram does show aperiodic energy, but the representation is easily distinguishable from that of the more or less horizontal and parallel harmonics displayed during the production of any of the phonated vowels in the spectrogram.

The bandwidth of the filter or filters used to generate narrowband spectrograms is usually somewhere between 30 and 50 Hz. To understand why the harmonics appear as they do on narrowband spectrograms, we must recall that resonators or filters that are more narrowly tuned respond to a limited number of frequencies. Because it is unlikely that the fundamental frequency of phonation will be lower than 50 Hz, a filter with that bandwidth (or a smaller bandwidth) will respond to and capture each harmonic separately as it scans through the frequencies in the speech signal. In addition, if we also recall that resonators or filters with narrow bandwidths are lightly damped, then we will understand that each successive puff of air emit-

ted during phonation will reach the analyzing filter before it has stopped resonating to the preceding puff of air. This means that the filter will respond continuously until sometime after phonation has ceased. The uninterrupted response of the filter is what underlies the continuous bands that represent harmonics. Finally, we should note that the light damping of the narrowband resonator or filter is complemented by a slow rise time. Taken together, these response characteristics explain why the harmonic display does not commence or cease until some time after the initiation or cessation of sound. Because of this, narrowband spectrograms are not used for making temporal measurements, such as the duration of acoustic segments and voice onset time. As we shall see, it is the wideband spectrogram that is used for temporal measurements.

Narrowband spectrograms have traditionally been used for making measurements of fundamental frequency and intonation. Variations in the first harmonic are often difficult to detect on a narrowband spectrogram. Assume that you are interested in measuring the peak in the fundamental frequency in a syllable and that the peak rises 10 Hz above the lowest value of the fundamental in that syllable. In a spectrogram with a frequency scale of 0 to 8 KHz or even of 0 to 4 KHz, a 10-Hz change will not result in very obvious deflection of the trace representing the first harmonic. However, because each harmonic in a series is a whole-number multiple of the fundamental frequency, a 10-Hz change in $f_0$ is easily observable in a higher frequency harmonic: A 10-Hz change in the fundamental frequency would correspond to a 100-Hz change in the 10th harmonic. Thus, because changes in fundamental frequency are visually more salient in higher frequency harmonics than in the fundamental frequency itself, measurements are usually made from the 10th (or a higher) harmonic. The procedure is simply to measure the frequency of a harmonic at a particular time and then to divide that frequency by the number of the harmonic. Such

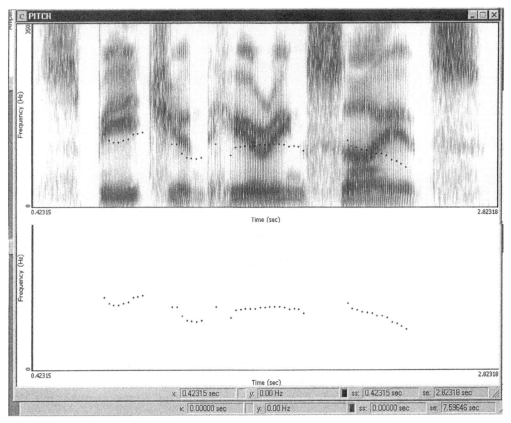

**FIGURE 13.5**   A computer software-generated fundamental frequency trace (bottom) paired with a time-linked wideband spectrogram (top) that also displays the superimposed fundamental frequency trace. (Courtesy of Kay Elemetrics Corporation.)

measurements are easily made in computerized analysis programs simply by positioning a cursor at the level of a higher harmonic and obtaining an instantaneous readout of frequency on the monitor.

It follows that the shapes of intonation patterns and the specific frequency values of intonation contours are also easier to detect in the higher frequency harmonics than in the fundamental frequency itself. For instance, terminal rises or falls in intonation and the relative degrees of such changes are more apparent in the 10th harmonic or in higher harmonics than in the first harmonic.

Although narrowband spectrograms can be used for measuring harmonic frequencies and observing continuous changes in intonation over the course of an utterance, analysis routines that isolate and depict varia-

tions in fundamental frequency as a function of time have become more available in recent years. Thus, it is possible to display variations in $f_0$ directly on a blank screen or superimposed on a spectrogram. Again, measurements are made simply by placing a cursor on any of the measured points of the display (Fig. 13.5) and obtaining a readout, eliminating the need to count harmonics, to measure the frequency of one, and to calculate the fundamental frequency by dividing the frequency by the number of the harmonic.

## The Wideband Spectrogram

As a practical matter, speech scientists studying phonetics (as opposed to those studying voice) are more often interested in the changing resonances of the vocal tract than in the harmonic structure of the speech signal. Although narrowband spectrograms do supply some information about formant frequencies, the information they display is not as useful or as relevant as that in wideband spectrograms. The precise (center) frequency of a formant is not easily observed in or measured from a narrowband spectrogram, especially when two formants lie close together on the frequency scale. Even the presence of particularly strong harmonics is not helpful, because they rarely coincide with the frequency of a peak of resonance. In addition, as we mentioned above, information about the timing of changes in vocal tract resonances is more reliably obtained from wideband spectrograms, and such changes often reflect articulatory distinctions (e.g., voice onset time) that are important to phonetic and phonologic analyses of language.

The most noticeable features of wideband spectrograms are the relatively broad bands of energy that depict the formants. The center of each band of energy is taken to be the frequency of the formant (the actual peak of resonance at a particular moment), and the range of frequencies occupied by the band is taken to be the bandwidth of the formant. As in the narrowband spectrogram, the relative degree of darkness of a band of energy can be used as a rough estimate of the intensity of the signal, and the relatively large horizontal blank spaces, in this case between the formants, represent troughs (zeroes, antiresonances) in the resonance curve of the vocal tract. Unlike a narrowband spectrogram, a wideband display effectively represents an aperiodic source that is being resonated in the vocal tract. The blank spaces in the temporal dimension of a wideband spectrogram indicate silence, including pauses and the silent gaps that are generated by voiceless stop closures, such as those for [p] in "speech" and excrescent [t] in "science", as shown in Figure 13.4.

The bandwidth of the filter used to generate wideband spectrograms is generally between 300 and 500 Hz. A filter with such a relatively wide bandwidth responds in the same way to one, two, three, or more harmonics that fall within its range. That is, the filter does not resolve the energy within its bandwidth into individual harmonics. The result is, as we have seen, the depiction of the resonance peaks in the acoustic signal. This lack of specificity with regard to harmonic frequency is, however, precisely what an investigator wants, because the formants that characterize a particular sound for a particular speaker will be essentially the same no matter what the frequencies of the fundamental or the harmonics or, indeed, even if there are no fundamental or harmonic frequencies at all, as when sounds are whispered.

There is a second important effect of the wideband filter in the generation of spectrograms. Because the wideband filter responds very quickly to the onset and termination of sound, it represents each glottal pulse separately. Each puff of air escaping from the glottis during phonation immediately excites the wideband filter, which stops responding as soon as the glottis closes and the airflow temporarily ceases. In other words, in contrast to the narrowband filter, the wideband filter responds intermittently rather than continuously. If you look closely at Figure 13.4, you will notice that the horizontal bands of energy that represent the formants are actually composed of individual vertical striations. Each of these striations represents one glottal pulse. (Each striation is darkest within the bandwidth of a formant and lighter or discontinuous in frequency regions that are not close to the peaks of resonance.) The rapid response of the wideband filter thus generates a display from which accurate temporal measurements can be made. Speech scientists who want to measure the duration of an acoustic event or the time separating different acoustic events will use wideband spectrograms.

## Amplitude and Power Spectra

It is often the case that an investigator might want a more specific, quantified representation of the amplitudes of the component

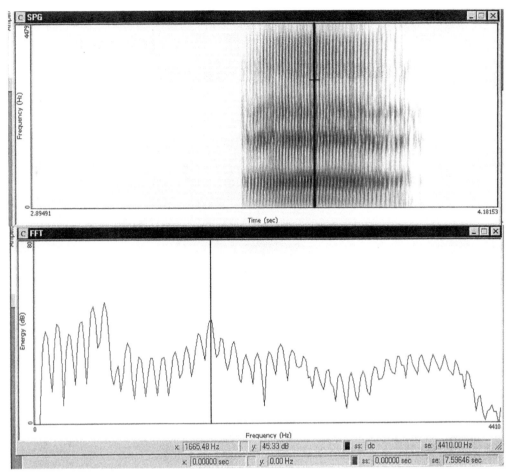

**FIGURE 13.6** Narrowband spectrogram (top) and corresponding narrowband amplitude spectrum (bottom) of the vowel [ɛ]. (Courtesy of Kay Elemetrics Corporation.)

acoustic features of the acoustic signal than the one provided by the varying degrees of darkness in a spectrogram. Analysis devices and computer programs permit the generation of an amplitude or power spectrum of the signal at any point in an utterance that is depicted in a wideband or narrowband spectrogram. The bottom portions of Figures 13.6 and 13.7 show narrowband and wideband amplitude spectra at the time indicated by the cursor in the spectrograms above them. Displays of this type are sometimes called amplitude sections.

Note that axes of these displays do not include any reference to time: The abscissa is scaled in frequency and the ordinate in some units of amplitude or intensity. There-

fore, in the narrowband amplitude spectrum, we can see the frequencies and relative amplitudes of each harmonic in the signal at the point in the vowel indicated in a spectrogram or a waveform; in the wideband amplitude spectrum, we can see the frequencies and relative intensities of the peaks of resonance (formants) at the same point in time. In most cases, the amplitudes of the harmonics or formants are scaled in decibels. Many researchers use a wideband power spectrum to determine formant frequency at a particular time because the peak of resonance is more objectively depicted on the frequency scale than it is in a wideband spectrogram. Generating a series of spectra at various points in the duration of an utterance can provide

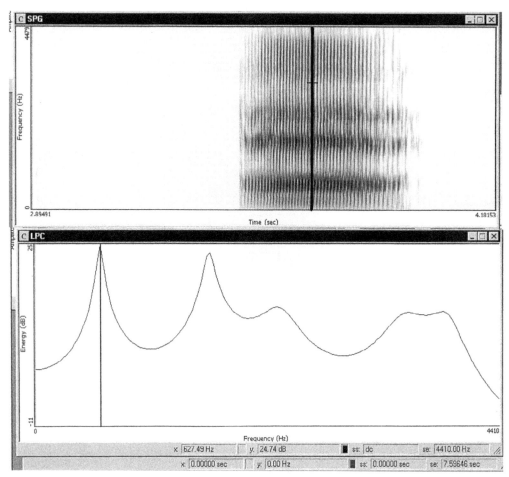

**FIGURE 13.7** Wideband spectrogram (top) and corresponding wideband amplitude spectrum (bottom) of the vowel [ɛ]. (Courtesy of Kay Elemetrics Corporation.)

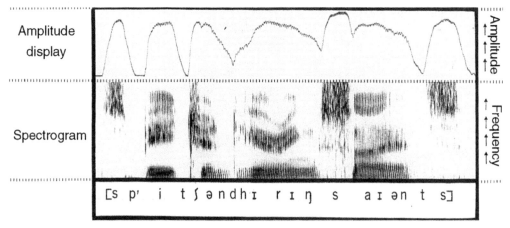

**FIGURE 13.8** Wideband spectrogram with the corresponding time-linked amplitude display shown above.

fairly accurate data specifying how the spectrum differs from time to time.

## The Amplitude Display

It is sometimes important to know how the overall amplitude of the acoustic speech signal varies with time (rather than looking at the individual amplitudes of component frequencies at a single point in time). Overall amplitude variation is depicted in an amplitude display (Fig. 13.8), also called the amplitude envelope. Like the direct representation of $f_0$ (described in the discussion of the narrowband spectrogram), this type of display is most often generated below or superimposed on a time-linked spectrogram.

## REFERENCES

### General Readings

#### Comprehensive

Baken, R. J., and Orlikoff, R. F., *Clinical Voice and Speech Measurement*. San Diego: Singular Publishing Group, 1993.

Baken, R. J., and Orlikoff, R. F., *Clinical Measurement of Speech and Voice,* 2nd ed. San Diego: Singular Publishing Group, 2000.

Flanagan, J. L., *Speech Analysis, Synthesis, and Perception*. New York: Springer-Verlag, 1965.

Holmes, J. N., *Speech Synthesis*. London: Mills & Boon, 1972.

Rosen, S., and Howell, P., *Signals and Systems for Speech and Hearing*. London: Academic Press, 1991.

#### Acoustic Phonetics

Abdelli-Beruh, N. B., The Stop Voicing Contrast in French Sentences: Contextual Sensitivity of Vowel Duration, Closure Duration, Voice Onset Time, Stop Release and Closure Voicing. *Phonetica 61,* 2004, 202–219.

Atkinson, J. E., Correlation Analysis of the Physiologic Features Controlling Fundamental Voice Frequency. *J. Acoust. Soc. Am. 63,* 1978, 211–222.

Baken, R. J., and Daniloff, R. G. (Eds.), *Readings in Clinical Spectrography*. San Diego: Singular Publishing Group; and Pine Brook, NJ: Kay Elemetrics Inc., 1991.

Borden, G. J., An Interpretation of Research on Feedback Interruption. Brain Lang. 7, 1979, 307–319.

Fant, G., Sound Spectrography. In *Proceedings of the Fourth International Congress of Phonetic Sciences. Helsinki Conference.* A. Sovijarvi and P. Aalto (Eds.). New York: Humanities Press, 1961, pp. 14–33.

Fodor, J. A., and Bever, T. G. The Psychological Reality of Linguistic Segments. *J. Verbal Learning and Verbal Behavior, 4,* 1965, 414-420.

Halberstam, B., and Raphael, L. J., Vowel Normalization: The Role of Fundamental Frequency and Upper Formants. *J. Phonet. 32,* 2004, 423–434.

Koenig, W., Dunn, H. K., and Lacy, L. Y., The Sound Spectrograph. *J. Acoust. Soc. Am. 17,* 1946, 19–49. Reprinted in *Readings in Clinical Spectrography of Speech.* R. J. Baken and R. G. Daniloff (Eds.). San Diego, CA: Singular Publishing Group; and Pine Brook, NJ: KAY Elemetrics, 1991, pp. 3–34.

Potter, R. K., Kopp, G. A., and Kopp, H. G., *Visible Speech.* New York: Dover Publications, 1966.

Raphael, L. J., Preceding Vowel Duration as a Cue to the Perception of the Voicing Characteristic of Word-Final Consonants in American English. *J. Acoust. Soc. Am. 51,* 1972, 1296–1303.

Stevens, K. N., *Acoustic Phonetics.* Cambridge, MA: MIT Press, 1998.

#### Instrumentation and Clinical Applications

Barlow, S. M. (Ed.), *Handbook of Clinical Speech Physiology*. San Diego: Singular Publishing Group, 1999.

Borden, G. J., Kim, D. H., and Spiegler, K., Acoustics of Stop Consonant-Vowel Relationships. *J. Fluency Disord. 12,* 1987, 175–184.

Casper, M., *Speech Prosody in Cerebellar Ataxia.* Unpublished doctoral dissertation, Ph.D. Program in Speech and Hearing Sciences, The Graduate School of the City University of New York, 2000.

Cooper, F. S., Speech Synthesizers. In *Proceedings of the Fourth International Congress of Phonetic Sciences. Helsinki Conference.* A. Sovijarvi and P. Aalto (Eds.). New York: Humanities Press, 1961, pp. 3–13.

Daniloff, R. G., Wilcox, K., and Stephens, M. I., An Acoustic-Articulatory Description of Children's Defective /s/ Productions. *J. Commun. Disord. 13,* 1980, 347–363.

Howell, P., and Williams, M., Acoustic Analysis and Perception of Vowels in Children's and Teenagers' Stuttered Speech. *J. Acoust. Soc. Am. 91,* 1992, 1697–1706.

Kent, R. D., and Rosenbek, J. C., Acoustic Patterns of Apraxia of Speech. *J. Speech Hear. Res. 26,* 1983, 231–249.

Kent, R. D., Netsell, R., and Abbs, J. H., Acoustic Characteristics of Dysarthria Associated With Cerebellar Disease. *J. Speech Hear. Res. 22,* 1979, 627–648.

Metz, D. E., Schiavetti, N., and Sacco, P. R., Acoustic and Psychophysical Dimensions of the Perceived Speech Naturalness of Nonstutterers and Posttreatment Stutterers. *J. Speech Hear. Disord. 55,* 1990, 516–525.

Read, C., Buder, E. H., and Kent, R. D., Speech Analysis Systems: An Evaluation. *J. Speech Hear. Res. 35,* 1992, 314–332.

Rubin, P., Baer, T., and Mermelstein, P., An Articulatory Synthesizer for Perceptual Research. *J. Acoust. Soc. Am. 70,* 1981, 321–328.

Sasaki, Y., Okamura, H., and Yumoto, E., Quantitative Analysis of Hoarseness Using a Digital Sound Spectrograph. *J. Voice 5,* 1991, 36–40.

# Research Tools in Speech Science for the Study of Speech Physiology

# 14

*The main cause of this unparalleled progress in physiology . . . has been the fruitful application of the experimental method of research, just the same method which has been the great lever of all scientific advance in modern times.*

–Dr. William H. Welch, Address to the United States Congress

## PHYSIOLOGIC MEASUREMENTS

In the last chapter, we saw how researchers and clinicians can use acoustic analyses to make inferences about the articulatory behavior of speakers. Such inferences, however, cannot provide a complete picture of speech articulation and physiology, mainly because a great deal about the behavior of the structures that generate speech is unknown. Moreover, there is no substitute for looking as directly as possible at the behaviors in which we are ultimately interested. Many devices and techniques developed during the past several decades allow us to specify speech articulation more or less closely. We shall discuss several of them, concentrating on those that are most widely used or that provide important information

that is not readily accessible without invasive techniques.

## MUSCLE ACTIVITY

Before going on to discuss instruments and techniques that are used in studying respiration, phonation, and articulation, let us look at a technique that has been used to investigate all three of these aspects of speech production: electromyography (EMG).

Movements of the structures within the speech production mechanism usually result from the combined effects of muscular, aerodynamic, and biomechanical forces. EMG provides information about the muscular forces by allowing us to record *muscle action potentials:* the electrical activity accompanying muscle contraction. In speech research, action potentials are recorded with bipolar electrodes. The two poles of these electrodes provide a measure of the difference in electrical energy at two points within a muscle as the electrical charge sweeps along the muscle fibers. Stronger muscle contractions result from the firing of more motor units and result in a greater difference in the electrical charge measured between the electrodes. Besides providing a measure of the strength of muscle contraction, EMG provides temporal measures of muscle activity. By inspecting the onsets and offsets of activity, we can specify the duration of muscle contractions as well as the relative timing of the activity of different muscles contributing to the movements of the structures used in the production of speech.

The most commonly used type of bipolar electrode used in speech research today is the hooked-wire electrode (Fig. 14.1). Hooked-wire electrodes are made of two very fine platinum–iridium alloy wires. The two wires are inserted through the cannula of a hypodermic needle, and the tips are bent back to form the hooks that give the electrode its name. The wires are then injected directly into the muscle to be studied, and the hypodermic needle is withdrawn (Fig. 14.2). The hooks anchor the wires in the muscle and prevent the electrode from moving while data are being gathered. At the end of the recording session, a sharp tug on the wires straightens out the hooks, and the electrode is easily removed.

Hooked-wire electrodes are most useful for muscles that are not close to the surface of an articulator (e.g., the genioglossus muscle). Another type of electrode that can be

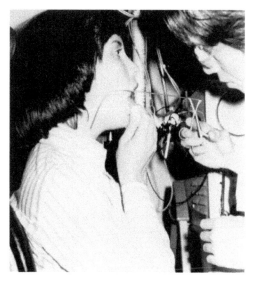

**FIGURE 14.2** Insertion of hooked-wire electrodes into the posterior cricoarytenoid muscle. The curved needle holder, shown in the physician's hand, is inserted orally. When the wires have been inserted into the muscle, the needle and needle holder are withdrawn. (Courtesy of Haskins Laboratories.)

used for muscles whose fibers are just below the skin (e.g., the orbicularis oris) is the surface electrode. The most commonly used type of surface electrode is created by applying some silver-based paint to the skin, placing two fine wires, whose insulation has been removed from the end, on the dab of paint, and then painting another silver dot on top to hold the wires in place. Surface electrodes are often not as muscle-specific as hooked-wire electrodes because they may be recording from a relatively larger area. This may cause them to transmit action potentials from more than one muscle, especially if several muscles are close to each other beneath the same area of the skin surface.

As we mentioned in Chapter 3, the EMG signal is an interference pattern (Fig. 14.3), the sum of the action potentials of many motor units. A *motor unit* consists of the muscle fibers innervated by a single motoneuron. An electrode records the electrical activity (action potential) of those motor units that are near it. Thus, the EMG signal from a

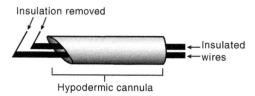

Insulation removed

Insulated wires

Hypodermic cannula

**FIGURE 14.1** Hooked-wire electrode used in electromyographic research.

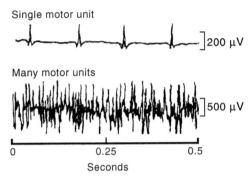

**FIGURE 14.3** *Top*: A raw (unprocessed) electromyographic signal. *Bottom*: An interference pattern that reflects the summed activity of many motor units.

single electrode does not necessarily represent the activity of an entire muscle. This means that the absolute amplitude of the EMG signal recorded on one occasion cannot be compared with that from another occasion, because the exact locations of the electrodes and thus the firing motor units they are recording may vary substantially from one day to another. It is, however, possible to inspect the relative EMG signal amplitudes recorded from the same electrode placement for differences between the timing and patterns of activity and to relate those differences to different phonetic events and to different conditions within the same experiment. For example, the activity of the orbicularis oris muscle for /p/ can be compared with that for /b/, or the action potentials for /p/, produced under different conditions of stress or speaking rate, can be compared with each other.

In most EMG studies, the raw signal of the interference pattern (Fig. 14.3) is modified in at least two ways. First it is rectified, so that all the negative values become positive. Second, the signal is smoothed to some extent so that the more or less gradual increases and decreases in action potentials (and thus muscular contraction) are more clearly depicted. In addition, the rectified and smoothed action potentials for many repetitions of the same utterance may be averaged together to reduce the variability in the data.

The results of these processing techniques can be seen in Figure 14.4.

## RESPIRATORY ANALYSIS

Because respiration underlies speech production, speech scientists are often interested in measures of basic respiratory function (air volume, pressure, and flow rate) during restful breathing. Such data are useful clinically, as they can determine possible causes of a number of speech disorders, especially those involving laryngeal function. Speech scientists and clinicians may therefore use information gathered by devices such as manometers and spirometers (Fig. 14.5) of various sorts. Even a cursory glance at the spirometer shown in Figure 14.5 reveals the obvious shortcoming of most such devices: They interfere with normal speech production. Therefore, the study of respiration and concomitant air pressure, flow, and volume during speech must be done with instruments that do not interfere with articulation and phonation. The miniaturization of sensing devices during the past several years has made the development of such instruments possible.

Air pressure varies throughout the respiratory system and the vocal tract during speech production. These pressure differences and changes, whether subglottal, intraoral, or nasal, can be studied by introducing pressure-sensing tubes to the area of interest. These sensing tubes, in turn, are attached to external pressure transducers that convert air pressure measurements to electrical signals that can be recorded and displayed in various ways.

Situating a pressure-sensing device subglottally is obviously a difficult and intrusive procedure involving a tracheal puncture. Measurements have also been made by placing a small balloon in the esophagus that is attached to a transducer, but pressure readings taken directly from the subglottal area are more accurate than indirect measures obtained from the esophagus. Measuring

Average EMG Signals

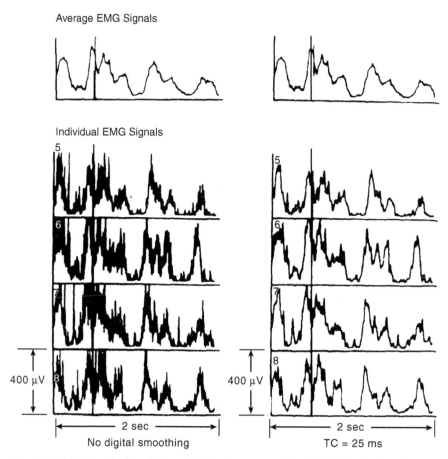

Individual EMG Signals

5

6

7

8

400 μV

400 μV

|← 2 sec →|  |← 2 sec →|

No digital smoothing  TC = 25 ms

**FIGURE 14.4** Rectified and integrated electromyographic (EMG) signals from the levator palatini muscle for the utterance "Jean Teacup's nap is a snap." Averaged signals of both unsmoothed (*left*) and smoothed (*right*) individual EMG signals are shown at the top. A time constant (TC) of 25 ms was used in smoothing the signals in the right-hand column. (Modified with permission from Kewley-Port, D., Data Reduction of EMG Signals. *Haskins Laboratories Status Report on Speech Research SR-50, 140,* 1971, 132–145.)

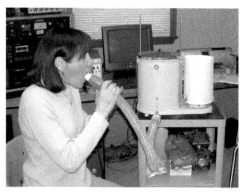

**FIGURE 14.5** A spirometer. (Courtesy of Adelphi University.)

intraoral air pressure is considerably easier and of great interest because intraoral air pressure changes in response to a wide variety of influences throughout the speech mechanism, including the articulation of speech sounds. Sensing tubes used to measure intraoral air pressure may be introduced through the nose so that they hang over the velum in the area of the oropharynx. Alternatively, they may be bent around the back molars of a speaker with the tube exiting the oral cavity via the buccal cavity and the corner of the mouth.

Measures of airflow, usually given in milliliters per second, can be made in a

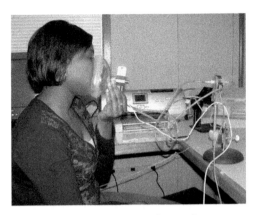

**FIGURE 14.6** A pneumotachograph. (Courtesy of Adelphi University.)

number of ways. Many of the devices used to measure airflow are appropriate for measuring air volume as well. This is because airflow and volume are related: Air volume is the result of flow multiplied by time. Most airflow measurements for speech are made using a device called a *pneumotachograph* (also called a Rothenberg mask after the researcher who devised it), which is attached to an airtight face mask large enough to allow the subject to speak with minimal interference to articulation (Fig. 14.6). The face mask may be divided into two chambers, permitting independent measurements of oral and nasal airflow. The pneumotachograph itself contains two pressure sensors separated by a resistor. The pressure drop across the resistor is fed to a transducer that generates a signal proportional to the airflow. A speech sound produced with relatively high air pressure and flow, such as /s/, may show a value of 7 cm $H_2O$ oral air pressure and about 500 mL/s of airflow. The data output of the pneumotachograph, as we indicated earlier, can also be converted to measurements of air volume.

Because of the relationships among sound pressure, the intensity of the speech signal, and airflow, it is possible to use acoustic information as a measure of nasal and oral emission of air. This can be done using a device analogous to the divided pneumotachograph, but which uses microphones instead

of airflow sensors and does not require the use of an airtight mask. One microphone is placed at the nares and separated by a baffle from the other, located at the lips. The acoustic strength of the nasal signal divided by the strength of the nasal plus oral signals has been termed a measure of "nasalance" that correlates fairly well with perceived nasality.

Measures of changes in lung volume during speech can be made with a *full body plethysmograph*. This type of plethysmograph is a completely sealed environment in which a speaker stands. As the thorax and the abdomen expand or contract during speech, air is forced out of or sucked into the plethysmograph. The volume of airflow can be measured and displayed as a graphic output by a transducer attached to the airflow sensors in the tubes that penetrate the walls of the plethysmograph.

Plethysmography can also be conducted with a *pneumograph*. Pneumographs may be used to record thoracic and abdominal movement associated with respiratory activity during speech. One type of pneumograph consists of coils of wire that surround the speaker's chest (thorax) and the abdomen. An electric current travels through the coils. During inhalation, the thorax and the abdomen enlarge, causing the wire coils to expand; the reverse happens during exhalation. Changes in the inductance of the current caused by the expansion and contraction of the wire coils are transduced, providing a record of inferred thoracic and abdominal movements. Figure 14.7 displays the graphic output obtained from a pneumograph.

Movements of the chest wall and the abdomen can also be monitored and recorded with a *magnetometer*. Magnetometers, essentially, comprise two coils of wire. An electric current passed through one of them generates an electromagnetic field that induces an electric current in the other coil. The strength of the induced voltage depends on the distance separating the coils. If one coil is placed on a subject's back and another directly opposite on some point along the

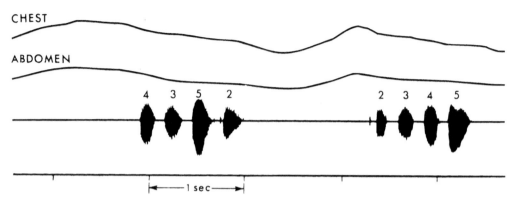

**FIGURE 14.7** Above the time line along the abscissa is the acoustic signal derived from a speaker saying two four-digit number sequences. *Top*: Two pneumographic traces, the top one recorded from a semihemispheric mercury-filled elastic tube placed on the chest; the bottom one is a trace recorded from the abdomen. Upward deflection indicates inspiration.

abdomen or thorax, the changes in the diameters of the rib cage or abdomen can be calculated as a function of the variation in the strength of the induced current. On the assumption that such changes in diameter (caused by the movements of the chest wall and abdomen) are positively correlated with changes in lung volume, it is possible to gain information about patterns of respiratory behavior. This technique presents virtually no risk to the subject and does not interfere with normal respiration during speech. We will note other uses of the magnetometer in the discussion of articulatory analysis.

## LARYNGEAL FUNCTION

Some of the instruments and techniques used to study the larynx and phonation allow us to look directly at the vocal folds; others provide indirect measures of laryngeal function. By using one or another of these instruments and techniques, we can gather information about how the vocal folds behave during phonation, about how they alternate between phonatory and nonphonatory states for the production of voiced and voiceless speech sounds, and about the area and shape of the glottis during speech.

The earliest device that permitted direct viewing of the vocal folds during phonation,

the *laryngoscope*, was developed in 1854 by Manuel Patricio Rodriguez Garcia, a Spanish singing teacher who had taught in Paris and in London. He fashioned a mirror that could be inserted into the mouth and angled in such a way that sunlight shining on it reflected down on the vocal folds, making them visible. Garcia's invention marked the beginning of modern laryngology, and his technique is still used today for laryngeal examinations (albeit without the need of sunlight). Garcia lived more than 100 years (1805–1906), and on his 100th birthday, he was honored with a dinner and received many accolades. It is said that his modest response to it all was, "It was only a mirror!"

Laryngeal activity can be recorded by making very high-speed motion pictures from modern versions of the laryngoscope. The movies can be replayed at speeds appropriate for frame-by-frame analysis. At most fundamental frequencies, however, it is not possible to introduce a cool light source that is sufficiently bright to resolve individual cycles of vibration. Alternatively, it is possible to observe the movements of the vocal folds by using a *stroboscope* (a light flashing at a fixed frequency). If the flash frequency is adjusted to be close to (but not the same as) the frequency of vocal fold vibration, the movements of the folds will appear to be slowed because the frames that appear to be

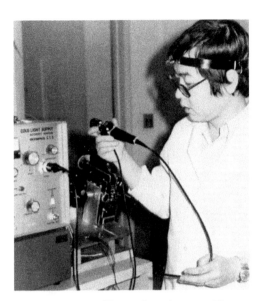

**FIGURE 14.8** A fiberoptic endoscope. The flexible fiber bundle with its objective lens, shown in the physician's left hand, is inserted into the nasal cavity. The larynx can be viewed with the eyepiece, shown in the physician's right hand. (Courtesy of Haskins Laboratories.)

from one cycle of vibration will have been "snapped" from successive cycles. This technique, however, depends on the speaker's ability to phonate at a nearly constant fundamental frequency so that the periods of successive cycles are virtually identical.

As useful as the laryngoscope and the stroboscope may be for viewing the vocal folds, they seriously obstruct the articulators and so they cannot be used effectively for studying glottal behavior during speech. In contrast, the *fiberoptic endoscope*, or *fiberscope*, can be used to view the folds directly during speech production (Fig. 14.8).

The endoscope conveys an image of the glottis through a thin, coherent bundle of glass fibers. The bundle is called coherent because of the way it is constructed: The relative positions of the fibers at both ends of the bundle are exactly the same. This allows each fiber to pick up a small portion of the image and deliver it to the same place within the reconstructed image that is formed at the other end of the bundle. Light is con-

veyed into the larynx from an outside source through additional glass fibers surrounding the coherent bundle. The overall bundle is quite thin (as small as 4 mm in diameter) and flexible. The size and flexibility permit direct viewing of the vocal folds during speech. The fiber bundle is inserted through the nasal cavity, over the top of the velum and down into the pharynx, where its objective lens is suspended above the glottis. The endoscope does not appear to significantly hinder either oral articulation or velopharyngeal closure.

The image that is conveyed can be viewed directly through an eyepiece or recorded on a videotape or film (see Fig. 4.6). It is possible, in the more advanced versions of the endoscope, to record images in color, using moderately high frame rates (which produce slow-motion pictures). The disadvantage of this technique is that the folds often cannot be lighted brightly enough for observation of individual vibratory excursions, as is possible with black-and-white high-speed motion pictures. The technique is, however, useful for direct observation of slower laryngeal adjustments, such as the phonatory repositioning of the vocal folds for voicing and devoicing gestures. It is also possible to obtain information about the shape and the area of the glottis during speech production.

There are two other techniques for obtaining information about variations in glottal states as an indirect measure of vocal fold adjustment. The first of these, *transillumination*, or *photoglottography*, is based on the straightforward notion that the amount of light shining through the glottis is directly proportional to its area (the degree of separation of the vocal folds). The source of the light is again a fiberoptic bundle, inserted though the nose and positioned just as the endoscope is. A photocell, positioned at the level of the "visor," the space between the thyroid and cricoid cartilages, registers the amount of light passing through the glottis at any moment. The changes in glottal area as a function of time are mirrored by the changing output of the photocell (Fig. 14.9). This

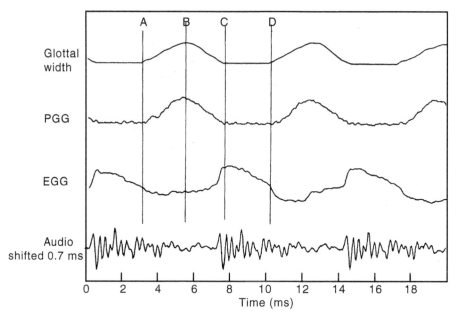

**FIGURE 14.9** Three cycles of vocal fold vibration in a male speaker. The photoglottogram (PGG), obtained by transillumination, corresponds closely to the glottal width measured from high-speed films. Peak deflections of the electroglottogram (EGG) correspond to maximum contact of the vocal folds. *A, D:* onset of vocal fold abduction; *B:* maximum abduction, onset of adduction; *C:* maximum adduction. (Modified with permission from Baer, T., et al., Laryngeal Vibrations: A Comparison Between High-Speed Filming and Glottographic Techniques. *J. Acoust. Soc. Am. 73*, 1983, 1304–1308.)

technique gives no information on the shape of the glottis, unlike endoscopic viewing, but does provide data on the extent of the glottal opening. It is, of course, also useful for providing information about the timing of the changes in glottal area. In addition, it allows resolution of individual vibratory cycles.

The *electroglottograph,* or *laryngograph,* is the second instrument that provides information about glottal states. In a sense, the output of the electroglottograph is the complement of the output of transillumination. Transillumination measures the degree of vocal fold separation, whereas electroglottography (*EGG*) measures the degree of vocal fold contact as a function of the relative conductance or impedance between two small electrodes placed on either side of the larynx. When the glottis is closed and a small electric current is conducted across the folds from one electrode to the other, the EGG signal peaks (Fig. 14.9). But, as the folds separate, the sig-

nal decreases because of the impedance created by the open glottis. The signal must be transmitted along the vocal fold tissue, then across the glottal airspace to the opposite fold, a journey that it fails to make efficiently because of the mismatch of impedances of muscle tissue and air. Hence, the electroglottograph indicates the amount of vocal fold contact during each vibratory cycle. It does not, however, tell us anything about the width or shape of vocal fold opening. Once again, timing information, this time with regard to vocal fold contact, can be obtained from the EGG signal. The EGG signal can also be used to determine the fundamental frequency of vocal fold vibration: The period of vibration (from which fundamental frequency can be calculated) is the time elapsed between two consecutive peaks in the EGG signal. Figure 14.9 illustrates the complementary relation between the measures of glottal width obtained from endoscopy or transillumination and those of vocal fold contact obtained from the EGG signal.

## ARTICULATORY ANALYSIS

Studying the movements of the supralaryngeal articulators presents a difficult challenge for speech scientists. The crux of the problem is the fact that the movements of the most important articulator, the tongue, are very fast, very complex, and, for the most part, not visible to an external sensor. Indeed, even the more slowly moving articulators, except for the lips and the mandible, cannot be observed externally during speech production. As a result, observation of the movements of various parts of the tongue, velum, and walls of the pharynx and oral cavity often require instruments and techniques that are sophisticated, expensive, and sometimes hazardous to use.

Perhaps the most obvious technique for studying articulatory movements, especially tongue shape and position, is x-ray photography. Although this technique was used fairly often for research in the 1970s, even the more recently developed x-ray microbeam system, which delivers relatively low doses of radiation, is no longer being used, partly because it is a complex and expensive system and partly because it carries some health risk. These considerations have led researchers to develop other, less costly, more risk-free techniques to study articulator movement.

One of those techniques is *ultrasound,* the sonar system of the vocal tract. As its name indicates, ultrasound is beyond the range of human hearing. The ultrasound wave that is used to image the vocal tract has a frequency of 1 MHz or more. The wave is emitted from a transducer in contact with the skin below the mandible. Waves of this sort are reflected whenever they cross a border between media of two different densities. Thus, as the sound wave passes from the tissue of the tongue to the less dense air above the tongue, it is reflected to a sensing device on the trans-

ducer. In effect, the sensing device detects an echo of the ultrasound wave. As in the case of the more familiar audible echoes of sound, the greater the time that has elapsed since the emission of the wave, the greater the distance between the transducer and the surface of the tongue.

A visual representation of the echoes can depict most of the oral surface of the tongue because the transducer rotates and so scans a given area with ultrasound waves. The current state of ultrasound technology allows speech scientists to make visual displays of the changes in the shape of the tongue surface at normal rates of speech production. In addition to the sagittal view of the tongue surface, the ultrasound wave can be directed in such a way that the shape of the tongue surface in the coronal plane can be observed (Fig. 14.10), a view that is essential for a complete picture of lingual behavior and one that was essentially unavailable in the past.

In addition to tongue shapes, phoneticians have long been interested in the points of contact between the tongue and the roof of the mouth during the articulation of speech sounds. Indeed, traditional articulatory classifications of consonant production have always included "place of articulation" as a descriptor. A place of articulation can, in most instances, be understood as a point of contact between the tongue and the hard or soft palate. Tongue–palate contact can be investigated by using a technique called *palatography*.

Speech scientists have been using palatography in one form or another for more than a century. In its earliest form, it could be used only to observe isolated, static articulations. A colored powder or paste was placed on a speaker's palate or on a prosthetic device fitted to his palate. The subject would then articulate a single sound (e.g., [s]), and then his palate or the prosthesis was photographed or drawn. The points where the powder had been removed by the tongue or where the smooth surface of the paste was disturbed indicated the points of lingual contact.

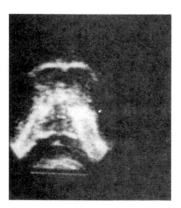 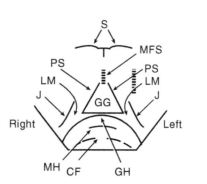 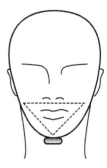

**FIGURE 14.10** *Left*: Coronal ultrasound scan of the surface of the tongue during speech production. *Center*: Schematic view of the ultrasound scan. S, tongue surface; GG, genioglossus muscle; GH, geniohyoid muscle; MH, mylohyoid muscle; MFS, median fibrous septum; LM, lateral muscle; J, jaw, inner aspect; PS, paramedian septum; CF, cervical fascia. *Right*: Diagram of the transducer placement. (Modified with permission from Stone, M., et al., Cross-Sectional Tongue Shape During the Production of Vowels. *J. Acoust. Soc. Am. 83*, 1988, 1586–1596.)

Contemporary palatography, often called *dynamic palatography* or *electropalatography* (EPG), allows investigators to monitor tongue–palate contact during running speech. This is accomplished by fitting the speaker with a palatal prosthesis in which transducers are embedded (Fig. 14.11). Each transducer generates a signal when the tongue touches it. The changing patterns of contact can be recorded and displayed later on a computer screen. They can also be observed as the speaker articulates speech sounds, enabling clinicians and patients to use EPG for instant feedback during therapy.

The EPG prosthesis imposes some limitations on the usefulness of the technique. No transducers are placed at the most anterior portion of the alveolar ridge, on the teeth, or on the velum, and so articulatory contact in these areas is not recorded. Furthermore, the amount of detail in the recorded data depends on the density of transducers in a particular region. A uniform distribution of the transducers on the surface of the prosthesis may thus provide less information than is desired from some areas and more than is needed from others, whereas an uneven distribution may provide a great amount of detail from the area where transducers are concentrated but very little about contact

in other locations. Finally, each EPG prosthesis must be either fitted individually for each subject (they are hard cast from a dental mold) or selected from a set of flexible reusable prostheses held in place with a dental adhesive. The individually fitted prostheses are expensive and may have to be recast if the dental structures of a subject or client undergo change. The reusable prostheses, on

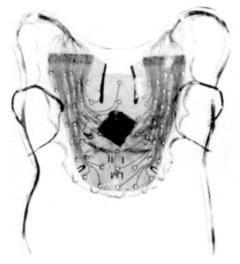

**FIGURE 14.11** An electropalate. (Courtesy of Rion Trading Co., Tokyo.)

the other hand, present the problem of exact relocation for a given subject from one use to the next so that data comparisons from one time to another are valid.

Movements of the jaw and changes in tongue shape have been investigated using magnetometers (discussed earlier under respiratory analysis). In the version of the magnetometer called EMMA (for electromagnetic midsagittal articulometry), generator coils are placed at the top and back of the speaker's head and on the speaker's jaw. The sensor coils are placed along the midline surface of the tongue and on other articulators.

It is possible to interpret the strength of the induced electrical current between the generator and sensor coils as a measure of distance between them, and thus, over time, as a measure of articulator movement. The EMMA system does not cause significant interference with normal articulation.

Movements of the velum can be monitored by using the fiberoptic endoscope. The endoscope is inserted nasally with the objective lens lying on the floor of the nasal cavity at a location appropriate for viewing the velum as it rises and falls during speech. Figure 14.12 displays endoscopic data

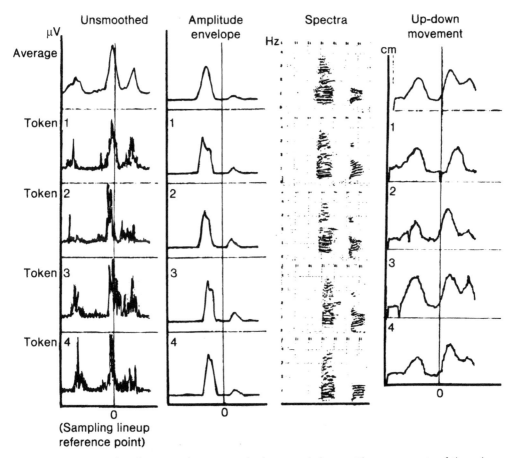

**FIGURE 14.12**  Results of an experiment on velopharyngeal closure. The movements of the velum, recorded by a fiberoptic endoscope, are shown in the rightmost column. Spectrograms and the audio envelope are also shown. The leftmost column shows electromyographic signals from the levator palatini muscle, after rectification. Four individual samples of each token are shown. The top waveform shows an average of 16 tokens. (Courtesy of Haskins Laboratories.)

along with simultaneous electromyographic and acoustic measures relevant to velar elevation.

Finally, we should note that a complete three-dimensional image of the entire vocal tract can be obtained using *magnetic resonance imaging* (MRI). The limitation of this technique is that current MRI machines are capable of producing images only at rather slow rates (although this situation is changing). Thus, although the technique has been used primarily to produce images only for static shapes of the vocal tract, it is valuable because it can provide information in almost any plane of observation. It should be possible, for instance, to clarify the nature of the transfer function of the vocal tract by comparing the calculated output of a static shape with the actual output produced by the speaker whose vocal tract is being imaged.

## MEASURES OF THE NERVOUS SYSTEM

The greatest impact on the study of speech and hearing of recent years is the development of new techniques for visualizing the activity of the brain in connection with normal and abnormal communication processes. Development of these techniques has given us insight into what parts of the brain are active for various normal "mental" processes and allows comparison of populations of speakers or listeners with different characteristics. In what follows, we will describe three techniques and present some typical results from each. We should point out that the equipment involved is generally very expensive, and, unlike some of the other methods we have described in this chapter, may not be found in some colleges or universities. The research we describe is more often (but not exclusively) carried out by a group of collaborating scientists working in a hospital or a specialized laboratory. In such venues, the equipment can be used for several types of speech disorders and the research can be funded by clinical applications. These techniques are undergoing extremely rapid development, with regard to both technology and the kinds of results they can produce.

## Event-Related Potentials

We know from earlier parts of this book that when a neuron fires, it creates an electrical field that travels along its axon. There are so many neurons in the central nervous system that they can, by firing simultaneously, create an electrical field that can be detected on the outside of the skull. For recording such activity, it is conventional to cover the surface of the subject's skull with equally spaced electrodes positioned as shown in Figure 14.13.

As much as 50 years ago, this technique was used to record the overall activity of the brain. It was found that the neuron aggregates of the brain display characteristic frequencies, changing from one rhythm to another, particularly during the stages of sleeping and waking. In different overall states, a Fourier analysis of the output of the cortical electrodes has different dominant frequencies. Thus, "alpha" activity (8 to 13 Hz) is dominant when the brain is at rest, but when

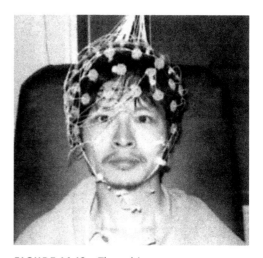

**FIGURE 14.13**   The subject wears a sensor net of electrodes used to record event-related potentials from the brain. (Courtesy of Valerie Shaeffer, City University of New York.)

the individual is in deep sleep, the dominant brain rhythm shifts to a "delta" rhythm of less than 4 Hz.

Although such analyses have been useful in diagnosing sleep disorders, it is more relevant to our purposes to study *event-related potentials,* or ERPs. If a stimulus is played into a subject's ear, it will evoke a response at the cortex that will be recorded by electrodes on the skull surface. Because the response to a single stimulus is quite small in electrical terms (1 to 10 μV), a signal-averaging method is used to increase the magnitude of the signal relative to the response of the overall background electroencephalogram. Figure 14.14 shows the effect on the signal of averaging an increasing number of responses to a single stimulus.

The response to a given stimulus is described in terms of the negative and positive peaks and their latency. Early components of the response to an auditory stimulus depend primarily on the intensity components of a stimulus, whereas later components (in particular, those occurring about 100 milliseconds after the stimulus, the N2 response) depend on whether or not the subject is attending to the stimulus (Fig. 14.15).

Although ERP techniques provide very precise information about the timing of a cortical response, it is difficult to be sure where the responsible group of neural elements is located in the brain. The techniques described below are far superior for describing the brain location of the events they record, but they do not record the time course of those events nearly as well.

## An ERP Experiment on the Categorical Perception of Speech Sounds

Anita Maiste and her colleagues (1995) at the University of Toronto studied the cortical response to a series of nine synthetic speech stimuli ranging from /ba/ to /da/, in equal frequency steps along an $F_2$ continuum. The listeners heard the first stimulus, at the /ba/ end of the continuum, 52% of the time, and each of the remaining eight stimuli was pre-

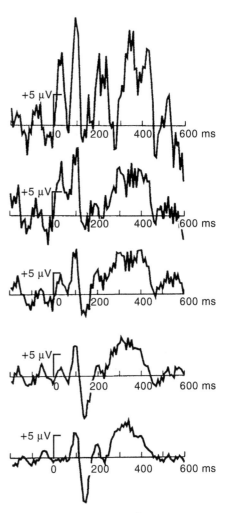

**FIGURE 14.14** Recordings from an event-related potential (ERP) experiment. Each waveform shows the averaged electrical activity recorded for 1 second after the presentation of a word. The number of waveforms averaged increases from top to bottom. *Top:* A single ERP trace. The common pattern is obscured by the noise in the signal, but it is quite clear in the bottom trace. (Reprinted with permission from Posner, M. I., and Raichle, M. E., *Images of Mind.* New York: Scientific American Library, 1997.)

sented 6% of the time. Thus, the subjects heard the first stimulus frequently and the other eight stimuli relatively rarely. (These stimuli are similar to those shown in Chapter 6, although the technique of stimulus

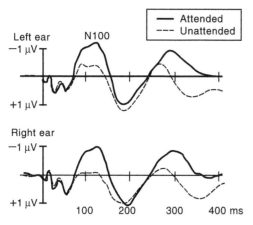

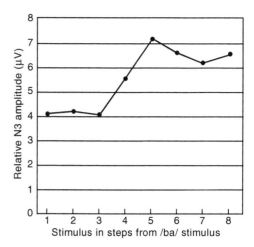

**FIGURE 14.15** Recordings from an event-related potential (ERP) experiment. The subjects heard sequences of tones in both ears but were asked to detect targets only in an attended ear. The negative wave, marked as N100, is larger in the attended than in the unattended ear. (Reprinted with permission from Frackowiak, R. S. J., Friston, K. J., Frith, C. D., Dolan, R. J., and Mazziotta, J. C., *Human Brain Function.* New York: Academic Press, 1997.)

**FIGURE 14.16** Relative amplitude of the N2 peak as a function of distance from the most frequently presented /ba/ stimulus. (Reprinted with permission from Maiste, A. C., Wiens, A. S., Hunt, M. J., Scherg, M., and Picton, T., Event Related Potentials and the Categorical Perception of Speech Sounds. *Ear Hear. 16,* 1995, 68–90.)

construction was different.) The subjects identified the first three stimuli of the continuum as /ba/, whereas the other stimuli were heard, in varying degrees, as /da/. The three stimuli identified as /ba/ evoked a small N2 response to the stimulus. The remaining six stimuli evoked a larger N2 response (Fig. 14.16).

In other words, the subjects responded to the three stimuli on the /ba/ end of the continuum as common and identical to each other, and provided a stronger N2 response to the stimuli on the /da/ end of the continuum because they were rarely presented. Thus, there was a clear discontinuity at the /ba–da/ boundary, and perception was categorical within each of the two categories.

## Positron Emission Tomography

A second technique in common use for brain visualization is positron emission tomography (PET). A similar technique is single-photon emission computed tomogra-

phy (SPECT). Both techniques are inherently invasive, and hence, they cannot be freely used on all subjects. Both, however, unlike ERP, allow the clear localization of the brain response to different experimental conditions.

The recording instrument for a PET study is a doughnut-shaped set of radiation detectors. The subject of an experiment is first injected in the arm with a small dose of radioactive-labeled water and is positioned lying down in a body-sized tube, surrounded by the round PET camera. During the minute after the injection, the radioisotope accumulates in the brain. The accumulation in a given brain region is proportional to the regional blood flow, which, in turn, reflects the amount of neural activity in the region. The PET camera records the amount of radioactive activity in the regions of a slice of the brain.

It is common to use the so-called "subtraction method" in studying the response to a given experimental condition. That is, a control condition is compared with an experimental condition by subtracting the

## CLINICAL NOTE

The instruments and techniques for the physiologic investigation of speech production have obvious clinical relevance, although it should be clear from our discussion that many of them are inappropriate for use in most clinical venues. There are several reasons for this: Some of the techniques (such as endoscopic examination of the larynx) are too invasive to be used outside of a hospital or laboratory setting. Other techniques, such as magnetic resonance imaging and magnetometry, require sophisticated instruments and technical support services that are well beyond the budget of the average clinic. But there are partial exceptions to this prohibition, even among some of the most invasive and costly techniques. For instance, if a clinician is seeking data about superficial muscle activity, it can be obtained relatively easily from the sort of "paint-on" electrodes that we have described above. Similarly, it is possible for a clinician to forgo the expense of making prosthetic palates when it is reasonable to use the reusable flexible palates to gather EPG information about tongue–palate contact.

Several devices and techniques, on the other hand, are very compatible with the resources, both technical and budgetary, of many clinics. Such tools are often commercially available at a reasonable cost and are backed up by PC-compatible, user-friendly software and by support services from the manufacturer. These include, among the techniques we have outlined, electroglottography, pneumography, and ultrasound. All of these tools (and some others which we have not had the space to include in this chapter) can be used to provide instantaneous feedback to clients about their respiratory, phonatory, and articulatory behavior.

response of the inactive brain condition, region by region, from the response in a condition for which the brain is active. For example, the control condition for a visual experiment might be gazing at a stationary point. The experimental condition might be gazing at a flickering checkerboard. The brain activity added by the checkerboard condition would be estimated by subtracting from it the brain images of the control condition. It is also common to use complex statistical techniques to normalize for differences in the size and shape of brain structures in different individuals. Statistical techniques also allow researchers who have gathered data in one plane to transform it to another. For example, views obtained in a coronal plane may be transformed to sagittal plane views by such statistical rotations.

## Some Experiments on Stuttering

A particularly significant clinical finding of recent years can be attributed to PET and SPECT studies of developmental stuttering. As you will recall from the early work of Penfield and Roberts, and the Wada test results, cited in Chapter 3, in normal individuals there is ordinarily greater brain activity for speech and language in the left cortex than in the right. An early study by a group of researchers at Callier Center showed a different result for individuals who stutter: Right hemisphere activity was greater than left in stutterers as compared with normal subjects in rest conditions. However, because of the limited time that SPECT experiments permit for the study of a given subject, it remained for PET studies to show similar results in multiple speech tasks using the same subjects for the series.

Braun and co-researchers (1997) showed left-hemisphere lateralization of activation in nonstutterers contrasted with relative right-hemisphere lateralization of stutterers in a variety of oral motor tasks. Fox and Ingham showed a similar pattern of aberrant activation for oral and choral reading for stutterers. Finally, in an ingenious preliminary study, Kroll and De Nil (1995) examined the pattern of brain activity in persons who had stuttered but had shown marked improvement after a standardized intensive course of fluency shaping. Even though the treated stutterers were using the techniques for controlling stuttering that they had learned in therapy, and therefore did not stutter during the oral reading task during the experiment, they still showed overactivity in the right hemisphere compared with normal subjects. The results thus suggest that treatment does not lead to a change in the underlying "normal" behavior. Although much of this work is preliminary with respect to identifying precisely the areas of the brain that show abnormal activity patterns in subjects who stutter, and under what conditions, these studies indicate the profound effects brain imaging studies can be expected to have on brain–behavior correlation in clinical populations in the future.

## Magnetic Imaging

The invasiveness of some of the imaging techniques (such as PET) developed by medical science and adapted for use by speech scientists has been a concern for many years. One of the earliest of these invasive techniques, developed about 1970, was x-ray tomography, or computed tomography (CT), also known as the CAT scan. The principle underlying CT is that if a highly focused beam of x-rays is passed through some bodily structure, such as the brain, it can create an image on a photographic plate, in which the darkness of the image varies with the density of the tissue. Thus, if the brain of a person who has had a stroke is exposed to x-rays, the damaged tissue will show up as a darker area, in contrast to the normal tissue. The CT scan is familiar to every aphasiologist or to any speech pathologist who deals with stroke patients. Although in recent years x-ray imaging techniques have proliferated, less invasive techniques have been developed, and it is hoped that they will be

valuable for studies of normal as well as disordered speech. At present, the technique with the greatest promise appears to be functional MRI (fMRI), a descendant of a slightly different predecessor, MRI. It has substantial advantages over both CT and PET, requiring neither the x-ray dosage for the former nor the injection of a radioactive isotope of the latter. Moreover, the MRI techniques offer superior temporal and spatial image resolution over PET.

For an MRI experiment, the subject is placed in an apparatus that looks rather like that used in a PET experiment, in that he is lying prone in a tube. In this case, a strong magnetic field surrounds the individual. It aligns atoms in the structures in a region of the brain. Radiofrequency pulses tip the atoms off their axes of spin, and, as they return to their previous axes, they give off a signal that can be recorded on a photographic plate. The image shows the distribution of hydrogen atoms in the pictured tissue. Whereas ordinary x-ray is sensitive to bone, MRI shows distinctions in soft tissues, such as contrasts among cortical white matter, cerebrospinal fluid, and gray matter. These images can reflect the structures of the brain almost as they appear in anatomy texts. The images shown by MRI depend on the precise way the scanning is done. A brain structure may be made more or less visible depending on the parameters of the scan. It is worth noting that PET and MRI images can be brought into alignment by special techniques, so that results obtained 10 years ago with PET can be confirmed by the more sensitive MRI.

## An fMRI Experiment

This experiment is one of a series by a number of laboratories seeking answers to questions about the subprocesses involved in recognizing words. We have had substantial evidence, since the time of the work of Wada, that speech production and perception are located primarily in the left hemisphere in most individuals. Modern brain imaging studies enable us to make this general finding far more specific.

A pair of experiments by Burton, Small, and Blumstein (2000) illustrates this kind of research. At issue was the question of what parts of the cortex are involved in different subprocesses of speech perception. In the first experiment, subjects were exposed in the magnet, with earphones on so that they could hear pairs of tones or words. The tones differed in pitch, whereas the words differed only in the voicing of the initial consonant, for example, "tip" versus "dip." For each pair of stimuli, the subject responded by pressing a button in one hand for "same" and in the other hand for "different." The result for words showed that there was brain activity along the top strip of the temporal lobe at one location anterior to the primary auditory area and at another posterior to it. Activity was always greater on the left side of the brain than on the right, as we would expect. There was no area where there was greater activity for tone discrimination than for speech stimulus discrimination.

In the second experiment, the tone stimuli and the subjects' task were the same, but the speech task was made somewhat more difficult. The pairs of speech stimuli differed not only in the first phone but in all three phones. For example, "tip" might be contrasted with "dean." The task of the subject was the same as in the first experiment, that is, to discriminate the voicing status of the initial phones as the same or different regardless of the differences between the other phones in the two words. The results of the second experiment were, in part, the same as those of the first one: no cortical regions showed more activity for the tone comparison than for the word comparison; activity was greater in the left hemisphere than in the right hemisphere; the same activity as in the first experiment was seen in the temporal lobe, in the same locations. There was, however, a new active area in the frontal lobe, Broca's area, an area heavily involved in articulation, although no articulation was required of the subjects.

The experimenters' explanation was that because the three phones in the stimulus pair were different, the listener was required to segment them perceptually, and this effort forced the subject to engage in articulatory recoding, hence the involvement of Broca's area. Other explanations, however, are possible, and further research will be required to decide which is most plausible.

The inventory of devices and techniques we have discussed for observing and measuring aspects of speech production is far from exhaustive. More complete listings and explanations are available elsewhere. Moreover, the state of the art in instrumentation is changing rapidly. Existing devices are continually being improved and modified, and new instruments and techniques appear with great frequency. Staying abreast of developments requires constant and careful attention to the research and clinical literature.

## BIBLIOGRAPHY

### General Readings

#### *Comprehensive*

Baken, R. J., and Orlikoff, R. F., *Clinical Voice and Speech Measurement.* San Diego: Singular Publishing Group, 1993.

Baken, R. J., and Orlikoff, R. F., *Clinical Measurement of Speech and Voice,* 2nd ed. San Diego: Singular Publishing Group, 2000.

Frackowiak, R. S. J., Friston, K. J., Frith, C. D., Dolan, R. J., and Mazziotta, J. C., *Human Brain Function.* New York: Academic Press, 1997.

Hardcastle, W. J., and Laver, J. (Eds.), *The Handbook of the Phonetic Sciences.* Malden, MA: Blackwell Publishers, 1999.

Posner, M. I., and Raichle, M. E., *Images of Mind.* New York: Scientific American Library, 1997.

Rosen, S., and Howell, P., *Signals and Systems for Speech and Hearing.* London: Academic Press, 1991.

Stone, M., Laboratory Techniques for Investigating Speech Articulation. In *The Handbook of the Phonetic Sciences.* W. J. Hardcastle and

J. Laver (Eds.). Malden, MA: Blackwell Publishers, 1999, pp. 11–32.

## Physiological Phonetics

Abbs, J. H., and Watkin, K. L., Instrumentation for the Study of Speech Physiology. In *Contemporary Issues in Experimental Phonetics*. N. J. Lass (Ed.). New York: Academic Press, 1976, pp. 41–78.

Atkinson, J. E., Correlation Analysis of the Physiological Factors Controlling Fundamental Voice Frequency. *J. Acoust. Soc. Am. 63,* 1978, 211–222.

Borden, G. J., An Interpretation of Research on Feedback Interruption. *Brain Lang. 7,* 1979, 307–319.

Farnetani, E., Coarticulation and Connected Speech Processes. In *The Handbook of the Phonetic Sciences*. W. J. Hardcastle and J. Laver (Eds.). Malden, MA: Blackwell Publishers, 1999, pp. 371–405.

Harris, K. S., Physiological Aspects of Articulatory Behavior. In *Current Trends in Linguistics*. Vol. 12, No. 4, T. A. Sebeok (Ed.). The Hague, The Netherlands: Mouton, 1974, pp. 2281–2302.

Maiste, A. C., Wiens, A. S., Hunt, M. J., Scherg, M., and Picton, T., Event Related Potentials and the Categorical Perception of Speech Sounds. *Ear Hear. 16,* 1995, 68–90.

Ong, D., and Stone, M., Three Dimensional Vocal Tract Shapes in /r/ and /l/: A Study of MRI, Ultrasound, Electropalatography, and Acoustics. *Phonoscope 1,* 1998, 1–3.

Orlikoff, R. F., Vocal Stability and Vocal Tract Configuration: An Acoustic and Electroglottographic Investigation. *J. Voice 9,* 1995, 173–181.

Perkell, J., Cohen, M., Svirsky, M., Mathies, M., Garabieta, I., and Jakson, M., Electromagnetic Midsagittal Articulometer (EMMA) Systems for Transducing Speech Articulatory Movements. *J. Acoust. Soc. Am. 92,* 1992, 3078–3096.

Sawashima, M., and Cooper, F. S. (Eds.), *Dynamic Aspects of Speech Production*. Tokyo: University of Tokyo Press, 1977.

Seaver, E. J., Leeper, H. A., and Adams, L. E., A Study of Nasometric Values for Normal Nasal Resonance. *J. Speech Hear. Res. 34,* 1991, 358–362.

Stone, M., Faber, A., Raphael, L. J., and Shawker, T., Cross-Sectional Tongue Shape and Linguopalatal Contact Patterns in [s], [ʃ], and [l]. *J. Phonet. 20,* 1992, 253–270.

Warren, D. W., Regulation of Speech Aerodynamics. In *Principles of Experimental Phonetics*. N. J. Lass (Ed.). St. Louis: Mosby, 1996, pp. 46–92.

## Instrumentation and Clinical Applications

Allen, G. D., Lubker, J. F., and Harrison, E., Jr., New Paint-on Electrodes for Surface Electromyography. *J. Acoust. Soc. Am. 52,* 1972, 124 (A).

Baer, T., Löfquist, A., and McGarr, N., Laryngeal Vibrations: A Comparison Between High-Speed Filming and Glottographic Techniques. *J. Acoust. Soc. Am. 73,* 1983, 1304–1308.

Baer, T., Gore, J., Gracco, L. C., and Nye, P. W., Analysis of Vocal Tract Shape and Dimensions Using Magnetic Resonance Imaging: Vowels. *J. Acoust. Soc. Am. 90,* 1991, 799–828.

Barlow, S. M. (Ed.), *Handbook of Clinical Speech Physiology*. San Diego: Singular Publishing Group, 1999.

Bless, D. M., Assessment of Laryngeal Function. In *Phono-Surgery: Assessment and Surgical Management of Voice Disorders*. C. N. Ford and D. M. Bless (Eds.). New York: Raven Press, 1991, pp. 91–122.

Braun, A. R., Varga, M., Stager, S., Schulz, G., Selbie, S., Maisog, J. M., Carson, R. L., and Ludlow, C. L., Atypical Lateralization of Hemispherical Activity in Developmental Stuttering: An $H_2^{15}O$ Positron Emission Tomography Study. In *Speech Production: Motor Control, Brain Research and Fluency Disorders*. W. Hulstijn, H. F. M. Peters, and P. H. H. M. van Lieshout (Eds.). Amsterdam, The Netherlands: Elsevier, 1997, pp. 279–292.

Burton, M. W., Small, S. L., and Blumstein, S., The Role of Segmentation in Phonological Processing: An fMRI Investigation. *J. Cogn. Neurosci. 12,* 2000, 679–690.

Cohen, K. P., Panescu, D., Booske, J. H., Webster, J. G., and Tompkins, W. J., Design of an Inductive Plethysmograph for Ventilation Measurement. *Physiol. Meas. 15,* 1994, 217–229.

De Nil, L. F., and Kroll, R. M., The Relationship Between Locus of Control and Long-Term

Treatment Outcome in Adults Who Stutter. *J. Fluency Disord. 20,* 1995, 345–364.

Fletcher, S. G., McCutcheon, M. J., and Wolf, M. B., Dynamic Palatometry. *J. Speech Hear. Res. 18,* 1975, 812–819.

Fourcin, A. J., Laryngographic Examination of Vocal Fold Vibration. In *Ventilatory and Phonatory Control Systems: An International Symposium.* B. Wyke (Ed.). London: Oxford University Press, 1974, pp. 315–326.

Gentil, M., and Moore, W. H., Jr., Electromyography. In *Instrumental Clinical Phonetics.* M. J. Ball and C. Code (Eds.). London: Whurr Publishers, 1997, pp. 64–86.

Gerratt, B. R., Haison, D. G., and Burke, G., Glottographic Measures of Laryngeal Function in Individuals With Abnormal Motor Control. In *Laryngeal Function in Phonation and Respiration.* T. Baer, C. Sasaki, and K. S. Harris (Eds.). Boston: College Hill Press, 1987, pp. 521–532.

Hardcastle, W. J., and Gibbon, F. E., Electropalatography and Its Clinical Applications. In *Instrumental Clinical Phonetics.* M. J. Ball and C. Code (Eds.). London: Whurr Publishers, 1997, pp. 149–193.

Harris, K. S., Electromyography as a Technique for Laryngeal Investigation. In *Proceedings of the Conference on the Assessment of Vocal Pathology (ASHA Reports 11).* C. L. Ludlow and M. D. Hart (Eds.). Washington, DC: American Speech-Language-Hearing Association, 1981, 116–124.

Hirano, M., and Ohala, J., Use of Hooked-Wire Electrodes for Electromyography of the Intrinsic Laryngeal Muscles. *J. Speech Hear. Res. 12,* 1969, 362–373.

Hirose, H., Gay, T., and Strome, M., Electrode Insertion Techniques for Laryngeal Electromyography. *J. Acoust. Soc. Am. 50,* 1971, 1449–1450.

Ingham, R. J., Fox, P. T., and Ingham, J. C., An $H_2O5$ Position Emission Tomography (PET) Study on Adults Who Stutter: Findings and Implications. In *Speech Production: Motor Control, Brain Research and Fluency Disorders.* W. Hulstijn, H. F. M. Peters, and P. H. H. M. van Lieshout (Eds.). Amsterdam, The Netherlands: Elsevier, 1997, pp. 293–307.

Kroll, R. M., De Nil, L., Kapur, S., and Houle, S., A Positron Emission Tomography Investigation of Post-Treatment Brain Activation in

Stutterers. In *Speech Production: Motor Control, Brain Research and Fluency Disorders.* W. Hulstijn, H. F. M. Peters, and P. H. H. M. van Lieshout (Eds.). Amsterdam, The Netherlands: Elsevier, 1997, pp. 307–320.

Lauter, J. L., Noninvasive Brain Imaging in Speech Motor Control and Stuttering. In *Speech Production: Motor Control, Brain Research and Fluency Disorders.* W. Hulstijn, H. F. M. Peters, and P. H. H. M. van Lieshout (Eds.). Amsterdam, The Netherlands: Elsevier, 1997, pp. 233–258.

Lester, D. S., Felder, C. C., and Lewis, E. N. (Eds.), *Imaging Brain Structure and Function.* New York: New York Academy of Sciences, 1997.

Lisker, L., Abramson, A. S., Cooper, F. S., and Schvey, M. H., Transillumination of the Larynx in Running Speech. *J. Acoust. Soc. Am. 45,* 1969, 1544–1546.

Pool, K. D., Devous, M. D., Freeman, F. J., Watson, B. C., and Finitzo, T., Regional Cerebral Blood Flow in Developmental Stutterers. *Arch. Neurol. 48,* 1997, 509–512.

Rothenberg, M., Measurement of Airflow in Speech. *J. Speech Hear. Res. 20,* 1977, 155–176.

Saito, S., Fukuda, H., Kitihara, S., and Kokawa, N., Stroboscopic Observation of Vocal Fold Vibration With Fiberoptics. *Folia Phoniatr. 30,* 1978, 241–244.

Sawashima, M., Abramson, A. S., Cooper, F. S., and Lisker, L., Observing Laryngeal Adjustments During Running Speech by Use of a Fiberoptics System. *Phonetica 22,* 1970, 193–201.

Stone, M., Sonies, B., Shawker, T., Weiss, G., and Nadel, L., Analysis of Real-Time Ultrasound Images of Tongue Configurations Using a Grid-Digitizing System. *J. Phonet. 13,* 1983, 189–203.

Unger, J., The Oral Cavity and Tongue: Magnetic Resonance Imaging. *Radiology 155,* 1985, 151–153.

Watkin, K. L., and Zagzebski, J. A., On-Line Ultrasonic Technique for Monitoring Tongue Displacements. *J. Acoust. Soc. Am. 54,* 1973, 544–547.

Watson, B. C., Pool, K. D., Devous, M. D., Freeman, F. J., and Finitzo, T., Brain Blood Flow Related to Acoustic Laryngeal Reaction Time in Adult Developmental Stutterers. *J. Speech Hear. Res. 35,* 1992, 555–561.

# The Phonetic Alphabet for American English

Based on the International Phonetic Alphabet

## THE SOUNDS OF AMERICAN ENGLISH[a]

| Vowel Sounds | Key Words |
|---|---|
| i | each, free, keep |
| ɪ | it, bin |
| e | ate, made, they |
| ɛ | end, then, there |
| æ | act, man |
| a | ask, half, past |
| ɑ | alms, father |
| ɒ | hot, odd, dog, cross |
| ɔ | awl, torn |
| o | obey, note, go |
| ʊ | good, foot |
| u | ooze, too |
| ə | alone, among |
| ɚ | father, singer |
| ʌ | up, come |
| ɜ, ɝ | urn, third |

| Vowel Combinations (Diphthongs) | Key Words |
|---|---|
| eɪ | aid, may |
| aɪ | aisle, sigh |
| ɔɪ | oil, joy |
| aʊ | owl, cow |
| oʊ | own, go |

| Consonant Sounds | Key Words |
| --- | --- |
| p | pie, ape |
| b | be, web |
| m | me, am |
| w | we, woe |
| ʌ | why, when |
| f | free, if |
| v | vine, have |
| θ | thin, faith |
| ð | then, clothe |
| t | ten, it |
| d | den, had |
| n | no, one |
| l | live, frill |
| s | see, yes |
| z | zoo, as |
| r | red, arrow |
| ʃ | show, ash |
| ʒ | measure, azure |
| j | you, yes |
| ç | huge, human |
| k | key, ache |
| g | go, big |
| ŋ | sing, long |
| h | he, how |

## Consonant Combinations (Affricates)

| | |
| --- | --- |
| tʃ | chew, each |
| dʒ | gem, hedge |

[a] Adapted from Bronstein, A. J. *The Pronunciation of American English*. New York: Appleton-Century-Crofts, Inc., 1960, pp. 28–30. Appendix.

# Nerves Important for Speech and Hearing

## Cranial and Spinal

## CRANIAL NERVES IMPORTANT FOR SPEECH AND HEARING

| | | | |
|---|---|---|---|
| I | Olfactory | Nose | |
| II | Optic | Eye | |
| III | Oculomotor | Eye | |
| IV | Trochlear | Eye | |
| [a]V | Trigeminal | Face | Motor to jaw muscles and to tensor palatini muscle; sensory from anterior two thirds of tongue |
| VI | Abducent | Eye | |
| [a]VII | Facial | Face | Motor to lip muscles |
| [a]VIII | Auditory | Ear | Sensory from cochlea with some motor fibers |
| [a]IX | Glossopharyngeal | Pharynx | Motor to pharynx; sensory from back of tongue |
| [a]X | Vagus | Larynx | Motor to laryngeal muscles |
| [a]XI | Accessory | Soft palate | Motor to levator palatini |
| [a]XII | Hypoglossal | Tongue | Motor to tongue muscles |

[a]Only functions related to speech and hearing are listed.

## SPINAL NERVES IMPORTANT FOR SPEECH

| | | | |
|---|---|---|---|
| [a]C1–C8 | Cervical | Neck | C3–C5 phrenic nerve to diaphragm |
| [a]T1–T12 | Thoracic | Chest | T1–T11 to intercostal muscles<br>T7–T12 to abdominal muscles |

[a]Only functions related to speech are listed. The dorsal roots (emerging from the back of the spine) are sensory. The ventral roots (emerging from the front of the spine) are motor.

# Glossary

**Abduct:** [L. "ab"–away, off.] To move away from the midsagittal axis of the body or one of its parts.

**Abscissa:** The $x$ coordinate of a point; its distance from the $y$ axis measured parallel to the $x$ axis (horizontal axis).

**Absolute Threshold of Audibility:** Magnitude of a sound detected by a listener 50% of the time.

**ABX Test:** Procedure for testing discrimination by requiring the listener to indicate whether the third stimulus presented (X) sounds more like the first or the second (A or B).

**Acceleration:** The time rate of change of velocity.

**Acoustic Reflex:** A bilateral reflex of the middle ear in response to loud sounds that alters middle ear impedance.

**Acoustic Resonator:** Air-filled structure designed to vibrate at particular frequencies.

**Acoustics:** [Gk. "akoustikos"–hearing.] The study of sound.

**Action Potential:** An electrical discharge that stimulates muscle activity.

**Action Theory:** A theory put forth by Fowler and Turvey that applies an ecologic view of motor coordination to speech production and perception.

**Adaptation Studies:** Tests of speech identification and discrimination administered after the listener has been repeatedly exposed to a particular stimulus, one that is usually the first or the last of an experimental continuum of stimuli.

**Adduct:** [L. "ad"–toward, to.] To move toward the midsagittal plane of the body or one of its parts.

**Afferent:** [L. "ferre"–to bear.] Bringing to or into; in the nervous system, neurons conducting from the periphery toward the central nervous system (sensory nerves, neurons).

**Affricate Sound:** A speech sound during which a stop closure is followed by a fricative release; one of the manners of consonant articulation.

**All-or-None Principle:** Principle stating that when a single nerve is stimulated at or above threshold, it fires at an amplitude independent of the intensity of the stimulus.

**Allophone:** One member of the family of sounds constituting a phoneme:–[pʰ] is an allophone of the phoneme /p/.

**Alpha (α) Motor Neurons:** Large efferent nerve fibers (8 to 20 μm in diameter) that innervate the skeletal muscles.

**Alveolar Process:** The inferior border of the maxillary bone or the superior border of the mandible; contains sockets holding the teeth.

**Alveolar Ridge:** The ridge behind the upper incisors with which the tongue apex makes contact to produce a variety of speech sounds in English.

**Amplitude:** (of a Wave) The absolute value of the maximum displacement from a zero value during one period of an oscillation.

**Amplitude Spectrum:** (pl. spectra.) A graphic representation of acoustic speech signal in which the abscissa (the horizontal axis) represents the component harmonic or resonant (formant) frequencies and the ordinate (the vertical axis) represents the amplitudes of the component frequencies.

**Analog-to-Digital Converter:** Electronic device that transforms continuous signals into signals with discrete values.

**Analysis-by-Synthesis Theory:** A theory which states that speech analysis or perception involves some form of rudimentary reconstruction or synthesis of the acoustic signal.

**Anterior Belly of the Digastric Muscle:** Paired muscle running from the mandible to the hyoid; aids in jaw opening.

**Anterior Faucial Pillars:** (also called the glossopalatine arch) Arch-like downward continuations of the soft palate containing the glossopalatine muscles.

**Antiresonance:** A filtering effect of the vocal tract characterized by loss of acoustic energy in a particular frequency region.

**Aperiodic:** Pertaining to vibrations with irregular periods. A waveform with no repetitive pattern.

**Aphasia:** [Gk. "a"–not + "phanai"–to speak.] Partial or total loss of the ability to use or understand language after damage to the brain.

**Apraxia:** Difficulty in the voluntary coordination of muscles that function normally for involuntary acts.

**Articulation:** Shaping of the vocal tract to produce speech sounds.

**Arytenoid:** [Gk. ladle shaped.] Triangular cartilages to which the vocal folds attach.

**Assimilation:** [L. "similis"–like, to become like.] A change in the articulation of a speech sound that makes it more similar to the articulation of a neighboring sound.

**Athetosis:** [Gk. "athetos"–without position or place.] A condition in which parts of the body constantly make slow, writhing involuntary motions.

**Audition:** Hearing.

**Auditory Agnosia:** ["a"–not + Gk. "gnosis"–knowledge.] Central auditory imperception of sound.

**Auditory Nerve:** Cranial nerve VIII. A sensory nerve with two branches: the vestibular, which carries information about bodily position, and the cochlear, which carries auditory information; also called the vestibulocochlear nerve and the acoustic nerve, respectively.

**Auricle:** [L. "auris"–ear.] The visible cartilage of the outer ear; also called the pinna.

**Autism:** [Gk. "autos"–self.] A syndrome characterized by difficulty in forming interpersonal relationships and in developing language.

**Autistic Theory:** A theory stating that children are internally rewarded for subvocal rehearsal of new words.

**Axon:** [Gk. "axon"–axis.] The part of a neuron that carries impulses away from the cell body.

**Babbling Stage:** The prelinguistic period during which infants produce sounds with no semantic reference.

**Basal Ganglia:** [Gk. "ganglion"–knot.] A collection of gray masses embedded in the white matter of each cerebral hemisphere (consisting of the corpus striatum, the claustrum, and the amygdaloid nucleus).

**Basilar Membrane:** Thin membrane forming the base of the organ of Corti that vibrates in response to different frequencies of sound and stimulates individual sensory hair cells in the organ of Corti.

**Bernoulli Effect:** The pressure drop caused by the increased velocity of a gas or liquid through a constricted passage.

**Body Plethysmograph:** An instrument in the form of a sealed box used to measure air displacement produced by respiratory movements.

**Brainstem:** The midbrain, pons, and medulla oblongata.

**Breath Group:** A segment of speech normally produced on a single expiration.

**Buccal Cavity:** [L. "bucca"–cheek.] The air space between the teeth and the cheeks.

**Carotid Artery:** [Gk. "karro"–sleep, stupor.] Principal artery of the neck supplying blood to the brain.

**CAT:** (Scan) See computed tomography.

**Categorical Perception:** The ability to discriminate (speech) stimuli only as well as one can label them.

**Catheter:** A slender tube inserted into a body passage or cavity.

**Central Nervous System:** (CNS) The portion of the nervous system consisting of the brain and the spinal cord.

**Central Tendency:** A value chosen as typical of a collection of measures.

**Cerebellum:** [L. diminutive of cerebrum.] A main division of the brain behind the cerebrum and above the pons; its function is to coordinate movement.

**Cerebral Hemispheres:** The two halves of the cerebrum; the main portion of the brain.

**Cerebral Palsy:** A group of disorders characterized by paralysis or muscular incoordination caused by intracranial lesion at or near the time of birth.

**Cerebral Vascular Accident:** (CVA, stroke) A clot or rupture of the blood vessels of the brain resulting in damage to the nervous system.

**Cerumen:** [L. "cere"–wax.] Earwax.

**Cervical Nerve:** [L. "cervix"–neck.] One of eight pairs of spinal nerves that arise from the segments of the spinal cord in the neck region.

**Cilia:** Hairlike processes found in the external auditory meatus, cochlea, and other parts of the body.

**Clavicle:** [L. "clavicula"–bolt.] The collarbone.

**Cleft Palate:** Congenital fissure in the roof of the mouth.

**Closed-Loop System:** A system operating under feedback control.

**CNS:** See central nervous system.

**Coarticulation:** A temporal overlap of articulatory movements for different phones.

**Cochlea:** The snail-shaped cavity of the inner ear that contains the sense organs for hearing.

**Cochlear Duct:** The membranous labyrinth of the cochlea that contains the organ of Corti; also called cochlear partition and scala media.

**Cognate:** (Voice) A pair of sounds, identical in place and manner of articulation, that differ only in that one is phonated and the other is not (e.g., /v/ and /f/).

**Collective Monologue:** Several people speaking as if alone but taking turns as if in conversation.

**Complex Tone:** Sound having more than one sine wave component.

**Computed Tomography:** (CT, also CAT) Radiographic imaging in a cross-sectional plane of the body. Each image is synthesized by computer analysis of x-rays transmitted in many directions in a given plane.

**Conditioned Response:** (CR) In classical conditioning, a response elicited by a previously neutral stimulus; in Pavlov's experiment, the salivation elicited by the bell alone after the bell was associated with meat powder.

**Conditioned Stimulus:** (CS) In classical conditioning, a previously neutral stimulus that comes to elicit a response; in Pavlov's experiment, the bell that elicited salivation.

**Contact Ulcers:** Points of erosion in the cartilaginous portions of the vocal folds apparently caused by forceful adduction.

**Continuant:** A speech sound that can be sustained while retaining its acoustic characteristics (e.g., /s/, /u/).

**Control:** A group in an experiment that is the standard of comparison to other groups in the experiment; often the control group is not subjected to the independent variable (e.g., the clinical treatment) that the experimental group receives.

**Conus Elasticus:** Membrane that continues the respiratory passageway upward from the cricoid cartilage to the vocal ligaments on either side of the glottis.

**Cortex:** [L. "cortex"–bark.] The outer or superficial part of an organ, as the outer layer of gray matter of the cerebrum.

**Costal Pleura:** (parietal pleura) The membrane lining the walls of the thoracic cavity.

**Cranial Nerves:** The 12 pairs of nerves that emerge from the base of the brain. (See Appendix B.)

**Creaky Voice:** See vocal fry.

**Cricoid:** [Gk. "krikos"–ring + "oid"–like.] The cartilage of the larynx that resembles a seal ring and forms the base on which the arytenoid cartilages rest.

**Cricothyroid Muscle:** Intrinsic muscle of the larynx that tenses the vocal folds.

**Critical Period:** (for learning language and speech) The period of life during which perception and production of a first language normally develop. It is believed that after this period, certain aspects of language learning are difficult or impossible.

**CT:** (Scan) See computed tomography.

**CVA:** See cerebral vascular accident.

**Cybernetics:** [Gk. "kybernetikos"–a pilot, to steer.] The study of self-regulatory systems.

**Cycle of Vibration:** One cycle of vibration is completed at the point where the motion of a vibrating body or a pressure wave begins to repeat itself.

**DAF:** See delayed auditory feedback.

**Damping:** The decrease in the amplitude of vibration over time.

**Decibel:** Unit of intensity; a ratio between the measured sound and a reference sound.

**Declination:** The decrease in fundamental frequency across a breath group or phrase.

**Delayed Auditory Feedback:** (DAF) A delay in hearing one's own speech, produced artificially.

**Dendrite:** [Gk. "dendron"–tree.] The branching process that conducts a nerve impulse to the cell body.

**Dependent Variable:** The variable in an experiment that is observed and that changes as a result of manipulating the independent variable.

**Descriptive Study:** A study in which the observer simply describes the behavior of subjects without trying to modify it.

**Detorque:** The elastic response to the twisting of a flexible body. More simply, the untwisting of a body that has been twisted.

**Developmental Aphasia:** Abnormal acquisition of speech and language in children caused by central nervous system impairment.

**Diaphragm:** The muscular and tendinous partition that separates the abdominal and thoracic cavities; a respiratory muscle.

**Digastric Muscle:** See anterior belly of the digastric muscle.

**Diphthong:** Phonetically, a vowel of changing quality; linguistically, a combination of two vowel sounds within a single syllable, interpreted as a single speech sound (phoneme). For example, [ɔɪ] as in "boy."

**Discrimination Test:** Type of test in which stimuli are presented in ordered groups. The listener determines similarities and differences among the stimuli. (See ABX Test.)

**Duplex Perception:** The perception of components of the acoustic signal as both speech and nonspeech.

**Dynamic Palatography:** See electropalatography.

**Dyne:** A unit of force; the force required to accelerate during 1 second a 1-g mass to a velocity of 1 cm/s.

**Dysarthria:** A disorder of articulation caused by the impairment of parts of the nervous system that control the muscles of articulation.

**Echolalia:** Automatic repetition of what is said by another.

**Efferent:** [L. "ex"–out + "ferre"–to bear.] Conducting from a central region to a peripheral region; refers to neurons and nerves that convey impulses from the central nervous system to the periphery (motor neurons, nerves).

**Egocentric Speech:** Talking aloud to oneself. (See monologue, collective monologue.)

**Elaborated Code:** Bernstein's term for the speech of those who do not assume that the listener shares the sociosemantic context of the message; explicit. (See restricted code.)

**Elasticity:** The force that causes a deformed structure to resume its original shape.

**Elastic Recoil:** Return of a medium to its resting state because of its structural properties.

**Electroglottograph:** An instrument used to measure impedance across the vocal folds. (See laryngograph.)

**Electromyography:** (EMG) Recording of the electrical potential accompanying muscle contraction by inserting an electrode into the fibers of a muscle or by applying an electrode to the surface of the skin.

**Electropalatography:** A technique for measuring patterns of tongue–palate contact using a prosthetic palate in which electrodes are embedded. When the tongue touches any of the electrodes, an electrical signal is recorded that can be used to depict the location and duration of the contact.

**Empiricist:** One who bases conclusions on experiment or observation rather than on reason alone; one who believes that experience is the primary source of human knowledge.

**Encoded:** (v., to encode) Transformed in such a way that the original elements are no longer discrete or recognizable.

**Endolymph:** The fluid in the membranous labyrinth of the inner ear.

**Epiglottis:** [Gk. "epi"–on + "glottis"–tongue.] A leaf-shaped flap of cartilage that closes the opening to the trachea, preventing food and liquids from entering.

**ERP:** See event-related potential.

**Esophagus:** [Gk. "eso"–within + "phagus"–food.] The hollow muscular tube extending from the pharynx to the stomach.

**Eustachian Tube:** [from Bartolommeo Eustachio, 16th-century anatomist.] Narrow channel connecting the middle ear and the nasopharynx. The open tube allows the pressure on opposite sides of the eardrum to be equalized.

**Event-Related Potential:** (ERP) Electrical activity of the brain (in response to a stimulus) recorded from electrodes placed on the scalp.

**Experimental:** (Study, Condition) The application of an independent variable to observe its effects on behavior.

**External Auditory Meatus:** Canal leading from the eardrum to the auricle; part of the outer ear.

**External Feedback:** A system's information about the consequences of its own performance; tactile and auditory feedback of speech. (See internal feedback, response feedback.)

**External Intercostal Muscles:** Muscles connecting the ribs and elevating them during inspiration.

**External Oblique Muscles:** Muscles of the abdomen coursing downward and forward in the lateral walls.

**Feature Detector:** A neural mechanism specialized to respond to a particular acoustic feature in the speech signal.

**Feedback:** Information about performance that is returned to control a system; positive feedback conveys error information, whereas negative feedback conveys the information that performance is as programmed.

**Fiberoptic Endoscope:** A flexible and coherent bundle of optical fibers used for direct visual examination of the interior of body cavities such as the glottis. Sometimes called a fiberscope.

**Fissure of Rolando:** A groove that separates the frontal from the parietal lobes of the cerebral hemispheres.

**Fissure of Sylvius:** A groove that separates the temporal lobes from the upper lobes of the cerebral hemispheres.

**Fluoroscope:** An instrument for direct visual observation of deep body structures by means of radiography.

**fMRI:** See magnetic resonance imaging.

**Forced Choice Test:** A perceptual test in which the number of permitted responses is limited.

**Forced Vibration:** Vibration caused by repeated applications of force to a vibrating body.

**Formant:** A peak of resonance in the vocal tract; formants are displayed in a wide-band spectrogram as broad bands of energy.

**Fourier Analysis:** The analysis of a complex wave into its sine wave components.

**Free Vibration:** Vibration caused by the single application of an external force.

**Frequency:** The number of complete cycles of vibration occurring in a second.

**Fricative Sound:** [L. "fricare"–to rub.] A sound produced by forcing the airstream through a narrow articulatory constriction (e.g., /s/); one of the consonant manners of articulation.

**Frontal Lobe:** The part of either hemisphere of the cerebrum that is above the Sylvian fissure and in front of the Rolandic fissure.

**Fundamental Frequency:** ($f_o$) The lowest frequency component of a complex periodic wave. The repetition rate of a complex periodic wave.

**Gamma ($\gamma$) Motor Neurons:** Small motor neurons that transmit impulses to the intrafusal fibers of the muscle spindle.

**Genioglossus Muscle:** An extrinsic tongue muscle that brings the tongue body upward and forward.

**Glide:** Sound whose production requires the tongue to move quickly from one relatively open position to another in the vocal tract; for example, /w/ and /j/ in English; one of the manners of consonant articulation.

**Glottal Attack:** A mode of initiation of voicing in which the vocal folds are tightly adducted at onset.

**Glottis:** The space between the true vocal folds.

**Gray Matter:** Unmyelinated areas in the nervous system; such areas consist largely of cell bodies that contrast in color with the whitish nerve fibers.

**Hard Palate:** The bony partition between the mouth and the nose; the roof of the mouth.

**Harmonic:** An oscillation whose frequency is an integral multiple of the fundamental frequency.

**Harmonic Series:** The fundamental frequency and harmonics of a complex periodic wave.

**Hertz:** The unit(s) of frequency. Equivalent to "cycles per second (c.p.s or $\sim$)."

**Homorganic (speech sounds):** Two or more sounds that are made in the same place of articulation (e.g., /t/, /n/, /l/).

**Hyoglossus Muscle:** An extrinsic muscle that can lower the tongue.

**Hyoid Bone:** [Gk. "hyoeides"–U-shaped.] A horseshoe-shaped bone at the base of the tongue above the thyroid cartilage.

**Hypernasality:** Voice quality characterized by excessive nasal resonance.

**Hyponasality:** Voice quality characterized by inadequate nasal resonance.

**Identification Test:** Perceptual test in which stimuli are presented separately to be labeled.

**Impedance:** Opposition to motion as a product of the density of the medium and the velocity of sound in it; the complex sum of reactances and resistances.

**Incisors:** The front teeth of the upper and lower jaw; eight teeth in normal dentition.

**Incus:** [L. "incus"–anvil.] The middle of the three ear ossicles; also called the anvil.

**Independent Variable:** The variable controlled by the experimenter in an experiment.

**Inertia:** 1. The tendency of a body in motion to stay in motion unless acted on by an external force. 2. The tendency of a body at rest to stay at rest unless acted on by an external force.

**Inferior Constrictor Muscle:** One of the three pharyngeal constrictor muscles. Its fibers act as a valve separating the laryngopharynx from the esophagus.

**Inferior Longitudinal Muscles:** Intrinsic tongue muscles that depress the tongue tip.

**In Phase:** Said of two signals with pressure waves that crest and trough at the same time.

**Intensity:** Magnitude of sound expressed in power or pressure.

**Intensity Level:** The power of a signal; decibels derived from a power ratio; the usual reference is $1,016$ W/cm$^2$.

**Interarytenoid:** Between the arytenoid cartilages; the transverse and oblique arytenoid muscles together compose the interarytenoid muscles. They function to adduct the vocal folds.

**Interchondral:** Between cartilages; used to refer to the parts of the intercostal muscles running between the cartilaginous portions of the ribs.

**Intercostal Muscles:** Muscles connecting the ribs; they act in respiration.

**Interference Pattern:** Display of a complex wave.

**Internal Auditory Meatus:** The canal from the base of the cochlea that opens into the cranial cavity; a conduit for cranial nerve VIII, the auditory veins and arteries, and cranial nerve VII, the facial nerve.

**Internal Feedback:** A system's information about its planned performance within the control center; the loops among the cerebrum, basal ganglia, and cerebellum during speech. (See response feedback, external feedback.)

**Internal Intercostal Muscles:** Muscles connecting the ribs. Most lower the ribs during expiration.

**Internal Oblique Muscles:** Muscles of the abdomen coursing downward and posteriorly along the lateral walls.

**Internal Pterygoid Muscle:** See medial pterygoid muscle.

**Intonation:** Changes in the fundamental frequency (perceived as pitch changes) during the course of an utterance.

**Intraoral Pressure:** Air pressure within the oral cavity.

**Inverse Square Law:** Law governing the fact that intensity of a sound varies indirectly as the square of the distance from the source.

**Isochrony:** The property of having equal time intervals between stressed syllables. (See stress-timed.)

**Joule:** One *joule* is the amount of work done by a force of one newton moving an object through a distance of one meter.

**Juncture:** The affiliation of sounds within and between syllables or words. Changing the location of a juncture can change meaning: "a + name" and "an + aim" differ in juncture placement.

**Kinesthesis:** [Gk. "kinein"–move + "aisthesis"–feeling.] Perception of one's own movement based on information from proprioceptors.

**Lag Effect:** More accurate identification of the delayed stimulus presented in a dichotic listening test.

**Laminographic Technique:** A radiographic method in which x-rays from several sources are focused in a plane, clearly defining soft tissues; same as tomography.

**Language:** [L. "lingua"–tongue.] The phonemes, and morphemes and the rules for combining them common to a particular group of people.

**Laryngeal Ventricle:** The space between the true and false vocal folds; also called the ventricle of Morgagni.

**Laryngograph:** Instrument used to measure impedance across the vocal folds. (Term used by Fourcin for the electroglottograph, q.v.)

**Laryngoscope:** A mirror and source of illumination for viewing the larynx.

**Larynx:** The cartilaginous structure, including the associated muscles and membranes, that houses the vocal folds. Commonly called the voice box or Adam's apple.

**Lateral Cricoarytenoid Muscles:** Muscles that compress the medial portion of the glottis by rotating the arytenoid cartilages.

**Lateral Inhibition:** The isolation of a stimulus on the basilar membrane because of the inhibition of response in the nerve cells surrounding the point of maximal stimulation.

**Lateral Pterygoid Muscle:** A paired jaw muscle; the superior portion elevates the jaw and the inferior portion lowers the jaw.

**Lateral Sound:** A sound in which the phonated breath stream is emitted primarily over and around the sides of the tongue; /l/ is an English lateral; one of the consonant manners of articulation. Also called liquids.

**Latissimus Dorsi Muscle:** Large, broad muscle on the back of the body on either side of the spine. It functions in forced respiration.

**Lax:** (Vowels) Phonetic property of vowels that are produced with lower relative tongue height than tense vowels and with shorter durations (e.g., [ɪ], [ɛ], [ʊ]).

**Levatores Costarum Muscles:** Twelve small triangular pairs of muscles that raise the ribs during inspiration.

**Levator Palatini Muscle:** Muscle running to and constituting most of the soft palate; its contraction elevates and backs the soft palate toward the pharyngeal wall.

**Linear Scale:** A scale in which each unit is equal to the next, permitting units to be summed by addition.

**Linguistic Competence:** What one knows unconsciously about one's own language; the ability to understand and produce the language.

**Linguistic Performance:** How the knowledge of a language is used in expressive behavior, such as speech or writing.

**Liquid Sound:** In English, /l/ and /r/, two of the semivowels produced with relatively prominent sonority and with some degree of lateral emission of air; one of the consonant manners of articulation. Also called approximants or laterals.

**Logarithmic Scale:** [Gk. "logos"– proportion + "arithmos"–number.] A scale based on multiples of a given number (base).

**Lombard Effect:** The increased vocal intensity of a speaker who cannot hear himself.

**Longitudinal Wave:** [L. "longitudo"– length.] A wave in which particle motion is in the same (or opposite) direction as wave movement.

**Loudness:** The subjective psychological sensation of sound intensity.

**Magnetic Resonance Imaging:** (MRI, fMRI [functional]) Three-dimensional tomographic imaging technique in which the magnetic nuclei, mainly protons, of the subject are aligned in a magnetic field, absorb tuned radiofrequency pulses, and emit radiofrequency signals that are converted to tomographic images.

**Magnetometer:** A device used to measure the distance or amount of contact between two structures (e.g., the tongue and the palate) by registering the strength of an electromagnetic field passing from one electric coil of wire to another.

**Malleus:** [L. "malleus"–hammer.] The outermost and largest of the three middle ear ossicles; also called the hammer. (See manubrium.)

**Mandible:** [L. "madere"–chew.] The lower jawbone.

**Manner of Articulation:** Classification parameter of consonant sounds based on the method used to obstruct or channel the airstream. For example, fricatives, produced by forcing the airstream through a narrow constriction formed by the articulators; stops, produced by a complete blockage of the airstream by the articulators.

**Manometer:** An instrument for measuring the pressure of liquids or gases.

**Maxillary Bone:** One of a pair of bones that form the upper jaw; the two together are often considered as one bone.

**Maximum Expiratory Pressure:** Combined active and passive forces available for expiration at a given lung volume.

**Maximum Inspiratory Pressure:** Combined active and passive forces for inspiration at a given lung volume.

**Medial Pterygoid Muscle:** A muscle on the inner side of the mandible that acts in speech to close the jaw. (Also called the internal pterygoid.)

**Medulla Oblongata:** The portion of the brain that is continuous with the spinal cord below and the pons above; it lies ventral to the cerebellum.

**Mel:** Unit of pitch; value of one-thousandth of the pitch of a 1,000-Hz tone.

**Metathesis:** A reversal in the order of two sounds in a word:–[æsk]→ [æks].

**Middle Constrictor Muscle:** The middle of three pharyngeal constrictor muscles that narrow the pharynx.

**Middle Ear:** Small cavity containing three ossicles: the malleus, incus, and stapes; functions as an impedance-matching transformer between air and cochlear fluid.

**Monologue:** [Gk. "monos"–single + "logos"–speech.] Speech by a single person. (See collective monologue.)

**Monophthong:** A vowel of unchanging quality.

**Morpheme:** The smallest meaningful linguistic segment. The word "books" contains two morphemes, "book" and "-s," which means "more than one."

**Morphology:** [Gk. "morphe"–form + "ology"–study.] Study of the form of words as affected by inflection or derivation.

**Motor:** Pertaining to movement. For example, a motor nerve or motor center of the brain that controls movement.

**Motor Neuron:** See efferent (neuron).

**Motor Theory:** A theory put forth by A. M. Libermanand colleagues that speech perception makes reference to speech production.

**Motor Unit:** An efferent nerve fiber and the muscle fibers that it innervates.

**MRI:** See magnetic resonance imaging.

**Muscle Spindles:** Specialized muscle fibers with sensory innervation that signal muscle length and changes in length.

**Myelin:** White fatty substance that sheaths many cranial and spinal nerves.

**Mylohyoid Muscle:** A thin, sheetlike muscle that forms the floor of the mouth and helps to raise the tongue.

**Myoelastic Aerodynamic Theory of Phonation:** Theory that vocal fold vibration is primarily caused by air pressure acting on the elastic mass of the folds.

**Narrowband Spectrogram:** An acoustic display in which the fundamental frequency and harmonics can be observed as they change over time.

**Nasal Sounds:** Sounds produced with an open velopharyngeal port, hence nasal emission of the airstream.

**Natural Resonant Frequency:** Frequency at which a system oscillates with greatest amplitude when driven by an external vibrating source. The strongest frequency component emitted when a vibrating body is set into free vibrations.

**Negative Feedback:** See feedback.

**Nerve:** A bundle of neuron fibers that convey impulses from one part of the body to another.

**Neuron:** One of the cells of which the brain, the spinal cord, and nerves are composed.

**Newton:** A newton is a unit of force equal to that required to accelerate a mass of one kilogram at a rate of one meter per second per second.

**Oblique Arytenoid Muscle:** Muscle that closes the glottis by approximating the arytenoid cartilages; with the transverse arytenoids, composes the interarytenoid muscles.

**Occipital Lobe:**  The most posterior lobe of the brain, behind the temporal and parietal lobes.

**Oddball or Oddity Test:**  Procedure for testing discrimination by requiring the listener to indicate which of three presented stimuli differs from the other two.

**Ontogeny:**  [Gk. "ontos"–being + "geneia"–origin.] The entire developmental history of an individual organism.

**Open-Loop System:**  A feed-forward system that operates without the benefit of feedback about performance.

**Open Response Set:**  Used in perceptual testing. Subjects have a free choice of response to any stimulus with which they are presented.

**Operant Conditioning:**  A process by which the frequency of response is increased depending on when, how, and how much it is reinforced.

**Oral Cavity:**  [L. "oris"–mouth; L. "cavus"–hollow.] The space inside the mouth.

**Oral Sounds:**  Sounds that are articulated and resonated in the oral cavity.

**Oral Stereognosis:**  The tactile discrimination or recognition of the shapes of objects placed in the mouth.

**Orbicularis Oris Muscle:**  The sphincter muscle of the mouth that contracts to purse, protrude, or close the lips.

**Ordinate:**  The $y$ coordinate of a point; its distance from the $x$ axis measured parallel to the $y$ axis (vertical axis).

**Organ of Corti:**  The sensory organ of hearing that rests on the basilar membrane and contains sensory hair cells that are stimulated by movements within the cochlear duct.

**Oscilloscope:**  An instrument that displays the magnitude of an electrical signal as a function of time; a cathode ray tube used to display waveforms.

**Osseous:**  [L. "os"–bone.] Bony; containing bones.

**Ossicles:**  Small bones; especially the small bones of the middle ear: the malleus, incus, and stapes.

**Ossicular Chain:**  Composite of the three middle ear bones: the malleus, incus, and stapes.

**Oval Window:**  Membrane between the middle and inner ear connecting and passing vibrations from the stapes to the cochlear fluids; also called the vestibular window, fenestra vestibuli.

**Palatoglossus Muscle:**  Extrinsic tongue muscle that raises the back of the tongue and can lower the soft palate; also called the glossopalatine muscle; the palatoglossus muscles form most of the anterior faucial pillars.

**Palatography:**  A method of measuring points of contact between the tongue and the palate.

**Parallel Processing:**  The coarticulation and assimilation of neighboring phones in speech production and the simultaneous decoding of neighboring phones in speech perception.

**Parietal Lobe:**  A lobe in the upper center of the cerebrum behind the fissure of Rolando and above the fissure of Sylvius.

**Parietal Pleura:**  See costal pleura.

**Pectoralis Major Muscle:**  The most superficial muscle of the chest wall; elevates the ribs in forced inspiration.

**Pectoralis Minor Muscle:**  A thin, flat, triangular muscle that lies under the cover of the pectoralis major. With the scapula fixed, it may elevate the ribs for inspiration.

**Perilymph:**  The fluid in the space between the membranous and osseous labyrinths of the ear.

**Period:**  The time taken for the completion of one cycle of vibration.

**Periodic:** Recurring at equal intervals of time.

**Peripheral Nervous System:** (PNS) Ganglia and nerves outside the brain and the spinal cord.

**PET:** See positron emission tomography.

**Pharynx:** [Gk. "pharynx"–throat.] The throat cavity made up of the nasopharynx, oropharynx, and laryngopharynx.

**Phon:** A unit of equal loudness.

**Phonation:** Production of sound in the larynx by periodic vibrations of the vocal folds.

**Phone:** A particular speech sound; an allophone, or variant of a phoneme; the aspirated [tʰ] and [t] are allophones of the phoneme /t/.

**Phoneme:** [Gk. "phone"–sound.] A family of sounds that functions in a language to signal a difference in meaning.

**Phonetic:** Relating to the production and perception of speech sounds.

**Phonology:** Study of the sound system of a language.

**Photoelectricity:** Electricity or electrical changes produced by light.

**Photoglottography:** See transillumination.

**Phrenic Nerve:** Motor nerve to the diaphragm composed of several cervical nerves.

**Pinna:** See auricle.

**Pitch:** The subjective psychological sensation of sound frequency; a low-frequency sound produces a perception of low pitch, and a high-frequency sound produces a sensation of high pitch.

**Place of Articulation:** Classification of speech sounds based on the location of articulatory contact or constriction and the articulators used. For example, the bilabial /p/ and lingua-alveolar /t/ have different places of articulation.

**Place Theory:** A theory which states that different frequencies activate the sensory nerve fibers at different places on the basilar membrane; higher frequencies closer to the base of the cochlea, lower frequencies toward the apical end.

**Plethysmograph:** Recorder of body volumes from which respiratory movements can be inferred.

**Plosive:** [L. "plaudere"–to clap.] A manner of consonant articulation made by sudden release of air impounded behind an occlusion in the vocal tract. Used synonymously with "stop."

**Pneumograph:** An instrument that records respiratory movements as changes in chest and abdomen circumference.

**Pneumotachograph:** Instrument for measuring respiration.

**PNS:** See peripheral nervous system.

**Poles:** An engineering term for resonances.

**Pons:** [L. "pons"–bridge.] A large transverse band of nerve fibers in the hindbrain that forms the cerebellar stem and encircles the medulla oblongata.

**Positive Feedback:** See feedback.

**Positron Emission Tomography:** (PET) Imaging technique using computer analysis of γ-rays produced after introduction of a radioactive isotope.

**Posterior Cricoarytenoid Muscles:** (PCA) Muscles that abduct the vocal folds by rotating and tilting the arytenoids, opening the glottis.

**Precategorical Acoustic Storage:** (PAS) Short-term auditory memory presumed to hold information during phonetic analysis.

**Pressure:** Force per unit area.

**Pressure Transducer:** A device that transforms relative pressure into an electrical signal.

**Primary Stress:** The heaviest stress or greatest emphasis placed on a syllable in a word. The second syllable of the word "because" bears primary stress.

**Proprioception:** The sense of the location, direction of movement, and speed of movement of the articulators (or, in general, of parts of the body).

**Prosody:** (adj., prosodic)–[Gk. "pros"–in addition to + "oide"–song.] The description of the patterns of speech relating to the stress, pitch, intonation, rhythm, and duration of syllables. (See Suprasegmental.)

**Pulmonary Pleura:** (also called visceral pleura) The membrane lining the lungs.

**Pure Tone:** A sound with a single sine wave (frequency) component.

**Pyramidal Tract:** (corticospinal) A major relatively direct pathway for transmitting motor signals from the motor cortex.

**Quantal Theory:** A theory put forth by K. N. Stevens that there are quantal discontinuities in the acoustic output of the vocal tract.

**Rarefaction:** Area in a wave between compression stages where the conducting medium is reduced in pressure; the reduction of pressure itself.

**REA:** See right ear advantage.

**Recency Effect:** Effect occurring when subjects tend to remember the last item (most recent) on a list more readily than others on the same list.

**Rectify:** To reverse the direction of alternating impulses or transform an alternating current into a direct current.

**Rectus Abdominis Muscle:** Major muscle of the abdomen running vertically along the midline of the anterior wall.

**Recurrent Nerve:** The branch of cranial nerve X (vagus) that innervates all intrinsic muscles of the larynx except the cricothyroid muscle; also called inferior laryngeal nerve.

**Relaxation Volume:** Amount of air in the lungs at the end of an exhalation during normal breathing; volume at which pressure inside the lungs is equal to atmospheric pressure, at about 40% vital capacity.

**Resonance:** Vibratory response to an applied force.

**Resonator:** Something that is set into vibration by an external vibrating source.

**Response Feedback:** Direct feedback from muscles. Part of the sense of movement and position of the articulators (or of parts of the body in general) called proprioception.

**Resting Expiratory Level:** (REL) See relaxation volume.

**Restricted Code:** Bernstein's term for the speech of those who assume that the listener knows the sociosemantic context of the message. (See elaborated code.)

**Retroflex:** Raising and retraction of the tongue tip; typical of the production of some allophones of /r/ in American English.

**Reverberate:** To be reflected many times, as sound waves from the walls of a confined space.

**Ribs:** Twelve pairs of bones extending ventrally from the thoracic vertebrae and enclosing the thorax.

**Right Ear Advantage:** (REA) The phenomenon that in dichotic listening tests, subjects usually more correctly identify stimuli delivered to the right ear than to the left.

**Rise Time:** The time an acoustic signal takes to attain maximum amplitude.

**Risorius Muscle:** A paired muscle radiating from the corners of the mouth; used in spreading the lips.

**Rugae:** The irregular ridges behind the upper incisors.

**Scalenus Medius Muscle:** One of three pairs of muscles on each side of the neck that may elevate the first rib for inspiration.

**Scapula:** Flat triangular bone on the back of the shoulder. Also called the shoulder blade.

**Secondary Stress:** The degree of stress intermediate to primary and weak stress. In the word "underneath," the first syllable bears secondary stress, the second syllable bears weak stress, and the last syllable bears primary stress.

**Section:** An acoustic display showing the frequencies and amplitudes of the components of a sound.

**Semantics:** [Gk. "sema"–sign.] The study of meanings and the development of meanings of words.

**Semantic Satiation:** The perception of the change in the identity of a word, or the loss of meaning of a word, after it has been heard many times in rapid succession.

**Semicircular Canals:** See vestibular system.

**Sensory:** (Nerve, Neuron) A peripheral nerve conducting impulses from a sensory organ toward the central nervous system; also called afferent nerve.

**Serratus Posterior Superior Muscle:** Muscle extending obliquely downward and laterally from the upper portion of the thoracic region of the vertebral column to the superior borders of the upper ribs. The muscles serve to elevate the ribs during inspiration.

**Servomechanism:** An automatic device that corrects its own performance.

**Sibilants:** [L. "sibilare"–to hiss.] The high-frequency fricative speech sounds of /s/ or /ʃ/ and their voiced cognates.

**Simple Harmonic Motion:** Periodic vibratory movement in which the vibratory body moves directly from one point of maximum displacement to the other point of maximum displacement, as, for example, in the motion of the tine of a tuning fork or of the seat of a swing.

**Sine Wave:** A periodic oscillation having the same geometric representation as a sine function.

**Sodium Amytal Test:** See Wada test.

**Sone:** A unit of loudness equal to that of a tone of 1 kHz at 40 dB above absolute threshold.

**Sound:** The vibrations of a sound source, transmitted through the air or another medium, that have the potential to stimulate the organs of hearing.

**Sound Pressure Level:** (SPL) With reference to sound, the pressure of a signal; decibels derived from a pressure ratio; the usual reference is 0.0002 dynes/cm$^2$.

**Sound Spectrogram:** A display of the components (harmonics or formants) of a sound as they vary in frequency and intensity over time. Frequency is shown on the ordinate, time on the abscissa, and intensity as relative darkness of the image.

**Sound Spectrograph:** An instrument that produces a sound spectrogram (q.v.).

**Sound Wave:** A longitudinal wave in an elastic medium; a wave producing an audible sensation.

**Source-Filter:** The source-filter theory of speech production accounts for the generation of speech sounds by positing that a source of sound (vocal fold vibrations, fricative noise, or both together) is filtered through the air spaces in the vocal tract.

**Source Function:** The origin of acoustic energy for speech; for vowels at the vocal folds, for voiceless consonants in the vocal tract, and for voiced consonants both at the folds and in the tract.

**Spasticity:** Involuntary contraction of a muscle or group of muscles resulting in a state of rigidity.

**Spectrum:** See amplitude spectrum.

**Spinal Nerves:** The 31 paired nerves arising from the spinal cord that innervate body structures. (See Appendix B.)

**Spirometer:** An instrument for measuring volumes of air taken in and expelled from the lungs.

**Spoonerism:** A transposition of the initial sounds of two or more words in a phrase; named after William A. Spooner.

**Stapedius Muscle:** Muscle of the middle ear that alters movement of the stapes in the oval window.

**Stapes:** [L. "stapes"–stirrup.] The innermost of the three ear ossicles; also called the stirrup.

**Sternocleidomastoid Muscle:** A paired muscle running diagonally across the neck that assists in forced inspiration by elevating the sternum.

**Sternohyoid Muscle:** An extrinsic laryngeal muscle that depresses the hyoid bone and may lower the larynx; one of the strap muscles.

**Sternothyroid Muscle:** An extrinsic laryngeal muscle that can lower the larynx; one of the strap muscles.

**Sternum:** The breastbone.

**Stimulus Onset Asynchrony:** (SOA) A time difference between the onsets of two dichotically presented stimuli.

**Stop Sound:** A manner of consonant articulation characterized by a complete blockage of the airstream for a brief period of time. Synonymous with "plosive" when the impounded airstream is suddenly released by the relaxation of the articulators blocking the airstream.

**Strain Gauge:** A transducer that converts movement patterns into patterns of electrical voltage.

**Stress-Timed:** Languages that are stress-timed are said to be produced with equal time intervals between stressed syllables. Used synonymously with isochrony.

**Stroboscope:** A device that emits brief flashes of light at a controlled frequency. Used to produce simulated slow motion pictures of vocal fold vibration.

**Styloglossus Muscle:** One of the extrinsic tongue muscles; lifts the tongue upward and backward.

**Subglottal Air Pressure:** Air pressure beneath the vocal folds.

**Superior Constrictor Muscle:** Uppermost of three pharyngeal constrictor muscles; narrows the pharynx in swallowing. May aid in velopharyngeal closure during speech.

**Superior Longitudinal Muscle:** Intrinsic tongue muscle that turns the tip of the tongue up.

**Suprasegmental:** Term for functions overlaid on the segments of speech, including stress, juncture, and intonation.

**Syllabic Consonant:** A consonant that functions as a syllabic nucleus.

**Syllabic Nucleus:** The major vocalic portion of a syllable.

**Syllable:** A unit of speech consisting of a single vowel or a vowel and one or more consonants.

**Synapse:** The region of juncture between one nerve cell and another.

**Syntax:** (adj., syntactic)–[Gk. "syn"– together + "tassein"–arrange.] Arrangement of the words of a sentence in their proper forms and relations.

**Taction:** The sense of touch.

**Tectorial Membrane:** Gelatinous membrane overlying the organ of Corti.

**Template:** A pattern.

**Temporal Lobe:** The lower lateral portion of the cerebral hemisphere, below the fissure of Sylvius.

**Tense:** (Vowels) Term used to describe vowels that are produced with extreme tongue position and longer duration relative to lax vowels.

**Tensor Palatini Muscles:** Muscles that open the eustachian tube and may tense the soft palate.

**Tensor Tympani:** Muscle that tenses the eardrum.

**Thalamus:** [Gr. "thalmos"–inner chamber.] A mass of gray matter at the base of the cerebrum; thought to be important to speech.

**Thoracic Nerves:** Twelve pairs of spinal nerves that arise from the segments of the spinal cord in the chest region. (See Appendix B.)

**Thorax:** The part of the body between the neck and the abdomen, separated from the abdomen by the diaphragm; the chest.

**Thyroarytenoid Muscle:** An intrinsic laryngeal muscle that can shorten and tense the vocal folds; consisting of external and internal parts (see vocalis); forms part of the vocal folds.

**Thyroid Cartilage:** [Gr. "thyreos"–shield.] The large shield-shaped cartilage of the larynx.

**Thyrohyoid Muscle:** A muscle running between the thyroid cartilage and the hyoid bone; it may lower the hyoid or change the position of the larynx; one of the strap muscles.

**Tidal Volume:** The amount of air normally inspired and expired in a respiratory cycle.

**Tomographic Methods:** See laminographic technique.

**Torque:** A rotational force; used to refer to the untwisting of the cartilaginous portions of the ribs.

**Trachea:** The windpipe, a tube composed of horseshoe-shaped cartilages leading to the lungs.

**Tragus:** Small cartilaginous flap that shields the opening to the external auditory meatus.

**Transfer Function:** The contribution of vocal tract resonance of the source function to the resulting speech sound. (See source function.)

**Transillumination:** A method of indirectly measuring glottal opening by measuring the amount of light transmitted through the glottis. (See glottograph.)

**Transverse Arytenoid Muscle:** See interarytenoid muscle.

**Transverse Muscles of the Tongue:** Intrinsic tongue muscles that narrow the tongue body.

**Transverse Wave:** A type of wave whose particle motion is perpendicular to the wave movement.

**Transversus Abdominis Muscles:** Muscles of the abdomen coursing horizontally across the walls and potentially active in respiration for speech.

**Traveling Wave Theory:** A theory which states that the cochlea analyzes incoming auditory signals into component traveling waves.

**Two-Point Discrimination:** The ability to perceive two discrete points in proximity as such and not as a single point.

**Tympanic Membrane:** The eardrum, a fibrous membrane at the end of the external auditory meatus; its response is transmitted to the middle ear ossicles.

**Ultrasound:** Ultrasonic waves (those above audible frequencies); a method of measuring the movement and shape of articulators by bombarding them with ultrasonic waves and displaying the reflections of the waves.

**Unconditioned Stimulus:** (UCS) In classical conditioning, a stimulus that naturally elicits a response; in Pavlov's experiment, the meat powder that elicits salivation.

**Uvula:** [L. "uvula" little grape.] Small fleshy mass that hangs from the back of the soft palate.

**Uvular Muscle:** The muscle within the uvula that may be active in velar raising.

**Velocity:** Speed in a certain direction.

**Velopharyngeal Closure:** The closing off of the nasal passages from the oral cavity by raising the velum against the back wall of the pharynx.

**Velopharyngeal Port:** The passageway connecting the oral and nasal cavities.

**Velum:** The soft palate.

**Ventricular Folds:** The false vocal folds; the folds above the true vocal folds.

**Verbal Transformation:** Changes in the auditory perception of a repeated utterance.

**Vertebrae:** (sing., vertebra) The segments of the bony spinal column.

**Vertical Muscles:** Intrinsic tongue muscle fibers that flatten the tongue.

**Vestibular System:** Three canals in the inner ear containing the sense organs for equilibrium.

**Vestibule:** The cavity at the entrance to the cochlea that houses the utricle and saccule, sense organs responsive to linear acceleration.

**Visceral Pleura:** See pulmonary pleura.

**Vital Capacity:** The total volume of air that can be expelled from the lungs after maximum inspiration.

**Vocal Fry:** (creaky voice) A vocal mode in which the vocal folds vibrate at such low frequency that the individual vibrations can be heard.

**Vocalis Muscle:** The internal portion of the thyroarytenoid muscle; the vibrating part of the vocal folds.

**Vocal Tract:** All cavities superior to the larynx used as a variable resonator; includes the buccal, oral, nasal, and pharyngeal cavities.

**Voiced, Voiceless:** The linguistic classification of a speech sound related to the presence or absence of phonation or to other articulatory or acoustic features.

**Voice Onset Time:** (VOT) The interval of time between the release of a stop consonant and the onset of voicing; conventionally given positive values if release precedes voice onset and negative values if release follows voice onset.

**Volley Theory:** Frequency information conveyed directly by the firing of neurons. At frequencies higher than the firing capacity of individual neurons, groups of neurons cooperate.

**WADA Test:** (Sodium Amytal test) A procedure to establish which side of the cerebrum is dominant for language.

**Watt:** A unit of electric power equivalent to 1 joule per second.

**Waveform:** A graphic representation of a vibratory event showing amplitude versus time.

**Wavelength:** ($\gamma$) The distance in space occupied by one cycle of vibration in a pressure wave. The distance between two consecutive stages of compression or of rarefaction in a pressure wave.

**White Matter:** Myelinated areas in the central nervous system.

**Whorfian Hypothesis:** The hypothesis that language can determine thought to some extent.

**Wideband Spectrogram:** An acoustic display in which the frequencies of resonances are depicted as they change over time.

**X-Ray Tomography:** See computed tomography.

**Zero crossing:** The place(s) where a waveform passes over the point of equilibrium or neutral pressure.

**Zeros:** An engineering term for antiresonances.

# Index

Page numbers followed by t and f indicate tables and figures, respectively